Fertility & Infertility

FOR

DUMMIES®

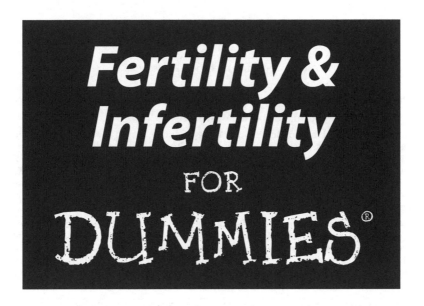

Fertility & Infertility FOR DUMMIES®

by Dr Gillian Lockwood, Jill Anthony-Ackery, Jackie Meyers-Thompson, and Sharon Perkins

BICENTENNIAL
1807
WILEY
2007
BICENTENNIAL

John Wiley & Sons, Ltd

Fertility & Infertility For Dummies®

Published by
John Wiley & Sons, Ltd
The Atrium
Southern Gate
Chichester
West Sussex
PO19 8SQ
England

E-mail (for orders and customer service enquires): cs-books@wiley.co.uk

Visit our Home Page on www.wiley.com

For general information on our other products and services, please contact our Customer Care Department within the U.S. at 800-762-2974, outside the U.S. at 317-572-3993, or fax 317-572-4002.

For technical support, please visit www.wiley.com/techsupport.

Wiley also publishes its books in a variety of electronic formats. Some content that appears in print may not be available in electronic books.

British Library Cataloguing in Publication Data: A catalogue record for this book is available from the British Library.

ISBN: 978-0-470-05750-6

Printed and bound in Great Britain by Bell & Bain Ltd, Glasgow

10 9 8 7 6 5 4 3 2 1

WILEY

About the Authors

Dr Gillian M. Lockwood BM BCh MA (Oxon) DPhil MRCOG is the Medical Director of Midland Fertility Services (www.midlandfertility.com). Gill was a late recruit to medicine. She read Philosophy, Politics and Economics at Oxford University and then worked as a Government Statistician. A television documentary encouraged her to change careers to Medicine and she qualified in 1986. A chance meeting with Professor Robert Edwards (the 'test-tube' baby pioneer) introduced her to the science of IVF and since 1990 she has specialised in Reproductive Medicine.

For 10 years Gill was Senior Clinical Research Fellow and Lead Clinician at the Oxford Fertility Unit, where her research interests included polycystic ovary syndrome, premature ovarian failure, and recurrent miscarriage.

She lectures and broadcasts on ethical and social issues in reproductive medicine, has chaired the British Fertility Society Ethics Sub-Committee, and is a member of the RCOG Ethics Committee. She is an Associate Editor of *Human Reproduction* and a member of the Editorial Board of *Human Fertility*. She has published over 30 'first author' articles in international journals and has contributed to many text books and review publications.

Since 2000 Gill has been the Medical Director of Midland Fertility Services (MFS), in the West Midlands. MFS is a 'nurse led' fertility unit at which the nursing staff perform all procedures required for IVF including surgical sperm retrieval (TESA), egg retrieval, and embryo transfer. MFS recently announced the successful delivery of the UK's first 'frozen egg' babies; a development that has given new hope of becoming 'genetic mothers' to the thousands of young women who each year have to undergo sterilising chemotherapy or radiotherapy.

Jill Anthony-Ackery BA (Hons) is the Communications Manager at Midland Fertility Services. Jill is a relatively recent entrant to the world of fertility treatment, with responsibility for the communications and marketing of MFS since 2003, initially as a consultant public relations director and then as a member of the clinic staff since 2004.

Her qualifications for such a role? A degree in art and film history (!) and 18 years' experience managing the reputations of client companies from a small UK trade association to international cosmetics, steel, and photographic equipment manufacturers. Oh! and also two years of ICSI treatment at MFS, during which she and her husband Gwyn conceived twins, suffered a miscarriage at around 12 weeks, then had an unsuccessful frozen embryo transfer, followed by a second full cycle, resulting in the birth of their daughter Connie in 2002.

When she returned to work in 2003, she combined her almost evangelical zeal about those miracle workers at MFS with her professional experience and patient perspective – and got paid for doing so! It's a dream job where she continues to be inspired daily by the team and patients.

Jill has written countless articles in a range of newspapers, consumer magazines, and trade publications from many industry sectors. She was also the original editor and a contributor to *Beyond the Lens*, the business bible for professional photographers. In 2006, her work at MFS won a gold award from the Chartered Institute of Public Relations and she works closely with national and regional press, television, and radio to satisfy the unquenchable media interest in assisted conception.

Jackie Meyers-Thompson is managing partner of Coppock-Meyers Public Relations/For Your Information Communications, and a 'professional' fertility patient.

Sharon Perkins is the nurse coordinator for the Cooper Center for In Vitro Fertilization in Marlton, New Jersey, one of the largest infertility centres in the United States. She previously worked in labour and delivery and neonatal intensive care.

Dedication

From Gill: This book is dedicated to my family. To my husband, Michael, who made it possible for me to study medicine; to my three sons, Nick, Jamie, and Sam, who remind me every day what a blessing children are; to my mother, Ivy, who makes it possible for me to work, travel, do research, give lectures, and still know my boys will be well fed and have their homework completed on time.

From Jill: This book is dedicated to my husband Gwyn who let me reveal so candidly some of the personal stories about our fertility treatment, and to our darling daughter Constance Lydia, who is the reason for my being able to contribute to this book.

From Jackie: This book is dedicated to my Darling Husband (DH!), Darren Thompson, who has loved me and believed in us, through it all. And to my mother, Larissa Meyers, and my father, the late Leonard Meyers, who taught me early and well that I could climb any mountain.

From Sharon: This book is dedicated to my father, who always believed I could do anything.

Authors' Acknowledgements

From Gill: This book is written with thanks to all the colleagues with whom I have worked since my first day as a clinical medical student in 1983. From the kind nurses who showed me how to take a blood sample without making a mess of the patient, to the patient professors who encouraged me to study for a PhD in Oxford when I'd discovered that reproductive medicine was the most exciting, rewarding, and interesting job ever.

My thanks also go to the patients. Being a fertility patient is tough but I have been fortunate to have the privilege of caring for a group of people who, almost without exception, have met the challenges of fertility treatment with patience, warmth, courage, and humour. And some got babies too!

From Jill: Gill and I have worked together at Midland Fertility Services since 2004 and while I learn something new/interesting/amazing/funny from her during every conversation, I thank her for the huge privilege of working together on this project.

My route to writing such a book was unplanned and a wonderful outcome to the dark moment, back in 1999, of being told 'you need fertility treatment'. Of course, our daughter Connie was the greatest result of that time and as the fertility experts at MFS are now my colleagues, I need to thank them *all* – mainly for helping us to have Connie, but also for the continuous learning process I enjoy from our work and which has helped me write this book – especially Su Barlow, Judith Baron, Heidi Birch, Jo Johnson, Anna Kavanagh, Vicki Robinson, and Linda Tanner.

Thanks to my parents David and Sheila Anthony (the oracles!) who made me believe I could achieve whatever I set my heart on. I hope to pass the same mind-set on to Connie, as unstinting belief in your child is a wonderful and lasting gift. They know how huge my thanks are.

While I have incorporated Gwyn's and my own personal stories into the book, I have also remembered the experiences of some of the MFS patients who have shared their stories with me over the last few years to re-tell through the media, including Vivian Barnes, Michelle Brookes, Shara Brookes, Elaine Eades, Julie Griffiths, 'Lucy', and Tom and Li McLoughlin-Yip. While their stories aren't explicitly included in the book, they have helped shape some of the content, so that readers in similar circumstances may find the best advice and a possible way ahead.

Also thanks to Mrs (Isobel) Watts – your influence continues!

Finally, to Samantha Clapp and Rachael Chilvers at Wiley – we took it to the wire, but we did it! Many thanks.

From Jackie: Thanks to Dr Jerome Check, Dr Jung Choe, and the Cooper Center for In Vitro Fertilization in Marlton, New Jersey. It was at the Cooper Clinic that I met my writing partner and friend, Sharon Perkins. Her humor, caring, and expertise make her as great of a nurse as it does a writer.

Thanks to Cousin Sandy, the Thompsons, the Jaffes, the Cicecklis, the Perlsteins, Melissa, Camille, Suzanne, Courtenay, Susan, Leslie, Sharon, and Nancy. Thanks too to Stephanie Smart and Jennifer R. Bloome.

From Sharon: Thanks to Jackie Meyers-Thompson; my husband, John; my children, John, Matt, Kim, Greg, Cindy, Ben, and Molly; Matthew Ryan, the most wonderful grandson in the world; my mother, Lois Orchard; my sister, Sue Collins; and my sister-in-law, Louise Kalmouni. My father, father-in-law, and mother-in-law would all have loved to see this book become a reality. As my mother says, they're having a book party in heaven!

Thanks to Dr Check, Dr Choe, Dr Nazari, Dr Krotec, and Carol. And to all the wonderful patients I've met over the years, this book is really for – and because of – you.

Publisher's Acknowledgements

We're proud of this book; please send us your comments through our Dummies online registration form located at www.dummies.com/register/.

Some of the people who helped bring this book to market include the following:

Acquisitions, Editorial, and Media Development

Project Editor: Rachael Chilvers

Development Editor: Tracy Barr

Copy Editor: Anne O'Rorke

Proofreader: Juliet Booker

Content Editor: Steve Edwards

Technical Editor: Dr Christian Becker, University of Oxford

Executive Editor: Jason Dunne

Executive Project Editor: Martin Tribe

Cover Photos: © GettyImages/ DAJ

Cartoons: Ed McLachlan

Composition Services

Project Coordinator: Jennifer Theriot

Layout and Graphics: Joyce Haughey, Stephanie D. Jumper, Barbara Moore, Laura Pence, Heather Ryan

Proofreaders: David Faust

Indexer: Aptara

Brand Reviewer: Jennifer Bingham

Publishing and Editorial for Consumer Dummies

Diane Graves Steele, Vice President and Publisher, Consumer Dummies

Joyce Pepple, Acquisitions Director, Consumer Dummies

Kristin A. Cocks, Product Development Director, Consumer Dummies

Michael Spring, Vice President and Publisher, Travel

Kelly Regan, Editorial Director, Travel

Publishing for Technology Dummies

Andy Cummings, Vice President and Publisher, Dummies Technology/General User

Composition Services

Gerry Fahey, Vice President of Production Services

Debbie Stailey, Director of Composition Services

Contents at a Glance

Table of Contents

Introduction

. . . .

*M*aking babies is supposed to be fun *and* easy. Most people want to make babies, assume that they can, and for a long time the big priority is avoiding making babies in the wrong place at the wrong time. But if you're part of the one in six couples who have problems making babies, then this is the book for you.

Infertility is a medical problem for about 3.5 million people in the United Kingdom. You are certainly *not* alone. But treatment is out of reach financially for some people and a tremendous personal strain on most. Many people (the 'just relax and you'll get pregnant' crowd) misunderstand fertility, and a few (the 'drink this vile potion and you'll get pregnant, guaranteed!' group) even exploit it. Clinical and scientific aspects of infertility continue to improve, yet the emotional considerations are often side-lined.

Fertility & Infertility For Dummies is the result of combining Sharon's expertise as an infertility nurse; Jackie's expertise as a patient; Gill's wealth of information as a leading fertility consultant; and Jill's experience of infertility as a patient and subsequently as the PR consultant for one of the UK's biggest fertility clinics. We wrote this book so that people trying to conceive will know when to seek help, what sort of help to seek (and avoid!) and what the emotional, financial, and medical considerations of assisted conception can be. We hope this book finds its way to the bookshelves and bedsides of everyone who needs emotional support or specialist help to have the baby they want.

About This Book

You can't pick up a magazine or turn on daytime television without hearing it: The great fertility debate over *when* women should have babies. But the quality of the information doesn't match the quantity of the coverage, because much of it is inappropriate or just plain inaccurate.

Meanwhile, for the 30,000 infertility patients being treated in the United Kingdom alone (which doesn't take into account the many people who haven't sought or can't afford fertility treatment), the question isn't 'when?' but 'if?'! Will they ever be able to conceive, carry, and deliver the child they are seeking, and will they be one of the fertility patients who sometimes pay up to £20,000 for the privilege of being told again, 'Sorry, the pregnancy test was negative'?

This book is intended to help you walk into a GP's or consultant's office and feel in control of the questions, investigations, and treatments for infertility. Our aim is to provide fertility patients – both those at the starting line and those close to the finish – with comprehensive information about the options available to them. We discuss topics ranging from the scientific to the spiritual, from the empirically proven to the fantasist, quasi-voodoo, providing a thought, an idea, or just a giggle along the way.

You can read through this book from front to back and feel confident that you can find the answer to just about any fertility issue, from natural family planning to cloning. But if you're like most people, you'll probably look through the table of contents, home in on the chapters that affect you, and jump directly to them. This book is a resource, to go back to whenever a new issue or question arises, to find the answer you need without reading through everything that goes before. It's good for people with every level of fertility expertise, from the novice to the jaded, been-there-done-that patient. The no-tech and low-tech fertility chapters come first, so you can skip them if you're already a veteran and move right into high-tech and *really* high-tech stuff found in the second half of the book.

We intersperse personal stories throughout the book; these (hopefully!) make interesting reading from the viewpoint of 'I did it, so you can too' stories.

How This Book Is Organised

Fertility & Infertility For Dummies is divided into seven parts. If you're just beginning to think about getting pregnant, you may want to start with the first couple of chapters. If you're familiar with infertility treatment, you may want to skip to the sections that apply to your current treatments, or to those you may be moving up to in the future. If you want to read through the entire book, you'll be well informed on all the latest infertility issues and the newest technological advances in the field.

The following sections explain the organisation of this book:

Part 1: Making Babies as Nature Intended

If you're a newcomer to the wonderful world of baby making, we suggest that you start reading here. In this part, we explain male and female anatomy (including everything you ever wanted to know about reproductive organs), look at the logistics and implications of getting pregnant, and review any habits and behaviour you could change – or not – before trying to get pregnant.

Part II: Planning a Pregnancy

This part helps you fine-tune your conception efforts using methods to predict ovulation, and helps you understand how complicated getting pregnant really is. We also assess the value of male and female fertility home-test kits, guide you through your first visits to your GP about possible infertility, and help you understand and deal with pregnancy loss. We also take a look at some alternative approaches to conception, from herbs to acupuncture.

Part III: Tests and Investigations

This part explains the tests you may be doing and those your GP may advise, to find out why you're not yet pregnant; we explain what the tests are and what the results may mean. We also accompany you on your visits to a consultant, and help you decipher what the doctor tells you, including the investigations that he or she may recommend. We explain tests for male infertility and what fertility treatments your hospital consultant can offer. We also take a look at the choices you have if you're told you need fertility treatment.

Part IV: Eureka! Possible Solutions

This part explains how to research and choose a fertility clinic and options for paying for your treatment, including possible NHS funding. We explain intrauterine insemination (IUI), in vitro fertilisation (IVF), and intracytoplasmic sperm injection (ICSI) and what each involves. We take you through the stimulation process, the egg retrieval, and look at how an embryo is created in a lab. We also look at embryo and egg freezing and at egg sharing treatments in this part.

Part V: Post-First Cycle: How You May Feel and What You Can Do

This part supports you through the two-week wait between IUI or embryo transfer before your pregnancy test and guides you through your options if the result is negative, including frozen embryo transfers, and considering another treatment cycle.

Part VI: Different Strokes for Different Folks: Options for Non-Traditional Families

This part considers third-party reproduction – the use of surrogacy or using donor eggs, sperm, or embryos to get pregnant. We also discuss parenting for 'non-traditional' families (gays, lesbians, and singles) and discuss fostering and adoption for every kind of family. Finally, we look at new – and sometimes controversial – treatments including fertility preservation and cloning.

Part VII: The Part of Tens

Want to read some tried and tested advice to keep you sane during your treatment? Want to know the difference between a gonadotrophin, an antagonist, and a recombinant? This is the part for you.

Icons Used in This Book

If either of us has a personal story that is funny, informative, inspirational, or otherwise interesting, we identify it with the Personal Story icon. These anecdotes are never essential reading, but they're usually entertaining!

If something's really important for you to keep in mind during your fertility treatment, we mark it with a Remember icon.

If something's technically interesting but not really essential to know, you see the Technical Stuff icon.

The Tip icon highlights practical information that may make the road to baby somewhat smoother.

If you see the Warning icon, pay special attention. It tells you about potential problems or difficulties.

Part I
Making Babies as Nature Intended

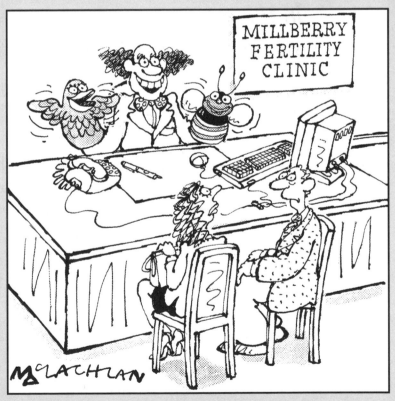

'Well, for a start, let's get back to basics.'

In this part . . .

You may not have given much thought to the difficulties of getting pregnant – more likely you've spent many years trying to avoid getting pregnant! However, after you make the decision to have a baby, you need to look at all the factors that go into having a successful pregnancy, from health issues to lifestyle changes. In this part we look at questions you need to ask before trying to get pregnant, and we give you some basic information on how human reproduction works – and how it will hopefully work for you.

Chapter 1

In the Beginning

. . . .

. . . .

*I*n the beginning of parenthood, there was Adam and Eve – who, after a bit of fun with a snake and an apple, had baby Cain. Another 62 children later and the first family was firmly established. No worries about not conceiving, no pressure to have more children than their brothers and sisters. Easy! Also, no stress of dealing with parents asking them when they were ever going to give them grandchildren. Lucky Adam and Eve.

This state of affairs didn't last forever. A few generations later, their descendant Abraham wanted a little Abe, but his wife didn't get pregnant, so his wife Sarah gave him her maid Haggar so he could have a child with her. Infertility had arrived in paradise, along with surrogacy. Now 5,000 or so years later, you're ready to start a family and probably thinking it's going to be easy. You want to have a baby – so have one! And that's exactly what may happen – no problems. But it's a fact that 10 per cent or more of the childbearing population all over the world, including about 1.75 million British couples, have problems getting pregnant or staying pregnant.

In this chapter, we look at some of the genetic realities you should be aware of as you think about adding to your family tree, and we discuss some personal and financial matters, too.

Making Babies: An Inefficient Process at Best

The path to pregnancy is an inefficient one even under the best of circumstances. For example, out of 100 couples under the age of 35 trying to conceive, only 20 will get pregnant in any given month, and of those 20, 3 will miscarry. In other words, if you're under 35, every month, you have a 17 per cent chance of walking out of the maternity ward with a baby nine months later. The chance is highest in the first few months of trying . . . babies do get made on honeymoon!

The good news is that for 100 couples under 35 trying to conceive, 85 couples will be pregnant within one year of trying. Of the 15 women not pregnant after a year of trying, 10, who may be subfertile or have mild infertility issues, will be pregnant after two years of trying without medical intervention. That leaves the other 5 per cent, who may never get pregnant without some help from the medicine (wo)man.

In the UK, the National Institute for Clinical Excellence (NICE) defines infertility as failing to get pregnant after two years of regular unprotected sex.

High-tech infertility treatments, such as in vitro fertilisation (IVF), claim a success rate of about 30 per cent for those under age 35 (see Chapter 12).

If you're over 35, you're in good company; 12 per cent of all first-time mums in the UK are over 35! Despite this, Mother Nature doesn't make it easy to become pregnant past age 35. By your late thirties, only 10 per cent of you will get pregnant in any given month and 17 per cent will miscarry. If you're over 40, the pregnancy rate, per month, slips to 5 per cent, with 34 per cent miscarrying. By age 45, your chance per month of conceiving is less than 2 per cent, and 75 per cent will miscarry.

Why the decrease in pregnancy and rise in miscarriage as you get older? A baby girl is born with all the eggs she will ever produce – approximately 1 to 2 million – and as she matures, the eggs reduce in number and increase in age, developing chromosomal abnormalities. Men make new sperm every day until their 70s and women are stuck with a dwindling supply of no-longer grade 'A' eggs, which may seem unfair, but that's biology!

Each embryo usually has 46 chromosomes arranged in 23 pairs (made up from an equal contribution from the egg and the sperm). The most common abnormalities are *trisomy*, the inclusion of a third chromosome of one type, instead of the normal two. At age 20, your chance of having a baby with a chromosomal abnormality such as Down syndrome (also called trisomy-21), or trisomy-13 or -18 (these usually result in newborn death shortly after delivery), is 1/526. By age 30, the risk is 1/385; by age 35, 1/192; by age 40, 1/66; and by age 45, 1/21. Over 70 per cent of early miscarriages are the result of chromosomal abnormalities in the egg, sperm, or both. Table 1-1 pulls all the numbers together.

Table 1-1	How Age Affects Fertility				
Age	**Under 30**	**30–35**	**36–40**	**41–45**	**Over 45**
Percentage of women who have difficulty conceiving (trying to conceive naturally for one year without success)	20%	20%	33%	66%	95%
Miscarriage rate	15%	15%	20%	40%	75%
Rate of chromosomal abnormalities	1/526	1/385	1/192	1/66	1/21

How Aging Affects Fertility

Whether you're dealing with fertility or fitness, age *does* play a role. Whether you *feel* 15 or 50, whether you look your age or not, your body knows how old you are, and your ovaries do too. Although women have more choices and control in their lives than ever before, our fertility age is pre-destined. Lifestyle issues, such as smoking and being overweight, can shorten our fertile years, but nothing can really increase them. It's all in the genes.

Calculating your fertility odds at different ages

For women, optimum fertility occurs when you're about 18 years old. It stays pretty constant in the early part of your 20s and then begins a gradual downward turn. By the time you turn 35, the process has accelerated. When you hit 40, the slide becomes even more dramatic; 33 per cent of women over 35 have some difficulty getting pregnant, and 66 per cent of women over 40 have infertility issues.

Men have it a little easier. Their peak fertility generally remains constant throughout their 30s. It does begin to decline over time, but at a slower pace than their female counterparts. Recent studies, however, do show a rise in chromosomal abnormalities in men over 35, and by age 50, most men show a 33 per cent decrease in the number of sperm produced. So although their problems may be less obvious when it comes to conceiving, the effects of age may play a significant role down the road.

You can keep yourself in better baby-making shape (and better overall health) through common sense 'healthy living', including nutrition and exercise. We touch on these topics in Chapter 3. But ultimately, you can't fool Mother Nature.

Now you may respond with the story of your 18-year-old cousin who couldn't conceive, your 45-year-old sister who did, or the 80-year-old movie star bouncing the newborn on his knee. Anything is possible. However, statistics provide information on the *likelihood* of conception, a healthy pregnancy, and babies. These numbers are a resource for determining the best plan of when and how you will conceive. But they're not a reason to review your life so far and regret not having your first baby before your GCSEs, spending too long with Mr Wrong, or choosing to travel the world before settling down.

Understanding how much age itself matters

We say this statement often throughout this book: Human reproduction is a very inefficient process *at any age*. When a woman is 35, one out of four embryos she produces is abnormal; this number increases to nearly one out of three at age 40, and five out of six at age 45. Although these statistics certainly show that age is a factor in conceiving, remember that you're an individual, not a statistic, and your odds may be better or worse than the statistics.

Separating fertility facts from media myths

How often do we read about those glamorous movie stars of 44, 45, and 47 with their new husbands or boyfriends and their new babies – or even twins – and think that Tinseltown must really have the magic key to overriding the incompatibility of fertility and being over 40. Could it be the water of the Hollywood Hills or the latest macrobiotic diet and 'yoga-lates' fad?

Or is it proof that if you are one of the 'beautiful people', your fertility age will endure? Actually, donor eggs and a good fertility clinic are likely to be the reality behind these fairy tales and, while any wanted baby is always news to celebrate, such media coverage can raise the hopes of us mere mortals who aren't privy to the whole story.

Ultimately, *you* are the only statistic that counts when you're trying to conceive. Again, the statistics provide probable outcomes, not facts. And if you remember only one piece of information in the field of fertility, remember that exceptions always exist. Consider that for all the reasons (including age) why you may not get pregnant, almost 20 per cent of women are diagnosed with unexplained infertility. This statistic certainly shows that while much is known, much is still not understood.

Use age as a suggested guideline – trying to turn Mr Right Now into Mr Right so that you can hit the 35-year-old cut-off is not sane thinking. Fertility usually decreases *over time*. You won't become infertile overnight. Indeed, studies have shown that many women experience *perimenopause* (the stage prior to menopause) and sub-fertility for as long as five to seven years before the onset of actual menopause (which *generally* signifies the end of your reproductive years). The average age of menopause is 51. You can still become pregnant during perimenopause, although it may be more difficult and require medical intervention because you ovulate less frequently and the quality of your remaining eggs isn't as good as it once was.

When is 40-something 'too old'?

Although the average age of women having their first baby has increased by 5 years in one generation you can't pick up a tabloid newspaper or watch daytime TV without hearing it: the great debate over when women should have babies. The average age of women having their first baby in the UK is now 29. But these aren't Bridget Jones 'lookalikes' who 'want it all'. A woman doctor of 62 becoming a mother causes outrage, but a popstar of 62 becoming a father for the seventh time heralds cries of 'Congratulations' and 'Whadda guy!' Unfortunately, much of the information in various debates in the popular media is either selective or just plain inaccurate. Recent statistics report an approximate 5 per cent chance in a given month for a woman over 40 to conceive. This number sounds frighteningly low, until you compare it with the statistic that shows that a healthy couple in their 20s has only a 20 per cent chance of success during any given month (after the first three months of 'trying'). This comparison is seldom brought up because the one isolated, surprising statistic often sells better than the facts.

Don't assume that everyone who offers up an opinion, even a public one, is experienced enough to comment on fertility and infertility. Instead, ask your doctor, ask your nurse, or read a book (like this one) written by people actually in the field. Ignore the hype. The next big story will take its place in no time.

Things to Think About Before You Conceive

The arrival of a baby has a huge impact on any couple's relationship – both positive and negative – and so pausing to consider the major changes a baby will bring to your life before you ditch those condoms or stop taking the pill is worthwhile. Here we consider some questions about the strength of your relationship and the affect of a baby on your income – and expenditure! However, as well as thinking about useful and responsible considerations, don't over-analyse! Taking too much time navel-gazing about whether everything in your life is perfect enough to have a baby means that you may never start trying, or when you eventually get round to it, your age may become a factor affecting your fertility.

Examining the state of your union

The state of your union is an issue we revisit throughout this book because this factor is one of the most important aspects in dealing with fertility, infertility, and baby makes three (or more). Although biology is a key issue in deciding when and if you're ready to conceive, maturity, financial security, and stability are equally important when you're deciding whether to try to become pregnant and raise your baby in a difficult and expensive world.

Many couples are anxious to seal the deal with a baby. This approach is fine for some couples, but others find that they need an adjustment period in the marriage before introducing someone new. Start out by talking with your partner about your hopes and expectations for children. Some couples find that although both partners want children, their timing may be different. You may need to come to a compromise, so that your partner can still fulfil his dream to see the world, and at the same time plan for a baby before your biological clock stops ticking altogether.

The quality of your partnership is the foundation for your family. Take time to make sure that your relationship is solid before moving on to the next level.

Don't just assume that a baby is the next logical step in a marriage. Babies are cute and cuddly *at times* (ask any parent about the alternatives of cranky and unmanageable), but they also require an enormous commitment of emotion, time, and money. If you or your partner struggle with the demands of your existing relationship, a baby will only make things more difficult. If both of you have trouble with joint decisions, finances, or future plans, a baby will more than likely increase those differences, *not* reconcile them. Teamwork is essential in raising Baby. Now is a good time to practise working together.

Some couples ease into the idea of having a new addition to the family by starting with a pet. Fido or Tiddles can serve as good indicators of your (and your partner's) sense of responsibility, discipline, and sacrifice. If you find yourself at each other's throats over whose turn it is to feed, walk, or bathe the pet, you may have a little work to do before planning and raising Baby.

Just keep talking! As with all other areas, communication is key in the decision to add to your family. If you find yourselves at an impasse, enlist the help of an outside party – a Relate counsellor, a therapist, or a doctor may be better able to guide both of you toward a decision that will ultimately benefit your entire family, however large or small that may turn out to be. But if you need counselling about a baby before you've even planned to conceive, the chances of things working out 'when you are three' are probably slim.

Pregnancy and work

How will getting pregnant affect your job? Both the Sex Discrimination Act 1975 and the Employment Rights Act 1976 confer statutory rights in relation to pregnancy and maternity, which means that employers can no longer refuse to employ women who are pregnant. Pregnant women are also entitled to the same leave period as anyone with a physical illness. As long as you're able to perform the main functions of your job, you can't be fired or not hired.

The pros and cons of a two-year honeymoon

My husband and I (co-author Jill) married when I was 29 years old and he was 42. We found out the month before we'd married that his vasectomy reversal had been successful – hurrah! – and decided to settle into our marriage for a few years before trying to conceive. When I was 32, we decided the time was right – he was in a better job, I had been promoted a couple of times, and we were buying a bigger 'family' home. Two years later, we were still trying for a baby. I questioned myself endlessly: 'Maybe we should have started trying right away' or 'If only I had those extra two years.' But that was pointless. We'd had great fun being a couple; we'd got to know each other even better, and had got to know how each other's families worked – a valuable insight into imagining how our yet-to-be family could be. Don't endlessly soul-search in that situation. But having come out of the other side, the single piece of advice I would give to girl friends in their early 30s who don't have children and who want children is to know what their fertility age is (see Chapter 10 for more information on ovarian reserve testing and calculating your fertility age). We're encouraged to know our cholesterol levels and blood pressure, so why not use the latest tests to have self-knowledge about your chances of conceiving naturally, and knowing approximately how long you might have to defer trying to get pregnant? Then if the news is good, go ahead and enjoy that 'couple time' together.

Women who are pregnant or have small children continue to be at a disadvantage when they are considered for promotion, because the workplace perception in many companies is that a mother will put her family before her job. And in most cases, that assumption is logical! So if you're a fast-track person who wants to stay on the fast-track, you may have to be 'better' at the job and more 'dedicated' than your childless female colleagues and all your male colleagues in order to convince your employer that your commitment to the job isn't going to change after you have a child.

Even though you may feel strongly *now* that your commitment to your career isn't going to change after you have a child, your feelings may change considerably after your baby arrives. One issue that may affect your situation is childcare. Good day care isn't always easy to find. Your working hours and the nursery's availability may not be compatible, or the childminder may be ill, leaving you at short notice, without childcare – and still a job to go to. The possibilities for disruption of even a well-planned childcare system are endless!

But thankfully more companies are learning that women own half the talent, intelligence, and ambition in their company. Consequently, some companies now offer on-site day care, flexitime, and enhanced maternity leave to keep the talent they have. In addition, the Government has increased the length of statutory maternity leave and the weekly benefit to £108.85 for a maximum of 39 weeks, and dads are also now entitled one or two weeks' paternity leave and Statutory Paternity Pay so that they can take time off work to care for the baby or support the mother following birth. Parental leave also brings mums and dads a right to take unpaid time off work to look after a child up to the child's 5th birthday (or 18th birthday for disabled children) or make arrangements for the child's welfare. It all helps.

Babies aren't superglue

Just as Baby's appearance won't repair a partnership in peril, it also won't put you on the personal road to happily-ever-after. Your child will not and *should not* be your antidote to a bad job, bad marriage, bad childhood, or bad life. This thinking sets up unrealistic expectations and virtually guarantees disappointment, both for yourself and your child. A baby will not solve your problems, and such an expectation has a negative impact on your child's emotional development. A baby brings not only joy but also sadness, anger, and all the emotions that you experience in your own daily life. Your child comes into this world with his or her own destiny and dreams to fulfil, not yours.

If your life is miserable without a child, chances are it will still be miserable after your child is born. So if you're looking to salvage your life by creating another one, consider making the changes you need to in order to create your own happiness *today*. Your future child, and everyone else, will thank you for it tomorrow.

The cost of a baby in pounds and pence

Research in November 2005 claimed that the average cost in the UK of raising a child to 21 was around £166,000 – or the equivalent of £657 a month. (In fact this sum is only slightly lower than the average cost of a house at the same time as the research). And this figure doesn't account for inflation! Childcare is the single biggest expenditure at around £46,000, followed by food at £15,630, and £12,055 on clothes. Even in the first year of their first child's life, parents spend about £7,716 on the child. Kids don't come cheap!

If you and your partner both are employed, you'll have the following financial and emotional factors to consider:

- ✔ Will you (usually the mother, but not always) stay at home for a few years?
- ✔ Will you use childcare?
- ✔ Do you prefer a nursery or a childminder? What's available in your neighbourhood?
- ✔ How will you feel if your baby cries for the childminder to pick her up rather than you?
- ✔ Will your mother babysit (a minefield arrangement that should never be assumed and only undertaken after very detailed discussion)?
- ✔ How will you deal with your mother-in-law giving the baby too many biscuits or putting too many clothes on her?
- ✔ If you find 'super nanny' can you also afford to pay for sick leave and holidays, and any maternity pay, as required by law for any employee?
- ✔ Can you afford not to work at all?

Ah, you say, but my child will go to school in a few years and then I can go back to work! Yes, but do you know how many days in a year school terms are *actually* in session? Do you know how often your child will get sick, fall down on the playground, or have a crisis at school requiring your presence? Do you understand that recorder practice starts at 4 p.m. and that every other child in year one is in the recorder orchestra? Do you know that children sometimes miss their bus and need to be picked up or dropped off at school?

How about the pre-teen years? Will you leave your child home alone for a few hours or do you try to convince her that after-school club is really cool? And if you think parenthood ever ends, well, think again. You're signing up for a lifelong job. Some 631,000 adults over 30 continue to receive significant financial help from their parents. That adorable, cuddly, newborn could turn into a multi-pierced, loudmouthed stranger before you know it, and you can't take this child back to the shop! And you wouldn't want to, because you'll love her – so much that it hurts sometimes, so much that her problems will break your heart, so much that you would give your life for hers. That's what parenthood is all about.

Be wise to both the fun and frustrations of parenthood, but don't think so long about it that you forever put off 'the month' you start trying for a baby. If we all thought about the enormity of parenthood, no one would ever become mum or dad. We'd all suffer paralysis through analysis and miss out on the most important, satisfying, difficult, and rewarding role of many people's lives – being a parent.

Timing Your Baby: The Big Picture

Timing is a major baby-making factor in several ways. Some baby stats for you to consider:

- ✔ **For how long will I be pregnant?** You probably think that nine months is the correct answer, but pregnancy is actually counted as 40 weeks, or ten months. This duration isn't as long as it seems. The first two weeks don't count, because they're the weeks before you ovulate, and the next two weeks are the weeks before you expect your period, so they don't really count either.

  Want to work out your due date? Take the date your last period started, count back three months, and then add one week. For example, if the date your last period started was July 1 and you count back three months, to April 1, and then add one week, your due date is April 8.

- ✔ **Am I equally likely to have a boy or girl?** As far as conception, boy babies outnumber girl babies 130 to 100, but by the time of birth, this ratio drops to 105 to 100, signifying the higher rate of miscarriage for baby boys.

Now that you're planning ahead, you want to know about the timing of . . . well, sex. We touch on this point a few more times, but the way to get pregnant is to have sex a day before or the day of *ovulation* (the release of your egg – Chapter 2 has more details). This interval gives the sperm time to get to the egg and meet in the Fallopian tube. Sperm, by the way, are pretty long-lived; they can hang around two or three days. Eggs, on the other hand, are more fragile – 24 hours is about their life expectancy.

Want a boy? Or a girl? One theory is that boy sperm (those that carry the Y chromosome, which, combined with the woman's X chromosome, creates a boy baby) are shorter lived but faster swimmers. Girl sperm (those that carry the X chromosome to create a girl) live longer but are slower. So if you want a girl, have sex two days before ovulation; if you want a boy, try to hit the day of ovulation straight on. (We discuss sex selection more in Chapter 23.)

Understanding the Long-Term Effects of Birth Control

You may not be quite ready to start baby-making yet; you may want to wait for promotion at work, or your sister's wedding to be over, or to move house. In the meantime, you want to use birth control, but you don't want to use it if it's going to make getting pregnant that much harder later on. So what method should you use?

- ✔ **Contraceptive pills:** The good news is that contraceptive pills aren't likely to impair your long-term fertility at all. Today's pills contain a fraction of oestrogen compared to pills from the 1960s. Most doctors say that you can start trying to get pregnant immediately after stopping the pill, without any problem. The pill is not advised for women over 35 who smoke, because it may increase the chance of blood clots and stroke. (By the way, don't smoke! See Chapter 3 for the impact of smoking on sperm and pregnancy.)

- ✔ **Intrauterine devices:** Intrauterine devices (IUDs) have had lots of bad press over the years, and with reason. They can increase the chance of *ectopic pregnancy* (a non-viable pregnancy that develops in the Fallopian tubes instead of the uterus) and can cause infection, sometimes quite serious. For this reason, an IUD is not the best choice if you want to become pregnant soon, especially if you have *endometriosis*, an outgrowth of uterine lining tissue into other parts of the abdominal cavity, or if you have a history of vaginal or cervical infection. (You can read more about endometriosis and ectopic pregnancy in Chapter 7.) In fact, some doctors recommend against using an IUD if you've never had children, because an IUD-related infection may make becoming pregnant much harder for you. And if you do get pregnant with an IUD in place, you face a significant chance of miscarrying.

- ✔ **The rhythm method:** The old rhythm method can actually be pretty successful; as long as you know what days you ovulate and avoid having sex on those days. But if you really, seriously, absolutely don't want to get pregnant right now, you're better off using a more reliable method. We have a name for couples who rely on the rhythm method: we call them parents!

- ✔ **Condoms and barrier devices (such as the diaphragm):** The old standbys are still fairly effective, at least 90 per cent if used consistently and correctly. Although they're not necessarily as easy or unobtrusive to use as the pill or an IUD, they don't have the side effects of their higher-tech cousins.

Gene Genie: Looking at the Family Tree

Before trying to get pregnant, you may want to know whether any hereditary diseases or genetic disorders occur on your family tree. These problems may be caused by a dominant gene that you could pass on, if you carry it, even if your partner doesn't carry it. The following sections tell you how to obtain the info you want and why even 'bad' news isn't necessarily cause for despair.

If you and your partner are blood relatives, you especially need to see a genetic counsellor before getting pregnant. You may carry more of the same abnormal genes than unrelated partners, which may make you more likely to have a child with a genetic problem. The risk for serious birth defects is 1 in 20 for second cousins and 1 in 11 for first cousins.

Gathering info

Ask the most talkative member of your family for a family 'birth history'. You may be surprised what you discover. Find out about the cause of infant or pre-adult deaths over the last few generations.

Researching your family history can provide other valuable information. For example, you may find out that everyone in your family took six months to get pregnant, a fact that may put your mind at ease, particularly around month number five of trying without success. Alternatively, the only thing you discover from family recollections may be non-specific, such as 'all the Smith boys died young'. Try and pin down why they all died young: Did they have haemophilia or muscular dystrophy, or did they all fall out of the same apple tree?

If your family tree reveals a genetic problem or a birth defect that shows up more than once, you'll probably want to have genetic testing done. A *gene map*, which can be done from a blood test, will show whether you carry abnormal genes that could cause problems for your child. If you're a known carrier of a disease such as thalassaemia, sickle-cell anaemia, or cystic fibrosis, you'll probably want to have your partner tested as well. These diseases are carried on recessive genes and are inherited only if both partners are carriers.

For couples at high risk of having an affected pregnancy (for example, where both partners are carriers of the cystic fibrosis gene, there's a 1 in 4 chance that any child they have together could have full-blown cystic fibrosis) the technique of *pre-implantation genetic diagnosis* (PGD) in which the genetic structure of embryos produced by *IVF* (the collecting of eggs and fertilisation with sperm in a laboratory) can ensure that only unaffected babies are made.

Before you panic

If you do uncover a 'bad' or questionable gene through testing, don't panic. This discovery is the reason for testing in the first place. Just remember:

- ✔ Not all gene mutations will cause disease. Some are merely benign changes. These differences are what make us all unique individuals.

- ✔ If you're a carrier of a recessive genetic disorder, you will not get the disease, but if your partner is also a carrier, your children could be seriously affected.

And remember, when looking at inherited diseases, medicine is constantly developing, which is good news: You have options that your grandmother and mother never had. You can receive pre-pregnancy genetic counselling or have early pregnancy testing of the fetus for abnormalities. Such problems are more common in women over 35, and no way existed to test for them during pregnancy in earlier generations.

Getting Pregnant: Was It Easier for Grandma?

Sometimes things seemed easier in Grandma's day. Large families were common, and everyone seemed to have children. In fact, getting pregnant may be harder today, for several reasons:

- ✔ People are having children later in life. Over the age of 25, you find a slight but definite decrease in fertility in women, a decrease that increases dramatically over age 35. Men are also less fertile at older ages.

- ✔ Due to better medical care, people are living longer and getting pregnant (or trying to) despite the presence of serious chronic disease, such as diabetes or lupus. In the past, just the *presence* of these conditions would have precluded the possibility of pregnancy.

- ✔ Male infertility, related to decreased sperm counts, has increased. Many theories circulate as to why this increase is occurring, with environmental factors being carefully studied.

- ✔ The incidence of sexually transmitted diseases has increased. Some of these diseases, such as chlamydia, cause serious damage to the reproductive organs.

- ✔ More men have had a vasectomy and women tubal ligation at a young age, and then decided to have another child. Needless to say, they immediately face fertility issues due to their previous choices.

- ✔ You may have the impression that everyone had children years ago, but start asking questions and you'll get a different story. You may find out that Uncle Charlie wasn't really Aunt Jo's son; he was her sister's child. Everyone may have been raising children, but many of those children may have been extended family members.

- ✔ People today talk more. Just because you never heard about your grandmother's stillborns or your mother's miscarriages doesn't mean that they didn't happen. Pregnancy talk today is big business, and this focus puts a constant in-your-face emphasis on pregnancy, which can make you feel as if everyone else is doing it better than you are!

Relax, this part is only the beginning for you, and we do our best to help you start baby-making with the best of them.

Chapter 2

Taking Baby Steps

*O*kay, you're officially trying to get pregnant. You've considered the alternatives (world cruise, new puppy, Ferrari) and have decided that you really, really want a baby. You've checked yourselves out financially, emotionally, and physically, and you're ready to get started. Undoubtedly, you think that you know how to get pregnant. Doesn't everybody? Our goal is to show you how to get pregnant in the shortest amount of trying time (not that trying isn't fun!) with the healthiest possible pregnancy. We take a close look at behaviour and habits (both good and bad) that can help or hinder your baby quest. In this chapter, we review a little basic biology and give you a list of do's and don'ts.

Biology for Baby Makers: Reviewing Male and Female Anatomy

Were you paying attention in science class? If you were, you probably learned hardly anything about reproducing one of your own kind, though you probably became well versed in the reproduction of birds and bees. The fact that all functional bees (workers and queens) are females and all male bees are drones and are doomed to die on their honeymoon always made us wonder why biology teachers were so obsessed with bees – they hardly set a good example! Most likely you suffered through the mandatory sex ed class, but because you were busy picking your nails and blushing (if you were a girl) or poking your mates and sniggering (if you were a boy), you probably didn't retain much. You probably took a quick peek at the film on the miracle of birth and announced loudly to all your friends, 'Yuk, gross, I'm never having kids!' And yet here you are, some undisclosed number of years later, completely changing your mind and wishing you had paid more attention back then. Don't worry; we're here to fill in the gaps in your reproductive education.

The human body is basically just a life-support system, a tool kit, and a transport mechanism for your brain. But it has one other very important role: it contains the kit for reproduction. Like all kits, your body contains both the basics and the accessories. When you buy an outfit, you can just buy the basics, but the accessories really pull your outfit together. When you're trying to have a baby, the parts that you don't see – the 'accessories' – determine whether you can get pregnant.

Looking at female accessories (besides shoes and handbags)

A naked woman is pretty unrevealing, from a reproductive viewpoint. You can't see the organs that count in childbearing, so you can't tell at a glance whether yours are present and functioning. Here's a look at what should be inside every woman, starting from the outside and working your way up. (See Figure 2-1.)

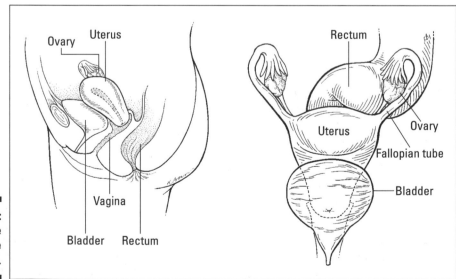

Figure 2-1:
The female reproductive organs.

The vagina

The vagina mostly serves as a passageway, first for the penis to deliver sperm to the cervix, the entrance to the uterus, and later for the delivery of the baby. If you have a very small vagina, intercourse may be uncomfortable. If your vagina is large, as it may be after having a baby, sex may be less pleasurable. Neither condition, however, should affect your ability to get pregnant.

The cervix contains glands that secrete fluid during sexual arousal, making the penis entering the vagina that much easier – and a lot more enjoyable!

The *hymen* is a non-functional piece of circular tissue found near the entrance to the vagina; the bleeding that women may have the first time they have sex comes from the tearing of the hymen. The hymen isn't a solid piece of tissue; 99 per cent of baby girls already have openings, or perforations, in the hymen. The hymen may also tear when a tampon is inserted the first time. An *imperforate hymen*, one that has no holes, can cause blood to back up behind the hymen and this blood can be forced back up into the Fallopian tubes. Women with an imperforate hymen have a higher incidence of endometriosis. (See Chapter 6 for more on endometriosis.)

The cervix

The *cervix* is the lower part of the uterus. It keeps the baby from falling out of the uterus when you're pregnant because it's a tight, circular ring of muscle. The cervix also guards against infection because it's filled with mucus that forms a barrier between your vagina and the inside of the uterus. If you have an *incompetent cervix*, your cervix doesn't stay tightly closed when you're pregnant but starts to open up from the weight of the growing baby. The first warning signs of an incompetent cervix may be premature labour itself and this occurrence is especially likely if you're carrying a multiple (twin or more) pregnancy. You're at a higher risk of incompetent cervix if you've had cervical surgery (such as a cone biopsy) for early cervical cancer. An incompetent cervix is usually stitched with a 'purse-string' suture called a *cerclage* or *Shirodkar* in early pregnancy to keep the baby where it belongs.

The uterus

The *uterus*, or womb, is a pear-shaped organ designed to hold and protect a baby for nine months. Every month the lining of the uterus, called the *endometrium*, thickens to make a nourishing bed for an embryo. If you don't get pregnant that month, the lining breaks down and is shed as your *menstrual flow*, or *period*.

If your body isn't making enough of the hormone oestrogen, your lining may not grow very much, and your periods may be light and scanty. Even though you may appear to pass buckets of blood each month, the average amount of blood lost with each cycle is only about four tablespoons (20 millilitres).

However, if you have very heavy periods (called *menorrhagia*) you may lose as much as 80 millilitres or more, in which case you should check your haemoglobin (iron levels) to make sure that you're not getting anaemic, as anaemia itself can cause infertility.

Many women have a uterus that doesn't conform to the standard upside-down pear shape you've all seen in pictures marked 'this is your uterus.' Most women have an *anteverted uterus*, which means it flops forwards, towards the pubic bone. And about 20 per cent of women have a *retroverted*, or backwards-tilted, uterus, which does not cause problems in getting pregnant.

Around 2 to 3 per cent of women have an abnormally shaped uterus. The most common variation is a *septate uterus*, which means that a band of tissue *(septum)* partially or completely divides the inside of the uterus. This tissue can be surgically removed. *Bicornuate* (two-horn) and *unicornuate* (one-horn) uteri have either one (uni) or two (bi) narrower-than-normal cavities. Women with T-shaped, bicornuate, and unicornuate uteri have higher-than-normal miscarriage rates.

A drug that was widely used in the 1960s to prevent miscarriage called Diethylstilbestrol (DES) was responsible for producing abnormalities in the genital tracts of daughters born to women who took it. The commonest DES abnormalities are a T-shaped uterus and a 'cocks comb' cervix.

It's also possible to have two separate uterine cavities, called a *didelphys uterus*; women with this condition usually also have a second cervix. You may need to have a caesarean section (a surgical delivery) if you have a double cervix (in gynaecology more isn't always better!). In addition, you could quite possibly get pregnant with twins, one developing in each uterus.

Even if the shape of your uterus is normal, it may contain some unwanted 'extras' – growths such as polyps and fibroids – which may decrease the chance of an embryo implanting and growing successfully in your uterus. *Polyps* (little outgrowths of endometrium) are readily removed by a minor operation called a hysteroscopic polypectomy and don't cause any complications after they're gone. *Fibroids* are circular 'knots' of dense muscle fibres that arise within the wall of the uterus (*intramural)*, project on a stalk outside the uterus (*subserous*), or encroach into the endometrial cavity (*submucosal*). Removing fibroids (also called *leiomyoma*) is more complex than removing polyps; sometimes they can't be removed without risking damage to your uterus. Removing fibroids can leave scar tissue in the cavity that can make it harder to get pregnant because the embryo won't be able to implant in the scarred area. You may also need a caesarean section after fibroid removal. Scar tissue can also form in your uterus after a *dilation and curettage* (D&C for short) – a common minor surgical procedure involving the scraping of the uterus lining. Where a lot of scar tissue exists, nearly filling the uterus, this condition is known as Asherman's syndrome. This scar tissue can also be removed surgically to make it easier for you to get pregnant.

The ovaries

Most women have two ovaries, which contain the most important accessory of all – eggs! How many eggs? Well, to look at a newborn baby girl, you would never guess that her ovaries already contain about 2 million eggs – and that's after a loss of 2.5 million eggs in the last three months before her birth! Every single day of your life, many eggs are lost through *atresia*, which means that they die off because they're not being stimulated to mature. By puberty, only 300,000 to 400,000 eggs remain, and every month, 500 to 1,000 are lost, along with the one or possibly two eggs that mature and are released each month. By age 50, only 1,000 or so eggs remain, and the majority are abnormal because the eggs are way past their 'sell-by' date.

What makes an egg develop and mature? The process goes like this:

1. **Follicle-stimulating hormone (FSH) is released from your pituitary gland in response to tiny regular pulses of gonadotrophin releasing hormone (GnRH) from the hypothalamus.**

2. **In the ovary, 10 to 15 eggs begin to grow.** The tissue surrounding each egg forms a follicle, a fluid-filled sac. Each follicle contains one egg.

3. **Luteinising hormone (LH) is released from the pituitary gland.** The follicle begins to produce oestrogen.

4. **One follicle becomes dominant, growing faster than the others.**

5. **As the dominant follicle grows, it produces more oestrogen that 'feeds back' to the pituitary to decrease the amount of FSH released and stop the smaller follicles growing.** This 'feed-back' loop is Mother Nature's way of ensuring that human babies are (usually) born one at a time. Although 'fertility treatment' babies often come in pairs, the 'natural' twin rate is only 1 in 80.

6. **A large amount of LH is released as the oestrogen rises.** This increase makes the egg inside the dominant follicle mature and ovulation is triggered.

7. **The follicle bursts, and the egg is released, hopefully to be wafted towards the Fallopian tubes by the frondy 'sea anenome' ends called the *fimbriae*.**

8. **The leftover, empty part of the follicle, now converts into the *corpus luteum* (a hormone-secreting structure), which produces progesterone to help an embryo implant.**

What exactly is in this egg?

You may wonder what eggs contain to make them into your potential scream-ing newborn. The answer is chromosomes – 23 chromosomes, to be exact. Each chromosome contains the genes that determine whether your baby is tall or short, blonde or brunette, and, to some extent, fat or thin. (Refer to Chapter 1 for more information on chromosomes and genes.)

Of course, an egg has more to it than chromosomes. Three protective layers surround the egg, starting with the *cumulus layer*. That's the nourishing and protecting fluffy layer of cells that completely surround the egg. Moving inward, looking down a high-power microscope you'll see the *corona radiata*, the protective single layer of cells covering the *zona pellucida*, the 'shell' of the egg. A mature, ready-for-fertilisation oocyte, or egg, has a small attachment called a *polar body*, which is the remnant left after the egg divides (a process called *meiosis*) so that it contains only 23 chromosomes.

All cells in the human body besides eggs and sperm have 46 chromosomes. Eggs and sperm have 23, so the baby they create when they come together has 46. Two of these 46 will be either 2 Xs meaning 'it' will be a girl or an X and a Y meaning 'it' will be a boy.

The ovaries 'take it in turns' to ovulate each month. If you have only one ovary, either because you were born that way or because one was surgically removed, your one ovary usually takes over egg releasing each month.

Determining whether it's a good egg

Making a mature, healthy egg is essential to getting pregnant. How do you know whether you're making good eggs? You can't be sure whether any month's egg is Grade 'A', but a properly matured egg, released at the right time of the month, when the lining of the uterus is ready to receive it, is needed for pregnancy to occur. Eggs deteriorate with age (hence the lower pregnancy rates and higher miscarriage rates experienced by women in their late 30s and early 40s) so age is quite a good guide to egg quality.

How can you tell whether you have eggs at all, much less good eggs? One sign of good egg production is a regular menstrual cycle. If you're very irregular, skip months, or have periods closer than three weeks apart, you may not be making good, mature eggs. Your periods should start about two weeks after your egg is released from the ovary (ovulation).

But how do you know when you ovulate? Some women always know, but others need the help of an ovulation predictor kit to be sure. We discuss ovu-lation predictor kits more in Chapter 3, but if you're lucky, your best sign of ovulation will be pain.

The Fallopian tubes

Fallopian tubes are vital accessories named after the 16th-century Italian anatomist Gabriele Fallopio. You should have two Fallopian tubes, one near each ovary. The tubes are kind of like a pickup bar – a place where sperm and egg should meet and hopefully go on to create something bigger and better – a baby! When an egg is released from the ovary, little projections called *fimbriae* on the end of the tube move back and forth to 'entice' the egg into the tube. When in the Fallopian tube, the egg needs a few days to travel down to the uterus. The egg is wafted on a carpet of mucus by millions of tiny hairs called *cilia* that beat synchronously. A bit like one of those travelators at the airport! Hopefully, along the way the egg meets Mr Sperm and fertilises, thereby transforming into an embryo by the time it reaches the uterus. Damaged tubes, usually due to an infection but sometimes from endometriosis or surgery, are a very common cause of infertility. We talk about this in depth in Chapter 7.

Putting all the parts together: Your menstrual cycle

The ovaries, uterus, and Fallopian tubes all need to function together for you to get pregnant. Here's what happens:

- **Days 1 to 5:** In the ovary, an egg begins to mature. This stage is called the early *follicular phase* of the cycle. In the uterus, the old lining breaks down and passes out through the vagina as your menstrual flow. This process takes two to five days.

- **Days 6 to 13:** In the ovary, one egg-containing follicle is growing and producing oestrogen. In the uterus, the oestrogen produced by the ovary is making the lining (endometrium) thicken. This stage is called the *proliferative phase.*

- **Ovulation (around day 14):** In the ovary, the follicle bursts, and the egg is released. It begins to travel down the Fallopian tubes where (hopefully!) fertilisation will occur. This journey takes several days. The endometrium is now thick enough to support the growth of an embryo.

- **Day 14 (approximately) to day 28:** In the ovary, the empty remnant of the follicle, the *corpus luteum*, produces progesterone. This stage is called the *luteal phase* of the cycle. The embryo floats in the uterus for several days slowly dividing to become a blastocyst. It can then 'hatch' through its shell and then implant in the thickened uterine lining and start to grow. This stage is called the *secretory phase*. If you're not pregnant, the lining will break down two weeks after ovulation, and your cycle will begin again.

Ouch! I think I've ovulated

About 20 per cent of women have pain called *mittelschmerz* (German for 'middle pain') when they ovulate. The pain seems to be caused by blood and fluid irritating the *peritoneum* (lining of the pelvis) around the ovary after it has released the egg from the follicle. Sometimes a small amount of vaginal bleeding occurs with ovulation, too.

Hanging out with the guys

Compared to women, guys let it all hang out, reproductively speaking. The testicles dangle the way they do to keep them at least one degree cooler than normal body temperature. Ideal clothing and lifestyle for a chap who wants to make babies would be a nice piece of bear skin loosely tied round his naked loins while he strides over the plain in search of a sabre-toothed tiger to hunt. Tight trousers, hot baths, laptop computers and long-distance driving are all bad news for sperm. Take a look at Figure 2-2 for a graphic portrayal of your average man.

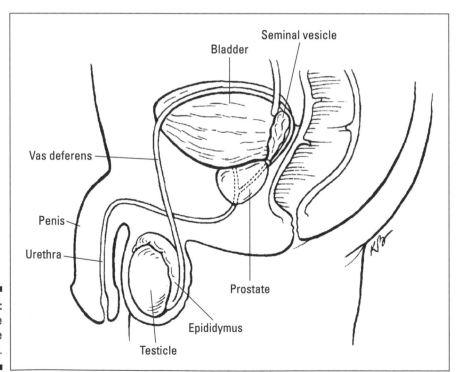

Figure 2-2: The male reproductive organs.

The penis: Does size matter?

How do I compare to everyone else? For those obsessed with the length of their penis, here are the standards: Normal length when flaccid, or limp, 10 centimetres (3.9 inches); stretched (still limp), 12.2 centimetres (4.8 inches); erect, 12.7 to 17.8 centimetres (5 to 7 inches). Hopefully that makes most of you fellows feel better. A small penis, less than 4.8 centimetres (1.9 inches) limp, is usually able to impregnate as long as it can get the sperm into the vagina, up towards the cervix. Size is rarely an issue in infertility.

Size may not matter, but function does. Your spam filter is probably working overtime getting rid of Viagra advertisements but you may be comforted to know that lots of men have problems with erectile dysfunction, also known as impotence. You may be comforted to know that you're not alone, but this condition can be an embarrassing detriment to getting pregnant. *Impotence,* the inability to have or sustain an erection, is more common as men get older; as many as 50 per cent of men between the ages of 40 and 70 have had problems with impotence. Impotence can be caused by diseases such as diabetes or arterial disease or by chronic conditions, such as alcohol abuse, or it can be a side effect of medications.

The opening that lets both urine and sperm out of the penis should be at the tip of the penis, located dead centre. Two types of variations can cause problems getting pregnant. One in around 300 men has *hypospadias,* which means that the opening is on the underside of the penis. In 20 per cent of cases, this problem is hereditary. In *epispadias,* the opening is on the top of the penis. Both conditions are associated with an unusual curvature of the erect penis; it curves up in epispadias and down in hypospadias. Both conditions can prevent the sperm from getting exactly where they need to be. Surgical correction is possible.

The testicles

Testicles are the sperm production and warehouse site. Here, as in many other places on the human body, nature has been generous and given two testicles, in case something happens to one. Testicles first develop inside the abdomen and gradually descend outside the body by the time a baby boy is born. At birth, about 4 in 100 boys have undescended testicles, properly called *cryptorchidism.* Testicles need to be kept a few degrees cooler than 98 degrees for sperm to develop properly, so to prevent future infertility, doctors usually recommend surgery to lower the testicles outside the body as soon as the baby is a year or two old.

The testicles are contained in a pouch of skin called the *scrotum.* In about 80 per cent of men, the left testicle is bigger and hangs lower. Sometimes the testicles are abnormally large, which can be caused by a *hydrocoele,* which is a collection of fluid inside the scrotum, or by a *varicocoele,* which is the condition of dilated or varicose veins in the testicle. These conditions can be surgically corrected. Untreated varicocoeles can raise the temperature of the testes and may cause infertility.

Sperm are produced every day, but it takes about 70 days for the new sperm to fully mature. Sperm production starts in the testes. FSH and LH, the same hormones that develop eggs (refer to the earlier section 'The ovaries'), are needed to begin sperm production. LH stimulates production of *testosterone*, another male hormone. The sperm mature in the *epididymis* (a duct behind the testis) and travel through the vas deferens, where they're bathed in the fluid known as *semen,* derived from the prostate gland. The fluid and sperm are then ejaculated through the urethra during male orgasm.

Sperm – 200 million of them!

Here comes one egg – or maybe two eggs, if it's a good month – drifting down the Fallopian tubes. The egg is the largest cell in the human body but it's still only about the size of a pencil point – in other words, barely visible to the naked eye. All of a sudden the egg meets up with about 200 sperm, the sole survivors of an ejaculation of over 200 million sperm a few hours before – talk about an embarrassment of riches. The sperm are much smaller than the egg, so small that all the sperm needed to re-populate the earth could sit on an aspirin tablet. There's enough room for all of them to attach their heads to the egg and try to beat down the door. Sperm have to hunt in packs but usually only one will succeed and the sperm head with the nucleus containing the DNA will be driven through the egg's shell and all the others will be shut out immediately.

Why are there so many more sperm than eggs? Because the journey through the uterus and up the tubes is a *long* way, and because only 50 per cent (of a *good* sperm sample) of the sperm know how to swim forward, *and* the majority of them are abnormally formed, so a tremendous number of sperm are needed to ensure that just a few hundred 'gold-medal swimmers' will get through to the egg. Their journey is like one of you trying to swim across the Atlantic Ocean. If there were 200 million of you, maybe a few hundred would make it. Imagine if you had to fertilise an egg when you finally got there!

Putting Male and Female Parts Together: Having Sex (At the Right Time)

Now that you know how all your parts work, are you ready to have a baby? Yes? Then it's time to have sex. No, not *right* now. It's important to have sex when the timing is right. How do you know when the timing is right? This moment is more than just mood lighting, an unexpected bunch of flowers, and foreplay. To become pregnant, you need to be close to ovulation.

You may be able to tell that you're ovulating in a few simple ways, just by watching the calendar, and being observant about how your body works.

If you're an on-the-dot, regular-as-clockwork type, with 28 days between the start of each period, you probably ovulate around day 14. You're also as rare as hen's teeth. Few women are that regular; most women usually have a few days' variation from month to month. But if your periods are regular, you can figure that you're ovulating about two weeks before your period starts, so if you have 32-day cycles, you ovulate around day 18.

Usually the mucus from your cervix increases around the time of ovulation. It also becomes very thin, clear, and stretchy; you can easily stretch it out a couple of inches (known in German as *Spinnbarkeit*). Rising oestrogen levels from a developing follicle create this mucus, which is easier for sperm to swim through than your usual thicker mucus and also has an alkaline pH, which helps the sperm live longer. At other times of the month, cervical mucus is acidic. Be sure that you're not confusing cervical mucus with semen from previous sex or increased secretions from sexual arousal.

If you're taking antihistamines, you may not notice a change in cervical mucus. Antihistamines are usually found in cold medications and allergy medicines, and dry up mucus everywhere, not just in your nose and chest.

If you have no objection to feeling around inside your vagina, you'll also notice that your cervix becomes softer, slightly open, and easier to locate with your fingers when you're about to ovulate. At other times of the month, the cervix is found farther back in the uterus, feels firmer to the touch, and is tightly closed.

Some women have headaches around the time of ovulation, and others complain of bloating or breast pain. You're probably already aware of your personal ovulation indicators, but you may have just never paid much attention to them. Now you should. They're a big help in choosing when to have baby sex.

Conceiving a Baby: How Sex Should Work

The time is right, the moon is bright, and it's time to get pregnant. Here's what needs to happen:

1. **You're near to ovulation; an egg is about to release from its follicle.** (Texting your partner to announce he must get home fast may work for some couples, but if he was just about to ask the boss for a pay rise, you may want to wait till he gets home.)

2. **You and your partner become aroused.** Your vaginal secretions increase allowing the now erect penis to enter the vagina much easier.

3. **During the man's orgasm, several million sperm are forcefully ejaculated into the vagina.** As they pass through the cervix into the uterus, the cervical mucus 'washes' the sperm so that they're ready to penetrate an egg.

4. Your egg is expelled from the follicle, is 'picked up' by the fimbriae, and enters one of your Fallopian tubes.

5. The sperm swim through the uterus up to the Fallopian tubes; they don't know which tube to choose and half get it wrong.

6. The next day your egg meets up with several hundred sperm (the brightest and best – it's 'survival of the fittest' in the great sperm race) in the Fallopian tube, and they all attach themselves to the egg.

7. The *acrosome cap* on the sperm's head contains a tiny packet of powerful enzymes that help one sperm to break through the outer layer of the egg, and the egg immediately becomes impenetrable to the rest of the sperm.

8. The genetic material of the egg and sperm combine, and the newly created embryo drifts down the fallopian tube to the uterus.

9. The embryo divides for a further 4–5 days until it becomes a *blastocyst* and then it can embed in the endometrial lining of the uterine wall. The developing embryo produces a hormone called human chorionic gonadotrophins (hCG), which sends a chemical message to the corpus luteum to keep making progesterone so that the endometrium doesn't break down and then, about a week later, you miss your period.

10. You're pregnant! Congratulations.

After sex, just lie there for a while. Don't jump up and go to the loo right away. Let gravity help those little swimmers get to where they need to be. Some doctors advocate placing a pillow under the hips during sex to give gravity a little edge in directing the sperm where they need to be. Doing so probably isn't necessary. Of course, the missionary position, man on top, is also an aid to gravity.

Figuring out how often to have sex

When you're trying to get pregnant, you need to strike a balance between too much sex and not enough. Too much sex lowers sperm counts, but if you have too little sex, you may miss the right moment for conception. Not having sex for more than five days may raise the number of sperm but decrease their motility (the active movement). Sex less than two days apart may decrease the sperm count. So how do you figure out when the right time is?

When you're close to ovulating, have sex at least every other day; some doctors recommend the two days before and the day you ovulate as the best time for conception.

Making Sure That You're Healthy – Before Conception

Even though you're probably anxious to get started on baby making, take a little time to make sure that you're in the best possible condition for conceiving a healthy baby. This consideration means making sure that you're not carrying an infection that could harm you or your baby and taking a look at your lifestyle habits, good and bad.

What you can't see: Common infections that may cause problems

The onset of the sexual revolution in the 1960s caused a lot of fallout, and some of it fell on future fertility. Sexually transmitted diseases, or STDs, have increased dramatically in the last 20 years. You may not even know that you have a sexually transmitted disease. Some STDs cause a vaginal or penile discharge, others cause itching or small sores, but some cause no symptoms at all. Most are easily treated with antibiotics. The problem is that many women don't realise they have an infection because most have no clear symptoms. The following sections describe a few of the most damaging STDs and provide some advice on how to avoid them.

You can be tested for sexually transmitted diseases, including HIV, before trying to conceive. If you suspect that you may have an STD, or have been exposed to one, you need to rule out this potential danger to your fertility and your unborn child.

Chlamydia: The most common STD

Chlamydia is the most common sexually transmitted disease in the Western world. The bacterium *Chlamydia trachomatis* is responsible for the infection and it is highly infectious. Both men and women can be infected, and both male and female fertility can be damaged. Chlamydia is easily tested for by swabbing the penis or cervix and sending the swab to a lab, or urine samples can be analysed using a special test. A blood test looking for chlamydia antibodies shows whether there has been a past infection and a high level may indicate active infection. Chlamydia is easily treated with antibiotics; doxycycline is the antibiotic of choice – hardly anyone is allergic to it and it's as cheap as chips! Make sure you're treated at the same time as your partner.

Here are some facts about the disease:

- ✔ Approximately one in ten sexually active adolescents has been exposed to chlamydia.

- ✔ Women with untreated chlamydia have a 40 per cent chance of developing pelvic inflammatory disease (PID), a major cause of damaged Fallopian tubes.

- ✔ Women with PID are seven to ten times more likely to have an *ectopic pregnancy*, a pregnancy that grows outside the uterus, usually in the tubes. (For more about ectopic pregnancies, see Chapter 5.)

- ✔ Most women (75 per cent) have no symptoms of infection; symptoms include lower abdominal pain, burning with urination, and vaginal irritation and discharge.

- ✔ Twenty five percent of men have no symptoms from chlamydia; 75 per cent have a discharge from the urethra, or pain and burning on urination.

- ✔ Men with untreated chlamydia can develop *epididymitis*, an infection in the testicles, where sperm are developed. This condition can lead to low sperm counts.

- ✔ Each year far too many women become infertile from chlamydia. With a first infection, 12 per cent of women become infertile; a second case increases infertility to 40 per cent. Eighty per cent of women who have had chlamydia three or more times are infertile.

- ✔ Fifty per cent of people with chlamydia also have gonorrhoea.

Untreated chlamydia when you're pregnant can cause blindness in your baby.

Gonorrhoea

Gonorrhoea is caused by the bacterium *Neisseria gonorrhoeae*, which can infect the genital tract, mouth, or rectum. It can be carried by males and females, and can be cured with antibiotics. Here are some other facts about gonorrhoea:

- ✔ Gonorrhoea is diagnosed second only in frequency to chlamydia.

- ✔ Like chlamydia, gonorrhoea in women can cause PID, leading to tubal damage. Most doctors test for gonorrhoea and chlamydia before doing common fertility tests such as a *hysterosalpingogram* (HSG), in which dye is injected into the uterus and fallopian tubes to see whether any irregularities exist. (We discuss HSGs in more detail in Chapter 7.) If you have gonorrhoea or chlamydia and push dye into the tubes and uterus, you may push the infection up also and end up with more tube or uterine damage than you had to begin with.

- ✔ Men with gonorrhoea usually have a discharge from the penis and a burning sensation; women may have no symptoms.

Syphilis

Syphilis is caused by the bacterium *Treponema pallidum*. The bacterium can be transmitted through genital, oral, or anal contact. Syphilis is easily cured with penicillin. Contrary to folklore, syphilis can't be caught from a toilet seat.

You may not get syphilis from toilet seats, but consider this: Syphilis can cause stillbirth, blindness, mental retardation, or chronic syphilis in your unborn child if you have this disease while pregnant. Syphilis is readily treated with antibiotics.

Ureaplasma and mycoplasma

Ureaplasma and mycoplasma are micro-organisms that can affect different parts of the body, depending on the strain. The genital tracts of both sexes can carry mycoplasma or ureaplasma. The following list gives some other information about the diseases:

- ✔ As many as 40 per cent of women and men are carriers of the bacteria ureaplasma or mycoplasma.

- ✔ Some controversy exists about whether certain strains of ureaplasma and mycoplasma cause problems in getting pregnant; some studies show that they increase the incidence of miscarriage and/or problems with the embryo implanting in the uterus. This risk seems to be related to either partner having the infection, which is easily passed between partners.

- ✔ New studies are questioning whether these bacteria really cause infertility or miscarriage; more studies will probably be done.

- ✔ As with other STDs, both partners are easily treated with a 14-day course of an antibiotic, such as doxycycline. Both partners must take the drug, or they'll probably continue to re-infect each other.

Genital herpes

Genital herpes is caused by the herpes simplex type 2 virus. The cold sores some people are prone to on their lips are caused by the herpes simplex type 1 virus. Scientists are working on a vaccine against herpes, which would work only for those not already infected with the virus.

Herpes can't be permanently cured because the virus tends to lie dormant and then return; outbreaks can be quite effectively treated with antiviral medications when treated in time.

If you have an outbreak of genital herpes at the time your baby is ready to be delivered, you'll need to have a caesarean section; if you deliver vaginally without treatment, your baby may suffer from mental retardation or may die.

HIV

Human immunodeficiency virus (HIV) causes the disease AIDS (acquired immune deficiency syndrome). At present, no cure for AIDS exists, although antiviral medications may keep the disease under control for some time. Here are some facts about HIV:

- ✔ Women with HIV can become pregnant and carry the pregnancy to term, but they risk transmitting HIV to the baby and must be delivered by caesarean section.

- ✔ The risk of transmission is about 25 per cent if you're untreated and may be as low as 2 to 5 per cent if you receive AZT, an antiviral drug, while you're pregnant.

- ✔ You will reduce the risk of transmission of the disease to your baby if you have a caesarean section rather than a vaginal delivery. Mothers who are HIV positive must not breast-feed their babies.

- ✔ You must wait 3 to 18 months after delivery to find out whether your baby is HIV positive, because during pregnancy your antibodies are passed to the baby. This means that all babies of HIV-infected mothers will test positive at birth. It can take as long as 18 months for all your antibodies to disappear from your baby's blood. After your antibodies are all gone, if the baby tests positive, the result means he is infected with the virus.

Behaving Yourself When Trying to Conceive

Because the best parents generally practise what they preach, setting up some good habits even *before* conception occurs is as good a start as any! Good nutrition is important at every stage of your life, but particularly when you're trying to conceive and maintain a pregnancy and ultimately deliver a healthy child. Although a perfectly tuned body isn't a necessity for having children, being fit certainly provides an ideal starting point. Nurturing your mind and heart is equally important. The following sections offer some tips on keeping your entire self in tip-top, baby-making shape.

Getting the proper nutrition

Although vitamins provide good supplementation, get as many nutrients and minerals as possible from the food you eat. So before ingesting supplements ranging from vitamin A to zinc, start instead with your diet. Eating three square meals a day, plus a snack, is a good place to begin. What should those meals be made of? If you consider chocolate a food group, read on to discover otherwise.

Look at your fertility diet in the shape of a pregnant woman's body. See Figure 2-3 for a visual of a pregnant you as a daily food chart. At the top, the smallest spot should be reserved for fats, oils, and sweets. This category includes jam, mayonnaise, margarine, sweets, and so on. Use these foods sparingly.

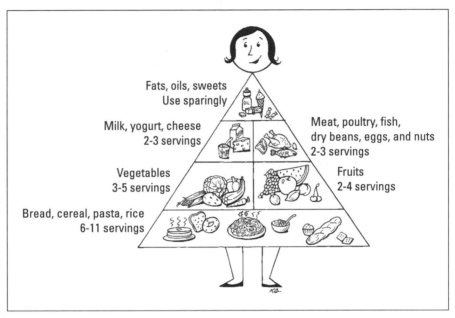

Fats, oils, sweets
Use sparingly

Milk, yogurt, cheese
2-3 servings

Meat, poultry, fish,
dry beans, eggs, and nuts
2-3 servings

Vegetables
3-5 servings

Fruits
2-4 servings

Bread, cereal, pasta, rice
6-11 servings

Figure 2-3:
A shapely reminder about what to eat – and how much.

The next step down on the chart consists of two slightly larger categories: the milk, yogurt, and cheese group and the group that includes meat, poultry, fish, dry beans, eggs, and nuts. Consume two to three servings from the milk, yogurt, and cheese group each day. In this category, a serving is considered 5 ounces (or 125 grammes) of milk or yogurt or 2 ounces (50 grammes) of processed cheese. Two to three servings (ounces) are recommended in the group that includes lean meat, poultry, fish, eggs, dry beans, and nuts. This daily intake provides you with calcium, riboflavin, protein, iron, and B vitamins.

The next level calls for three to five servings of vegetables and two to four servings of fruit per day. A serving size of vegetables consists of 1 cup of raw leafy vegetables, 5 ounces (125 grammes) of cooked vegetables, or 8 ounces (200 grammes) of vegetable juice, and a serving size of fruits consists of one medium apple, banana, or orange, 5 ounces (125 grammes) of chopped cooked or canned fruit, or 8 ounces (200 grammes) of fruit juice. Notice that the recommended servings have increased from the higher level of this food chart. Pay attention to this recommendation. Vegetables and fruits are your most important source for fibre, vitamin A, vitamin C, and carbohydrates.

At the bottom of the pregnant-woman daily food chart, you find the largest food group, which contains bread, cereal, rice, and pasta. Consider this part as the abdomen! The recommendation is that you eat six to eleven servings of this group per day. But before you wolf down a plate of pasta, remember your serving sizes. A serving in this group consists of one slice of bread, half a bagel, 1 ounce of ready-to-eat cereal, 5 ounces (125 grammes) of cooked rice or pasta, three to four small, plain crackers, or one 4-inch pancake.

If this chart seems like any other food plan you've ever seen, well spotted – it is! Healthy eating is a standard practice; few tricks exist when it comes to eating healthy. When trying to conceive, eat enough but not too much and use your calories for healthy foods and not empty ones (such as chocolate). If you're not lactose intolerant, you may want to up your dairy intake; if you're *lactose intolerant,* which means that you can't properly digest milk products, you can get calcium from oral supplements.

Be careful of health foods such as soy, sunflower seeds, or herbs that promise to raise your oestrogen level. (You can read more about herbs in Chapter 3.) Your body – more specifically, your ovaries – should be producing oestrogen. By introducing an outside source, you're not assisting your body in manufacturing its own supply; you're only supplementing it artificially. This addition doesn't change the quality of your eggs or their output of oestrogen. You'll only confuse any measurement of oestrogen, because trying to distinguish what your body makes on its own from that which you gain from outside sources is impossible. Skip any supplement or food that claims to increase your oestrogen level.

Another practice to avoid is dieting, particularly fad diets. Conception is an act of incredible balance and timing. You don't want to throw your body off with the latest diet that promises to help you lose 5 pounds fast. More than likely, such a diet is a method that probably won't help your weight or your health any more than it will help your fertility.

If you're significantly overweight or underweight, you may want to consult your doctor before trying to conceive and especially if your periods are irregular. Either extreme can cause problems in fertility, particularly if your weight is symptomatic of another condition such as diabetes, polycystic ovary syndrome (PCOS), or amenorrhea. Twelve per cent of all infertility is a result of weighing too much or too little. In an Australian study of 3,500 women, very obese women were half as likely to conceive when compared to their healthier peer group. The researchers also concluded that no good comes of being underweight, either: Women who are below moderate weight also have less chance of becoming pregnant.

The good news is that 70 per cent of all women diagnosed with infertility related to being overweight or underweight conceive spontaneously when their weight becomes normal.

If weight loss or weight gain is in order, consider addressing this matter before trying to conceive. Check with your GP and ask for a healthy diet and exercise plan. If you must lose – or gain – weight simultaneously with your baby-making efforts, make sure that your GP is aware of *both* goals.

Ways in which extremes of weight can affect fertility include menstrual disturbance, disturbance to the lining of the uterus, inability to ovulate (anovulation), and increased risk of miscarriage.

Taking vitamins

Multivitamins are a good way to supplement your diet, but they're not a substitute for good nutrition. While you're trying to conceive and when you're pregnant, you need both. Much has been written about the importance of folic acid in early pregnancy. Folic acid has been shown to reduce the risk of neural tube defects (defects of the spinal cord) such as *spina bifida* and *anencephaly*. (Check out Chapter 3 for more information on multivitamins.)

'Pre-natal' multivitamins contain adequate amounts of folic acid and suffice while you're trying to conceive. As with everything else, moderation is key. Mixing and matching individual vitamin supplements can result in too much of a good thing, which translates into *not* such a good thing. Let the drug manufacturers figure out the dosages. Just stick with the basics.

Finding Information

The best answers to pregnancy related questions come from your GP. After you have your GP's opinion on whatever you're concerned about, then by all means expand on this knowledge by looking in books by writers suitably qualified, or on the Internet.

Turning to books and the Internet for information

Reading is good. Reading about pregnancy is better, particularly if you choose books and other materials that focus on areas that you *do* have control over, namely nutrition, exercise, and good self-care. Take the time to read about and make the changes that you can do to create a healthier you, which in turn will make you a healthier *two*.

Books are always a great source of information, but the Internet can also provide an abundance of resources. Log on to a search engine such as Google or Yahoo! You'll be rewarded with a plethora of possibilities on everything to do with pregnancy.

Be a careful consumer. When visiting a Web site, check out the source providing the information. Chat rooms are wonderful for support and referrals, but act on medical advice only from a professional.

Talking to friends

Ooooooh, a toughie! Support is a wonderful thing, but pressure isn't. If you decide to share with your friends that you're trying to conceive, don't turn your efforts into a quest or a competition. You may want to inform your friends that you're trying and that you'll let them know if and when you succeed. This approach can help prevent the 'Are you there yet?' questions that are asked in the right spirit yet often result in a feeling of pressure.

Old wives' tales

When people know you're trying to get pregnant, not only do they give words of support and reassurance, they often slip into the wise old woman mode and offer you 'tried and tested' received wisdom. (Cue spooky music from *The Twilight Zone*). Here are some examples of folklore or old wives' tales (try at your own risk!):

✔ Honeymoons are a really good time to become pregnant . . . with twins! You may think this outcome is related to sex, but no, according to one tale, a couple will have twins if they see a film during the first three days of their honeymoon or go swimming on the first day of their marriage.

✔ If you can't manage a honeymoon just now, you might consider having a messy friend come to your house and leave a nappy under a bed. Doing so is supposed to ensure a birth in your house.

✔ If you'd rather be the one leaving things about, go to a strange house and lay your coat or hat on a bed there; doing so is also supposed to help you get pregnant. Maybe you could visit all the open houses in your area and lay your coat all over town to make *sure* that this method works.

✔ Make love on any of Britain's ancient fertility symbols, including the Cerne Abbas giant in Dorset or the Fertility Stone near Pateley Bridge in North Yorkshire. If you fancy the open-air and the chance of being caught, it may add a little frisson to your love-making.

✔ Sniff! Sniff! Smelling behind a pregnant woman's ear will cause you to conceive.

✔ If you sleep with a pink ribbon under your pillow and sleep on the right, you'll get a girl. If you sleep with a red ribbon under your pillow and sleep on the left, you'll get a boy.

Friends who have had children or have tried to conceive can be incredibly helpful in lending perspective to your monthly challenge and can also offer suggestions on everything from doctors to nappies, reading materials to relaxation techniques. You may also find that you get an enormous amount of support from friends who are neither married nor with children. Those faced with the challenge of searching for Mr or Ms Right may turn to the same elements of luck and timing that also apply to making a baby. Single friends can be incredibly supportive in helping you remember that you have a lovely partner to cherish even if you're not quite pregnant yet!

Through my own fertility treatment, I (co-author Jill) confided in some good friends and also in a colleague whom I learned was also considering fertility treatment. These friendships became even stronger and will be lifelong as a result of sharing my experience. They also made coping when treatment didn't work much easier, as they had been part of my fertility journey from the start and I didn't have to recount the whole saga to explain why I was in pieces at certain times.

Listening to the old wives

The good news about letting your friends and family know that you're trying to conceive is that everyone has an idea. The bad news is . . . everyone has an idea. And although most of these ideas are well meaning, many of them also weigh in at downright wacky. But if you're game for a different approach, you might give an old-wives' tale a whirl (see the sidebar 'Old wives' tales'). If you'd rather stick with the more proven method, you may still enjoy reading about some of the superstitions and stories that others swear by. If doing so only gives you cause to smile, just remember another old adage: laughter is the best medicine.

Part II
Planning a Pregnancy

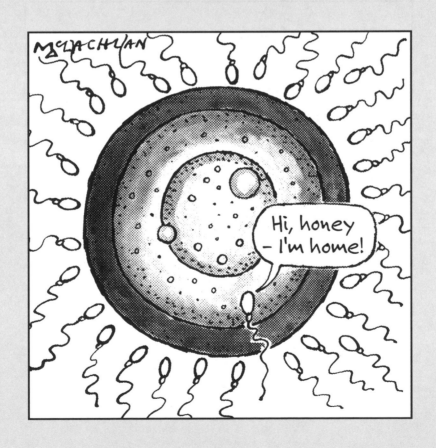

In this part . . .

In this part we look at some simple methods of improving your chances of pregnancy, as well as some alternative choices such as herbs, reflexology, and acupuncture. We also look at predicting ovulation to help you get pregnant and guide you through the first visit to your GP about possible infertility. In this part we give you emotional help in handling a pregnancy that ends too soon and explain why this can happen.

Chapter 3

We're Trying! We're Trying! (to Get Pregnant)

*A*fter you start trying to get pregnant, you expect results – that's human nature. But Mother Nature isn't always working to your timetable, and you may find yourself still trying after a few months, and anxious to step up the pace a bit with some scientific help. In this chapter, you can find out about some low-tech but helpful methods of trying to pin down that elusive positive pregnancy test.

A number of testing methods are available to help you identify exactly when you're ovulating; they test everything from urine to saliva. Some have been in use for decades, and others are brand new.

Predicting Ovulation: Kits, Sticks, and Software

Maybe you've been trying to get pregnant for a few months and you're beginning to feel frustrated and even a little anxious that you're never going to get pregnant. Flick back and read the statistics in Chapter 1 to remind yourself that nature is inefficient, or remember that everyone in your family took six months to get pregnant. Maybe you can try something more scientific that will prove to be more successful. You thought that you hit all the 'right' days to have sex for the last few months, but maybe you're missing the 'real' right day or misinterpreting your body's ovulation signs. This section covers a few ways to monitor your ovulation cycle that are more scientific than counting calendar days. Hopefully, one will work for you!

Ovulation is the monthly release of an egg from your ovary. Ovulation is the one time during the month that you can actually get pregnant. Your window of opportunity is approximately three days.

Be careful how you spend your money – buying expensive ovulation and sperm test kits is no substitute for having regular unprotected sex to try and make a baby!

Using an ovulation predictor kit

Ovulation predictor kits (OPKs) are a popular way to test if and when you ovulate. The tests measure the amount of LH (luteinising hormone) found in your urine. LH generally rises 24 to 36 hours before ovulation; the rise of LH is called your *LH surge*. You should have sex one or two days before ovulation and on the day of ovulation to improve your chance of getting pregnant.

OPKs are easy to find; every chemist or pharmacy sells them. They use your urine, a cheap and abundant substance, to test for ovulation, and the sticks are small enough to carry around with you.

Positive levels of some urine OPKs

Many brands of urine ovulation predictor kits are available. We've listed a few samples in the table. The number listed is the amount of luteinising hormone needed to make the stick register a positive surge. Sensitivity is measured in units called *mIU/ml,* which means milli-International Units per millilitre.

Brand	Sensitivity	Number of Sticks	Length of Test Time
Boots	40 mIU/ml	5	3 minutes
Clearblue	40 mIU/ml	7	3 minutes
Clearblue Digital	40 mIU/ml	7	3 minutes
First Response	50 mIU/ml	5	3–5 minutes
Superdrug	40 mIU/ml	5	3 minutes

The OPKs, or 'pee sticks' as they're called, have some drawbacks. Certain women, such as women with polycystic ovaries (see Chapter 7), may have a high LH all the time, so the kits will always be positive. Women over 40 or those in premature ovarian failure (POF) may also have a higher than normal LH, because LH and FSH (follicle-stimulating hormone) both rise in POF. Some tests are also difficult to read, require several steps that need to be carefully done for good results, or start to show positive only when the LH reaches 40 mIU/ml (milli-International Units per millilitre), the International Standard for an LH surge.

Some women may not have a surge that registers as high as 40 mIU/ml; so look for kits that register positive at 25 mIU/ml.

Most kits show a positive result as a line as dark as or darker than the control line. Read the test at exactly the time indicated; sometimes the lines darken for a few hours, but that doesn't mean you're having a surge.

The kits are harder to use if you don't have regular cycles; unless you know approximately when you ovulate each month, you may use up a lot of sticks trying to figure out when your surge starts. If you have regular cycles, you can start testing about 16 days before you expect your next period, but if your cycles are irregular, you need to test every few days to make sure that you don't miss the big 'O' day. Table 3-1 can help you determine when to start testing.

Table 3-1	Counting Days, Saving Sticks																	
Length of Normal Cycle	22 23 24 25 26 27 28 29 30 31 32 33 34 35 36 37 38 39 40
Start Testing This Many Days After Your Period Starts	5 6 7 8 9 10 11 12 13 14 15 16 17 18 19 20 21 22 23

OPKs aren't cheap; they cost about £15–£20 for five or seven sticks. You'll use one stick each time you test, and you need to test every 12 to 24 hours around the time of ovulation to accurately 'catch' your surge. Resist the urge to buy the cheaper kits. They may not register lower LH levels, and they may be much harder to read. As a result, you use up more sticks because you're showing all your friends and asking their opinion on which line is darker. In addition to using up a lot of sticks, you may use up a lot of friends, too!

OPKs register only when your surge has begun, so you won't be able to time sex as accurately for the two days immediately before ovulation.

Also, OPKs tell you only when you're *about* to ovulate – they can't show you whether you've actually released an egg. Women with LUFS, or luteinised unruptured follicle syndrome, may produce an egg, have an LH surge, and yet not release the egg. Of course, you can't get pregnant if the egg isn't released.

Adding computer power with a fertility monitor

If you want to go a little higher tech than the OPKs, you may be interested in a fertility monitor – such as Persona or the Clearblue Fertility Monitor – which works a little differently than the standard OPK. These monitors are actually small computers that store data about your cycle to tell you when you're going to ovulate. They're more labour intensive; you need to start testing the first day of your period and test every day around the same time. Morning is the recommended time to test. Because they test both oestrogen and LH levels, fertility monitors can better predict ovulation about five days before it occurs, giving you a better chance to have sex one or two days before ovulation.

Unlike some of the one-use OPK urine tests, which are reliable only in natural cycles, the fertility monitor can be used if you're taking fertility medications, such as gonadotrophins. This devices also 'sets' itself to your cycle if you're somewhat irregular.

These monitors can be expensive – from £23 to £100 – and you also need to buy the sticks. Like the less expensive OPK kits, monitors may not be accurate if you're menopausal or breast-feeding, have polycystic ovaries (see Chapter 7) and a normally higher than usual LH level, or are taking tetracycline antibiotics, so they won't be able to tell if you've released an egg.

Just spit here – the saliva test

Salt content in your saliva increases as your oestrogen levels rise. Saliva ovulation kits test your salt levels and provide an alternative if constantly peeing on a stick isn't for you. The method has several advantages:

- ✔ The entire kit is contained in what looks like a tube of lipstick, so carrying this item around isn't too conspicuous.
- ✔ Because the lens can be washed and reused, this kit is a one-time purchase.
- ✔ The method claims about 98 per cent accuracy.

✔ Unlike urine ovulation kits, these kits can be used any time, anywhere. You can use the saliva kit on the bus, which is out of the question with urine-based OPKs!

✔ The saliva kit costs about the same as a urine ovulation kit (about £15–£20), but can be used many times over.

But disadvantages include:

✔ The saliva kit is slightly more complicated than an ovulation kit to use. You have to take the lens out and put it back properly or you won't read it correctly. You also risk the possibility of breaking or scratching the lens.

✔ Also, as with urine OPKs, this kit tells you only when you're about to ovulate. It won't confirm that you have actually release an egg.

The saliva test can be done every day starting at day one of your cycle; at first you'll see only little dots (of salt) when you look through the viewing piece. As ovulation gets closer, you'll see what look like ferns (see Figure 3-1); when the ferns cover the whole slide, you're about to ovulate. The test takes about five minutes for the slide to dry before you can accurately read it.

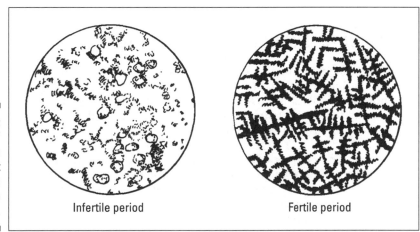

Figure 3-1: 'Ferning' appears on a saliva test when you're close to ovulation.

Infertile period   Fertile period

Tracking your fertility with software

Chances are that if you're reading this book, you've been trying to conceive for a while and may be already keeping track of all the details of your menstrual cycle and when you're having sex. You may have a fertility notebook by now, but you may also write everything down on little pieces of paper and lose them. If you'd like a more scientific approach, however, books and software are available that are specifically designed to keep track of all kinds of fertility information. If natural, non-interventionist conception is important to you, tracking your fertility with high-tech software may be a better prospect than the possibility of high-tech assisted conception.

A variety of PC software titles are available on the Internet, including *TCOYF (Taking Charge of Your Fertility)* Software (and also known as *Ovusoft*) found at www.tcoyf.com and *Hormonal Forecaster* available from www.hormonalforecaster.com. Like all such software, these will identify when you should 'have sex now'!

Both include complete charts to record menstruation, basal body temperature, cervical mucus observations, cervix position, and other custom indicators using a calendar interface. The software calculator will use data to generate ovulation charts and predict ovulation. You can interpret your ovulation charts yourself or let the programme do it for you.

Hormone-tracking software to predict when you're ovulating so you can conceive is also used by women who prefer natural family planning to avoid pregnancy.

Taking your morning temperature

Recording your basal body temperature (BBT) is one of the oldest methods of predicting ovulation. *BBT* is just a long-winded way of saying 'your individual normal temperature'. To get this statistic you use the same type of thermometer that you use to take your temperature to find out whether you have a fever when you're not feeling well.

This method of predicting ovulation is simple but requires a certain amount of determination and a good memory. You need to remember to take your temperature every morning *before* you get up. You need to take your temperature before you get up, eat, drink, or smoke (but you should have quit this habit by now!) because any activity at all will raise your temperature, and eating or drinking will raise or lower it, depending on what you consume.

You may want to buy a special BBT thermometer, which has larger numbers to make it easier to read each one-tenth of a degree, which you need to record. Alternatively, you could use an instant in-the-ear digital thermometer – a bit more expensive than the standard glass thermometer, but so much quicker and possibly more accurate.

Many charts are available to help you plot your temperature, but you can easily make one yourself. All you do is mark down your morning temperature to the exact one-tenth of a degree and then connect the 'dots.' You're looking for a subtle drop in temperature, followed by a sustained rise in temperature for more than three days, during which your temperature should rise at least

0.5 degrees Celsius. The drop occurs just before ovulation, and the rise indicates an increase in your progesterone levels – progesterone increases only after you've ovulated. Your chances of conceiving are improved at the point where the temperature drops – or ideally the day before that! This result means 'have sex now'! This method has a few drawbacks. The most obvious one is that you need to be scrupulous about taking your temperature and recording it so that you don't forget it. Also, you have to keep your chart for a whole month for the temperatures to be meaningful. In addition, the drop in temperature is sometimes difficult to detect.

Factors other than hormones can cause an increase or decrease in your temperature. If you're sick, even small temperature fluctuations may make your chart inaccurate, and you'll think you've ovulated when actually you have flu. Alcohol, too little or too much sleep, and subtle illnesses can all change your temperature.

Your BBT can also indicate whether you're pregnant. If your temperature stays elevated more than 15 days, there's a good chance that you're pregnant – unless, of course, you have flu. If your temperature starts to drop after ten days or so, you may have a *luteal phase defect*, which means that your progesterone may be too low to sustain a pregnancy.

Home sperm tests

You can buy over-the-counter sperm home-testing kits from high street chemists and even supermarkets. These tests don't give laboratory detail about shape or movement, but can indicate the number of sperm in any sample.

FertilMARQ is a sperm test available to buy online. The test won't give you detailed information regarding the shape *(morphology)* or movement *(motility)* of the sperm, but it will let you check out two semen samples to see whether the concentration of sperm meets the accepted fertility level of 20 million/ml. For more information visit www.sperm.test.com.

Fertell offers both male and female fertility testing kits in a single purchase. The male kit not only tests the number, but also the motility of the sperm, via an ingenious column of fluid that acts as artificial cervical mucus. If enough sperm pass through the fake mucus, you may carry on trying to get pregnant the old-fashioned fun way. If the test indicates the motile sperm concentration is below the cut-off level for 'normally expected values', you should see a doctor. See www.fertell.co.uk for more information.

Weigh up the cost of these tests with the cost of similar tests with your GP or at a fertility clinic. Chances are that if you have a problem with the sperm, you'll end up paying again for even more sensitive tests, which also give you the benefit of getting the results first-hand from a fertility specialist.

Practice Makes Perfect

Although sex on eight or ten consecutive days may be fun at first, and a dream for many of your friends, as the months go by, even your partner may get jaded at the summons to 'baby dance right now'!

Before the thought of conceiving via a sterile Petri dish without the presence of you or your husband becomes an attractive alternative, remember that regular sex (that is, every other night from the end of one period to the start of the next) will increase your chance of conceiving, avoid the robot-like mechanics of baby-making sex, and help keep the romance alive.

Regular sex may also help avoid the increasingly common relief of 'we'll never have to have sex again' that some couples feel when they have had to work really hard to conceive naturally and find out they're finally pregnant!

Positive Thinking – Home Pregnancy Tests

If you think that you used a lot of ovulation predictor sticks, wait until you start using home pregnancy tests (HPTs)! Home pregnancy tests are available in every chemist or pharmacy. These tests give fast results, usually in 2 to 5 minutes. Most tell you to not urinate for 4 hours before you test so the concentration of the hormone will be high. Some kits suggest that you urinate in a cup and dip the wand into it, and other kits suggest peeing directly on the stick.

The rabbit died

Home pregnancy tests have been available since the 1970s; earlier tests had to be done by GPs. The earliest tests were available in the late 1920s and gave rise to the sweetly whispered phrase, 'The rabbit died', in movies for the next 40 years. The urine was collected in the doctor's office and then sent off to the lab, where it was injected into a virgin rabbit (or sometimes a frog). A day or two later, the rabbit was killed and her ovaries examined to see whether they contained bulging masses called *corpora hemorrhagica*. If they did, you were pregnant! So if you ever get sick after months of 'peeing on a stick', be thankful we don't still use the rabbit!

All the tests, from the 1920s on, measured hCG (human chorionic gonadotropin), the hormone released by the implantation of the embryo and the growing placenta. The newest tests are very sensitive; the most sensitive tests on the market detect concentrations of 25 mIU/ml, which usually occur around the time you would miss your first period. (The unit *mIU/ml* means milli-International Units per millilitre.) Other kits don't test positive until the hCG level is 50 mIU/ml, so read the box before you buy. Some tests claim to be accurate a few days *before* your period is due, but any results one to four days before your period is due may not be accurate. You may have had a late implantation, or you may have ovulated a day or two after you thought you had. Another test should be done a few days later if your period still hasn't started.

The average level of hCG ten days post ovulation is 25 mIU/ml then 50 mIU/ml 12 days post ovulation, and 100 mIU/ml 14 days after you ovulate. Keep in mind that these numbers are averages; your number may be higher or lower and still be perfectly normal.

Blood tests can also measure hCG, detecting concentrations less than 5 mIU/ml. Blood tests give an exact number, so only with blood tests can you tell whether your hCG levels are doubling every two to three days, as they do in most normal pregnancies.

Table 3-2 lists the common brands of pregnancy testing kits – costing between 99p and £11.99 – that show the lowest hCG number they claim will register a positive result.

Table 3-2	Common Home Pregnancy Tests		
Brand	**Sensitivity**	**Day to Test**	**Length of Test Time**
Boots	50 mIU/ml	Day your period is due	1 minute
Clearblue	50 mIU/ml	Day your period is due	3 minutes
Clearblue	25 mIU/ml	From 4 days before your period*	2 minutes
Clearblue Digital	25 mIU/ml	From 4 days before your period*	3 minutes
First Response	25 mIU/ml	From 4 days before your period*	3 minutes
Predictor	50 mIU/ml	Day your period is due	4 minutes
Quik-Check	25 mIU/ml	Day your period is due	3 minutes
Superdrug	50 mIU/ml	Day your period is due	1 minute

* Results on days three or four before your period have an accuracy of between 53–83 per cent depending on the brand, compared to a claimed accuracy of 99 per cent when tested on the day your period is due, so be aware of the inaccuracies of early-testing!

Some tests show a positive as a little + sign; others want you to drag all your friends back in to the bathroom (if you still have any friends left after ovulation) and have them compare the control line to the test line to see whether they match. Usually, a positive is indicated by a test line that's as dark as or darker than the control (see Figure 3-2).

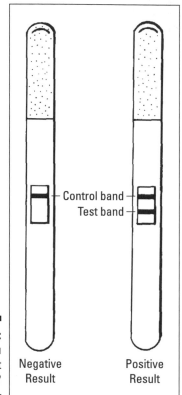

Figure 3-2:
Are you
pregnant
or not?

Control band
Test band

Negative
Result

Positive
Result

Don't let the test sit around before looking at it, as some test results will change after an hour or two and will not be accurate.

Dealing with a false positive

False positive results are rare in home pregnancy tests, but you may have a false positive if:

✔ You're taking injections of the hormone hCG to induce ovulation or for any other reason; it takes 5–7 days for 10,000 U of hCG (a standard dose) to completely clear your system.

✔ You recently had a miscarriage or ectopic pregnancy, and the hCG levels have not dropped to a negative range yet.

✔ You have developed a rare condition called a hydatydiform mole (or a 'molar pregnancy'), which may go on to become a cancer called chorio-carcinoma. This cancer usually follows a full-term birth, miscarriage, or other pregnancy loss.

A hydatydiform mole is a fast-growing cancer, so if you recently had a pregnancy loss of any kind and have a positive home pregnancy test and heavy bleeding, you *must* see a doctor immediately. This cancer is usually treated with methotrexate, which can avoid the need for a hysterectomy.

Coping with That Time of the Month Again: The Pain of Not Getting Pregnant

It's negative . . . again. That word reminds you of just how hard you're trying and how painful a negative result has become. In the beginning, the negative results were easier to take and you looked at the next chance of having sex and getting pregnant as a bit of fun, and that next time would be 'the one'. But, as the months pass and the number of negative results increases, the process of starting all over again grows more difficult.

Sometimes a home pregnancy test can occasionally be wrong, but most positive results are usually picked up by these simple tests. So how do you deal with those results that are less than positive? Here are a few suggestions to make the process a little easier:

✔ Test once and forget it. Our bodies are beautifully timed so that if you are indeed pregnant, you'll know soon enough. Although not every pregnant woman misses a period, other symptoms and signs pop up. If you're still not sure, test again in a week (not to be confused with an hour). If you're truly not satisfied then, visit your GP for a pregnancy blood test (also known as a *beta hCG*).

✔ Try not to drown your sorrows in copious amounts of alcohol or drugs or engage in other reckless behaviour. You still may be pregnant, and that type of negative celebration isn't the best start for baby. Even if you're not pregnant, you want to stay in tip-top shape so that you can get there. A glass of wine is fine; a bottle is not.

✔ Feeling sad is okay and sharing this news with friends and family can help. You may experience a feeling of loss, and for some women, it is. Just remember that you have done nothing wrong. Human reproduction relies on chance and this month, the odds were against you.

Looking at medications and your work environment for answers

Have you overlooked something that could be interfering with your getting pregnant? Think back a few months, especially when thinking about sperm production; the sperm being ejaculated today have been over two months in the making, so anything your partner was taking a few months ago could be affecting his sperm count today. Ask yourself the following questions about a few possible deterrents you may not have thought about:

- ✔ Has your partner taken antibiotics, such as erythromycin or gentamycin, or antifungal medications, such as ketoconazole, or been treated for psoriasis? Has he taken anabolic steroids, cimetidine, marijuana, or cocaine? These medicines can all affect sperm production.

- ✔ Does your partner have high blood pressure? Sometimes, when you've been taking a medication for a long time, you almost forget the serious side effects it can have. Men who take certain types of antihypertensives called calcium channel blockers may produce sperm that can't penetrate eggs well; or they may have *retrograde ejaculation,* a condition in which the semen is pushed backwards into the bladder instead of being ejaculated out; or they may have an inability to get and sustain an erection. Other antihypertensive drugs are available that don't have these effects. Suggest that your partner talk to his doctor about switching medications if possible.

- ✔ Are you using a vaginal lubricant for sex? Even though substances such as KY Jelly don't contain spermicides, they can slow down sperm in their race to the egg. If you have to use a lubricant, try plain baby oil.

- ✔ Where do you work and what substances are you exposed to there? For instance, if you're a builder, painter, welder, or solderer, you may be exposed to large amounts of lead. You run the same risk if you're renovating an old house and scraping old paint off the walls. Lead exposure in men has been linked to low sperm count and decreased motility of sperm. In women, lead exposure may cause low birth weight in babies, high blood pressure during pregnancy, damage to a baby's nervous system, and developmental delays.

  Healthcare workers are exposed to a number of potentially dangerous drugs, as are pharmacists; exposure to chemotherapy drugs, radiation from X-rays, or inhaled anaesthetics used in the operating theatre all can contribute to infertility. Reps, lorry drivers, and chefs are all at the mercy of overheating around their groin that can raise the temperature of their testes and harm the quantity and quality of sperm.

Changing your job isn't always practical, but both men and women should consider potential exposure to dangerous substances or other, seemingly benign, workplace conditions that can harm your chance of conceiving and having a baby.

Considering religious practices

You may not have thought much about your religious beliefs causing problems with fertility, but at times, religious practices can interfere with your getting pregnant. For example, if your beliefs place restrictions on when you can have intercourse; remember that not everyone ovulates on day 14, and skipping days before day 12 may mean that you miss your fertile time each month.

Synchronising calendars

In today's age of conflicting schedules, many of you may find that you and your partner are spending far more time apart than together. As a gentle reminder for those trying to conceive, being in the same place at the same (ovulation) time is a necessity!

If you're not one of the few women whose ovulation is both predictable and consistent, having a partner that travels can be a problem. You're not alone. Couples who are separated by work/travel schedules or who find themselves on different work shifts have an inherent difficulty in baby making. Because of these erratic schedules, determining whether the problem is timing or something more serious is often difficult. Many couples end up in their GP's surgery when the only adjustment they need is to their diaries.

Ever wonder why so many women get pregnant on vacation? Sure, relaxation is part of it, but for others it may signify the rare occasion of actually being with your significant other at just the right time.

If you fall into this 'too busy' category, figure out, as best you can, when you might ovulate, and schedule a time for you and your partner to be together. OPKs, basal body temperature, and other predictors can help you pinpoint the time of ovulation. However, as far as being in the same place at the right time, you may need a little more creativity. Joining your partner on a business trip, even for a night, may be just what it takes. An afternoon rendezvous, rather than lunch, can also help make two become three. Finding time together – alone – may not only get you on the road to parenthood but also give you plenty of practice for it along the way!

Looking at Your Lifestyle

Now is probably the time to look close to home for other reasons that could prevent you conceiving – take a good look at yourselves! 'Everything in moderation' is certainly a good motto for habits, good and bad. Too much exercise can have a less than desirable effect, while coffee, drunk in moderation, can be benign. But, without insisting that you introduce a totally regimented routine, consider some things that are best eliminated entirely from your lifestyle, particularly when you're trying to conceive.

Giving up smoking

Smoking is bad for you. You all know it. Yet 30 per cent of women in the UK still smoke. Need some good reasons to quit? Here are a few:

✔ Smokers are 50 per cent more likely to miscarry.

✔ Smokers are two to four times more likely to have an *ectopic* pregnancy (one that implants in the fallopian tube rather than in the uterus, a topic we discuss in detail in Chapter 7).

✔ Smokers go through the menopause earlier, decreasing the number of years in which pregnancy can occur.

✔ Smokers' eggs have more genetic abnormalities.

✔ Smokers' eggs are prone to *polyspermy*, where two or more sperm enter an egg. The embryos that result are chromosomally abnormal and will not grow.

✔ Smokers' children have reduced fertility.

If you've quit but your partner hasn't, he may want to consider the following:

✔ Men who smoke have a lower sperm count.

✔ Men who smoke have a 20 per cent decrease in sperm motility.

✔ The risk of childhood leukaemia is higher if Daddy smoked.

✔ Smokers' sperm have more abnormal shapes. Abnormally shaped sperm have a higher rate of chromosome abnormalities.

Eliminating alcohol

Studies show that even moderate drinkers (that is, less than three units of alcohol a day) have more trouble getting pregnant.

Continuing to drink while pregnant increases the chance of miscarriage and also can cause fetal alcohol syndrome (FAS). FAS babies have learning and behavioural problems and typically have small heads, a flat midface, small eye slits, and a low nasal ridge.

Even though you may think that more babies get made because of alcohol than because of avoiding it, a Danish study shows that teetotallers conceived more quickly than even 'light' social drinkers (those who drink less than five units of alcohol per week).

Say 'no' to drugs

All illegal drugs are strictly out of order when trying to conceive and when you're pregnant. There's a higher incidence of death amongst new-born babies of women who have taken illegal drugs during pregnancy and an increase in the number of babies born with problems with their growth or mental development. Babies born to drug addicts also experience withdrawal symptoms, which are both painful and distressing. These are the problems that two common illegal drugs can cause when you're trying to get pregnant, but all illegal drugs can cause similar problems:

- ✔ **Cocaine:** Cocaine causes constriction of the blood vessels, which can result in early miscarriage, premature birth, and problems with the *placenta,* the organ that nourishes the baby. In addition, cocaine can cause menstrual irregularities, complicating the possibility of you becoming pregnant.

- ✔ **Marijuana:** Marijuana lowers sperm count, decreases sperm motility (the ability to move forward), lowers the amount of testosterone in males, and results in an increased number of abnormal eggs and sperm.

Cut back on caffeine

Evidence now shows that caffeine is associated with an increased risk of miscarriage. In addition, other studies show that drinking several cups of coffee a day may increase the risk of developing *endometriosis,* abnormal tissue growth that can affect your uterus or fallopian tubes as well as cause increased difficulty becoming pregnant and early miscarriage. A cup of coffee contains twice the amount of caffeine found in one can of cola. Limit caffeine to less than 200 milligrammes a day, which is two cups of coffee, or, better yet, cut it out completely! Tea also contains caffeine, but much less than coffee – 12 to 100 milligrammes per cup.

Stay out of the sauna

Anything that raises the temperature of a man's testicles can decrease sperm production and motility. Hot tubs, saunas, steam rooms, and tight underwear are out for men who are trying to conceive!

And in case you're thinking of jumping in the tub without him, high temperatures have also been associated with egg damage and miscarriage. Find another way to relax when you're pregnant – or trying to be.

Exercise with caution

So your partner decided to work out stress by bicycling or playing rugby. This exercise should be a good thing, right? Wrong! Prolonged cycling can cause damage to the groin from constant pressure of the bike seat, and contact sports can lead to injury to the testicles and can damage sperm production. The temperature that builds in those tight lycra cycling shorts is also detrimental to sperm.

Women who exercise a great deal may find that their periods have stopped. This condition is called *amenorrhea* and is common among women who are very thin and exercise daily (think ballet dancers and marathon runners). Obviously, you can't get pregnant if you're not having periods because you're not producing any eggs. So what can you both do to reduce stress that won't cause fertility problems? Knitting is nice. If knitting isn't enough for you, exercise in moderation is fine – for both of you!

Avoid anabolic steroids

Some studies show that as many as 6 to 7 per cent of all men have used anabolic steroids before age 18 to build muscle mass.

Anabolic steroids suppress the body's ability to make testosterone, which is necessary for normal sperm production. This damage can be permanent, so stay away from the steroids.

Dump the douche

Douching – a procedure in which water or a medicated solution is used to clean the vagina and cervix – is a bad idea whether you're trying to get pregnant or not.

Women who douche regularly have a 73 per cent increase in pelvic inflammatory disease (PID), which can cause damage to the Fallopian tubes and uterus. The ectopic pregnancy rate is about 75 per cent higher in women who douche regularly. For women between the ages of 15 and 44, the risk of developing cervical cancer is about 80 per cent higher for those who douche than those who don't. Dump the douche!

Eating for Two? Sampling a Fertility Diet

Good nutrition is something that you should *not* ignore. The healthier your body is, the healthier all its systems perform – including the reproductive system – which makes both common and medical sense. Nutrition is part of the bigger picture that also includes such basics as getting enough sleep, exercising, and nourishing your body as well as your mind. Although good nutrition is rarely the sole factor that brings about a baby, it does help to better preserve your overall health so that you may enjoy your future child as well, and as long, as possible.

Here's a brief look at some foods and our recommendations:

- ✔ **Red meat:** Studies show that red meat can neither help nor hurt your chances of getting pregnant. Trim all visible fat and cook the meat thoroughly. Red meat is also a good source of iron. Women with a strict vegetarian diet can experience sub-fertility through iron deficiency and anaemia, which can be corrected with an OTC iron supplement.

- ✔ **Dairy:** Many women trying to conceive cut dairy products from their diet, but there's no conclusive medical or scientific data that supports the notion that dairy foods compromise fertility. Also remember that calcium is needed for growing babies' bones. Use organic products if possible. If you're lactose intolerant, dairy products can create havoc in your reproductive system, so be aware of your personal dietary needs.

- ✔ **White flour and processed sugar:** No studies have proven that refined sugar or processed flour decreases fertility. But a well-balanced diet requires limiting their intake.

- ✔ **Artificial additives:** Despite hot debate, no definitive studies prove that additives such as aspartame and MSG are harmful. But limit or eliminate these additives from your diet if the controversy worries you.

- ✔ **Omega-3 fatty oils:** Studies are underway to evaluate the use of omega-3 oils in male infertility and in women with endometriosis. Omega-3 oils, present in oily fish, soybeans, flaxseed oil, canola oil, wheatgerm, and walnuts, have been shown to reduce heart disease. We recommend that you avoid fresh tuna, swordfish, and shark (all of which can contain tiny amounts of heavy metals, such as mercury) in favour of salmon, mackerel, or sardines, and limit canned tuna to two servings a week.

Don't eat raw or undercooked fish, meat, or poultry when trying to get pregnant or during pregnancy. These products have a higher than normal chance of carrying listeria, a bacteria that may make a mum-to-be somewhat ill but wreak havoc on an unborn child's nervous system. Listeria has also been linked to an increased rate of spontaneous abortion.

For those looking for a moderate approach, consider planning your diet around the major food groups that we discuss in Chapter 2. You may also choose to consult a nutritionist to make sure that you get the proper balance of vitamins and minerals. A good diet is a good idea whether you're trying to conceive or not.

If you choose to opt for a complete nutritional overhaul, realise that this option is a long-term commitment and is unlikely to produce a quick fix for your fertility issues. For most people, changing diet is a major lifestyle change and may lead to better overall health. On the fertility front, however, keep your expectations in check; diet changes alone are unlikely to get you pregnant.

Looking at Supplements – Vitamins, Minerals, Herbs, and More

Dietary supplements are very popular; one survey shows that over 40 per cent of adults in the UK use some form of supplement. Dietary supplements include herbs, vitamins, minerals, amino acids, enzymes, and extracts.

Vitamins are essential nutrients needed by our bodies in small amounts and available for most people through consuming a normal diet; consequently most people don't need vitamin supplements. Vitamins are divided into two groups:

- **Water soluble:** Vitamins B-complex and C need regular replacement in the body because they dissolve in water before being eliminated in urine. You need a continuous supply of these vitamins in your diet.

- **Fat soluble:** Vitamins A, D, E, and K aren't needed by the body everyday and are stored in the liver and fatty tissues and eliminated much more slowly than water-soluble vitamins. Huge doses of these vitamins can be toxic and lead to health problems. You can obtain all the vitamins your body requires through a normal healthy diet.

Because vitamins and other supplements are sold over the counter, without a prescription, they are often viewed as harmless. But studies have shown that some supplements are far from harmless: some supplements, such as ephedra, have been implicated in causing death, and others, such as comfrey, can cause severe liver damage.

Yet, Traditional Chinese Medicine (TCM) and many naturopaths (those who employ a drugless approach to healthy living) and herbalists offer supplements as a way to help get (and stay) pregnant. Internet sites are full of happy mums claiming that supplements were responsible for their pregnancies.

If you choose to try both Traditional Chinese Medicine (TCM) and Western medicine simultaneously (despite our advice to the contrary), make sure that all of your practitioners, doctors, and nurses, are aware of what you are taking. Not revealing this information is an ideal way to confuse the people whose goals are to help you conceive. Also keep in mind that some TCMs contain high levels of compounds that work like steroids and which can interfere with hormone results and fertility treatment.

So who do you believe, and are there any supplements that you absolutely should not take? For answers, read on.

Multivitamins have got it in one

Are certain vitamins, taken in greater (or lesser) quantity, more likely to result in increased fertility? At the time of writing, no clinical evidence supports this possibility. We advise you to stick to a standard multivitamin or pre-natal vitamin. Your local pharmacist can recommend a good OTC brand.

Multivitamins versus prenatal vitamins

A good multivitamin has the correct amount of the vitamins you need, so you rarely need to supplement them with additional vitamins. Your body takes in only what it needs from water-soluble vitamins (generally the maximum recommended daily dose found in most multivitamins) and urinates out the rest.

A *pre-natal* vitamin, which is simply a multivitamin with a greater concentration of folic acid and iron, is recommended to help prevent neural tube defects, such as spina bifida, and compensate for the loss of iron after you get pregnant. An excess of iron *can* result in constipation, which can be remedied through the introduction of additional fibres, fruits, and vegetables in your diet – a good thing no matter where you are on the baby-making quest.

Some studies have shown that liquid prenatal vitamins are better absorbed than pills. They may also be less likely to make you nauseated after you become pregnant.

No empirical evidence exists to support many of the anecdotal claims of the effects of individual vitamin and herb supplements in improving fertility, even for supplements such as wheatgrass and *l-arginine* (a non-essential amino acid found in wheat, rice, seeds, grapes, and other foods, and believed to help improve the quality of eggs). Although vitamins won't get you pregnant, they *will* help you keep your body in the best nutritional shape possible, along with proper diet, exercise, and general care. This balanced state is the best place for babies to come from!

Too much of a good thing: Overdosing on vitamins

Overdoing your intake of some vitamins can cause adverse reactions in your system. Excess amounts of fat-soluble vitamins, such as vitamins A, D, E, and K are stored in your body instead of being excreted. Although adequate levels of vitamin A help to preserve your vision and immune system, an excess can result in liver disease and birth defects when taken by pregnant women.

Overdosing on vitamins *through foods alone* is highly unlikely. Because most foods contain small amounts of any individual vitamin or nutrient, you would have to eat bushels of bananas, oranges, or spinach to get too much. Overdosage of any particular vitamin, mineral, or nutrient is generally only a danger if you consume it in a concentrated form, such as vitamin pills or powders.

However, when you're pregnant, avoid liver and liver products, because they contain high levels of vitamin A, which can be harmful to your baby.

If you're taking a standard multivitamin rather than a pre-natal vitamin while pregnant, make sure that it doesn't contain extra ingredients such as herbs. Many health food stores sell blends that contain herbs. Don't take these types of vitamins during pregnancy.

Herbs

Although herbs have been used for centuries, studies on their safety and benefits have been few. Herbs aren't benign, and someone with some knowledge of their interactions should oversee their use. Practitioners in this area may include chiropractors, osteopaths, nutritionists, homeopaths, and naturopaths.

Remember that even if the right herbs are prescribed, it's difficult for a non-herb specialist to distinguish between a bag of genuine herbs and a bag of leaf dust.

Here's a look at some of the more popular herbs used in the treatment of infertility. This list represents a small sample of herbs that can be used and represents herbs that are both Western in origin as well as Chinese:

- **Black cohosh:** A herb with oestrogenic qualities, black cohosh is often used to relieve the discomfort associated with menopause (hot flushes, for example). Studies have been mixed on whether black cohosh is effective. Black cohosh is also recommended to boost oestrogen production, although no proof exists that this works. Side effects of black cohosh are dizziness, nausea, low pulse rate, and increased perspiration.

- **Dong quai:** Dubbed the 'ultimate herb' for women, dong quai is used for everything from restoring menstrual regularity to treating menopausal symptoms. Dong quai is a blood thinner and should not be taken during an IVF cycle or by women who have very heavy periods.

- **False unicorn root:** Native Americans used this herb to improve menstrual irregularities and to alleviate problems associated with menopause and problems with infertility due to irregular follicular formation.

- **Nettle leaves:** This herb is considered to be an overall uterine tonic that better prepares the uterus for implantation of the embryo.

- **Primrose oil:** A fatty acid, primrose oil may increase cervical mucus to make the route easier for sperm to get to the egg. An unwanted side effect of primrose oil may be thinning of the uterine lining, making implantation more difficult.

- **Red clover:** This herb is often used to boost oestrogen in a woman's body. This *exogenous,* or outside the body, form of oestrogen may raise your oestrogen levels artificially; however, raising your oestrogen levels artificially is meaningless if the rise isn't caused by the production of a mature egg.

- **Red raspberry leaves:** Another uterine toner, this herb reportedly increases the uterine lining thickness (in order to make the uterus more receptive to the embryo). Red raspberry causes uterine contractions and absolutely should not be used in early pregnancy.

- **Vitex:** Also known as chaste tree berry, this herb has been used by herbalists for many years to help regulate women's hormones. Some use Vitex to increase luteinising hormone levels and help an egg release. According to others, Vitex can also increase progesterone levels and should be used only after you ovulate – not before. If taken earlier, it may keep you from releasing an egg. If taken in the luteal phase, after you ovulate, it may regulate and lengthen your cycle to give the embryo a chance to implant. Vitex is slow acting, so it may take several months for any effect to occur.

- **Wild yam:** In large doses, wild yam is used as a contraceptive (the first oral contraceptive pill was synthesised from yam extract); in smaller doses, it may promote progesterone production. Don't take wild yam until after ovulation occurs.

The following herbs stimulate the uterus so you absolutely should not take them after you get pregnant:

- Black cohosh
- Dong quai
- False unicorn root
- Feverfew can help migraine and painful periods. Feverfew may have the potential to harm an unborn baby.
- Golden seal may boost the immune system, but is dangerous if you have blood clotting disorders or high blood pressure and has been known to cause uterine contractions.
- Pennyroyal may alleviate digestive disorders, liver and gallbladder disorders, colds, and skin diseases. However, if taken in large quantities pennyroyal has been reported to cause abortion.
- Red raspberry leaves

In addition, avoid these supplements if you get pregnant:

- Blue cohosh: May cause fetal heart defects
- Mugwort: May cause fetal abnormalities

Herbal treatment of infertility is not a do-it-yourself approach! Let all your doctors know whether you're taking any kinds of herbs, whether they're the over-the-counter variety or from a complementary therapist because they may all cross-react with the drugs prescribed by your GP or fertility specialist.

Folic acid

Folic acid, a B vitamin, is essential when trying to get pregnant. Many studies have shown that 0.4 milligrammes of folic acid a day cuts the chance of having a baby with neural tube defects by 50 per cent. Neural tube defects occur in 6 of 10,000 births in the UK and include problems with the spine and brain. Neural tube defects develop very early in pregnancy, in the first four weeks, so taking a good multivitamin containing this amount while trying to get pregnant is essential. Many foods, including leafy green vegetables, fortified cereals, orange juice, and lean beef, contain folic acid, but overcooking can destroy folic acid, so take a folic acid supplement, even if you eat well.

Supplements for better sperm production

Fertility isn't just a female issue. In fact, 30 per cent of the time, male factor is responsible for a couple's failure to conceive.

So, women aren't the only ones who may venture onto an alternative path for treating medical problems related to infertility. Keep in mind that studies have been mixed as to the efficacy of taking supplements. Also remember that in male problems where surgery is deemed necessary (to fix a varicocele or any other structural issue), diet and/or supplements won't do the trick. These tips, however, can benefit overall health, which can contribute to better reproductive health. A new sperm takes 70 days to develop into a mature swimmer, so what you do today can affect conception down the line. The following supplements have been shown in some studies to benefit sperm count and movement:

- **Zinc:** May increase sperm motility and sperm count
- **Vitamin B12:** May increase sperm count
- **Vitamin C:** May increase sperm count
- **Vitamin E:** May increase sperm motility
- **Selenium:** May increase sperm motility
- **L-Carnitine:** May increase sperm motility and sperm count
- **L-arginine:** May increase sperm motility and sperm count (but not to be used by people who suffer from cold sores or herpes)
- **Folic acid:** May increase sperm motility and sperm count
- **CoQ10:** May increase sperm motility and sperm count

A good multivitamin should contain an adequate amount of all these elements.

Hair-brained or crowning glory?

Hair analysis promises to identify the mineral status of the body and to correct any imbalance with a programme of vitamin and mineral supplements and a wholefood – preferably organic – diet. Some people are almost evangelical about the results, others remain wholly sceptical. Hair analysis is expensive, and OTC multivitamins and a well-balanced diet are common sense, DIY alternatives that can give the same results. The programme is usually a minimum of six months; time which could be better spent consulting a fertility expert, especially where a woman's 'fertility age' is an issue.

Turning to Complementary Therapies

So much of getting you through this time of 'working at' and waiting for a positive pregnancy test is about positive thought, de-stressing, and finding ways to cope. Some people place huge faith in complementary therapies. This information is not an exhaustive analysis of all that is available, but a summary of some of the alternative approaches to increasing your chances of conceiving.

All complementary therapies cost – and sometimes, a lot! Unfortunately, no definitive formula exists to separate the well meaning but ineffectual, those who can have a positive impact on your chances of conceiving, and the quacks or the crooks. Rule of thumb – take a personal recommendation, but remember that what worked for your friend's cousin may be a costly no-hoper for you, and her success may have been due to a combination of other clinical, lifestyle, and emotional factors.

On pins and needles – acupuncture for infertility

Acupuncture is a 5,000-year-old traditional Chinese practice that's most often used to relieve chronic pain by inserting needles into a variety of pressure points on the head and body to balance the flow of energy (qi) in the body.

In April 2002, the prestigious medical journal *Fertility and Sterility* cited evidence that acupuncture, when used in conjunction with in vitro fertilisation, notably improved pregnancy rates. In the study involving 160 patients, acupuncture was performed just before the transfer of embryos into the uterus and again after the transfer took place. Needles were inserted along the spleen and stomach meridians, as well as other sites, to stimulate blood flow to the uterus. Forty-two per cent of the acupuncture group got pregnant, compared to 26 per cent of the non-acupuncture group. The sedative effect of acupuncture is also believed to assist in relaxing a woman, 'quietening' her uterus, and making it more receptive to embryos.

Although this study requires a follow-up to make sure that the previous results were not psychosomatic and are indeed repeatable, the findings were certainly of great interest.

Whether its effects are actually physiological or not, acupuncture works well with a fertility routine. However, be sure that those performing the treatment are fully trained. Many fertility clinics work in conjunction with an acupuncturist and/or can recommend someone who specialises in fertility based treatment.

Saying 'Om': Meditation and yoga

For those who need a little more help than self-help, consider the structure of a class such as meditation or yoga. Although they're not cure-alls, these ancient arts can go a long way in easing your body and spirit.

Both meditation and yoga can carry you through your pregnancy as well. Meditation can help relieve the discomfort and pain of everything from morning sickness to labour, and yoga can keep your pregnant body fit and focused all the way through.

Massaging away what ails you

Consider massage or reflexology as healthy, low-fat, guiltless ways to reward yourself as you go through the fertility process (or any other stress-producing activity for that matter!). If the hormones, either naturally produced or artificially added, are getting you down, schedule a relaxing Swedish massage or a reflexology session. Although relaxation itself won't get you pregnant, it certainly makes the fertility process a little more tolerable.

If you opt for massage therapy or reflexology, keep these important points in mind:

✔ Although massage and reflexology can be very beneficial, make sure that the therapist knows that you're trying to conceive. Massaging certain areas of your body or feet can be harmful during pregnancy. Your massage therapist should be aware that you may be pregnant during this process, and she should be skilled in what areas to focus on and what areas to avoid.

✔ If you think that you may be pregnant, consider skipping the massage or reflexology treatment from anyone other than an experienced pregnancy specialist professional, familiar with massage or reflexology during pregnancy, who knows which oils are safe to use with pregnant women.

✔ Some clinics claim high success rates with the practice of deep muscle massage and internal massage to reduce or eliminate scar tissue such as endometriosis and other types of structural anomalies that might prevent pregnancy. Little proof supports these claims, as no one has shown that it's possible to massage away excess or scar tissue. Take great care if pursuing this type of treatment. Internal massage can be detrimental, if not just painful, expensive, and altogether unnecessary.

Chapter 4

You, Your Fertility, and Your GP

....

In This Chapter

▶ Knowing when to see your GP

▶ Listing FAQs for your first visit

▶ Coping with first tests and what to expect

▶ Understanding the truth about OTC remedies

....

*Y*ou've revised your lifestyle! Everything is now 'in moderation' – exercise, diet, alcohol, caffeine, and multivitamins. Everything, that is, except sex, which has entered the 'bunnies' stage of every other night and is already losing some of its spontaneous passion.

But you're still not getting pregnant. If you've been trying for a while and you've still got nothing to show for it but a weary partner and months of fertility charts, you're probably ready for the next step: Seeking fertility treatment. In this chapter, we look at the first tentative steps towards being a fertility patient and provide information to help you cope with the many questions and tests that lie ahead.

Deciding When the Time is Right to See Dr G Practitioner

Most fertility experts – including us – say that you should visit your GP if you aren't pregnant after one year of regular unprotected sex, if you're under age 35, or after six months if you're over 35. However, a year – *a whole year* – seems an awful long time if you're under 35 and every month you have the disappointing 'no-blue-line' result.

Seeking medical help to get pregnant is a big step. You always thought you were an average sort of person, and now you find that you're part of the 10 per cent of women who don't get pregnant in a year of trying. For the first few months, you could pretend it wasn't a big deal, but now, well, it's time to make an appointment with your GP.

When not to wait – even a few months

Sometimes it's just not a good idea to wait six months or a year before seeing a doctor about not getting pregnant. You should also see a doctor earlier if:

- You're a woman over age 38. You should see a doctor once you start trying to get pregnant; you have fewer months to succeed because your aging ovaries are making fewer good eggs.

- You've had a previous ectopic pregnancy or more than one miscarriage.

- You've had or have any sexually transmitted disease, such as chlamydia or gonorrhea. Such diseases may have damaged your Fallopian tubes making conception either difficult or impossible without IVF.

- Your periods have stopped or are very irregular – that is, less than 21 days or longer than 35 days. You may require help regulating your cycles so that you produce an egg every month.

- You have very painful periods, which could be a sign of endometriosis. If you do have endometriosis, you may need treatment to get pregnant.

- You experience deep pain in the vagina during intercourse – possibly indicating pelvic infection or endometriosis.

Similarly, if your partner has had any of the following, which may have caused damage to his sperm, visit your GP for a semen analysis sooner rather than later:

- Any history of trauma to the testicles

- Had undescended testicles as a small boy

- Any sexually transmitted infection

- Any sexual problems, such as premature ejaculation

- Works with radiation or chemicals

- Knows that he had mumps as an adolescent

Of course, if you've had your tubes tied or if your partner had a vasectomy, you need to see a specialist to discuss either reversal of the surgery (see Chapter 8) or in vitro fertilisation (which we discuss in detail in Chapter 12).

First Visit to your GP

In the UK, you don't usually shop around for an NHS GP – you go to whoever you're registered with. If you live in a one-GP town, your access to a GP with current knowledge, or much experience of treating infertility may be restricted. If so, go for the first visit but encourage the GP to refer you to a specialist as soon as possible. If your GP practice is medium to large, ask which GP at the surgery has a particular interest in infertility. This doctor may not be your personal GP, but you may save time by making your first appointment with him or her.

Your general practitioner (GP) may use the letters 'DRCOG' after their name, which means that they've passed the diploma examination of the Royal College of Obstetricians and Gynaecologists. This examination recognises a GP's interest in women's health although the diploma isn't a specialist qualification.

So, should you encourage your partner to attend your first why-aren't-we-pregnant GP appointment? That depends on a few things:

- **Will he feel horribly out of place?** Some men don't like to go to the doctor, ever, for anything. You probably know by now whether your partner will do well at the GP's surgery. If you're going to sit there (half naked, no less) worrying about how he feels, go by yourself for that first crucial visit.

    On the other hand, if your partner is the person in your relationship who remembers detail, writes things down correctly, asks sensible questions, and provides moral support, by all means, take him to your first GP visit. Chances are that he'll probably need to have his own testing done, so he may as well get familiar with the doctor right from the start.

- **Are you going to have to share information with your GP that you don't want your partner to know?** For example, did you have a termination of pregnancy, give a child up for adoption, have a sexually transmitted disease, or do any other thing you'd rather your partner didn't know about? Then go to the first visit by yourself, explain the situation to the GP, and take your partner to the *next* visit.

- **Are you going to be embarrassed about undergoing an examination with your partner there?** Some women aren't comfortable having other people, even a partner, present for a gynaecological examination. If this situation is going to make you uneasy, maybe your partner can stay in the waiting room until the examination is over and then come in when you're dressed. (Although if you eventually have to have fertility treatment and/or actually give birth, get used to him being around while you're on your back being prodded and poked – it's all part of the experience and one that he should 'share'!)

Thinking About FAQs for Your First Visit

Whether you go alone or as a couple to your GP's appointment, prepare a list of questions ahead of time so that you won't forget anything. Here's a starter list (you'll probably have other questions specific to your own situation):

- ✔ What tests are you able to do to check our fertility and chances of conceiving?

- ✔ Can any of these tests be done today or do we need to return on a specific day of my period?

- ✔ Are you able to prescribe fertility drugs that could increase our chance of conceiving? If so, which drugs?

- ✔ In your experience, have these drugs ever helped someone to conceive or are they simply a stepping stone – and a time-delay – to assisted conception?

- ✔ How long should we try this method before we do further testing? (Some doctors start you on drugs for a few months before putting you through more invasive testing. Others may do blood tests and a semen analysis before starting you on any medication.)

If your doctor shrugs and gives you the impression that she would do simple methods forever, you can request – even insist – on being referred to a consultant for further tests and investigations.

Dr G Practitioner is going to have some questions for you, too. She'll want to know the following, so come prepared with the answers:

- ✔ How long you've been trying to get pregnant

- ✔ How often you have unprotected sex

- ✔ Whether you use any lubricants

- ✔ Whether you engage in any unusual practices that could affect your fertility (don't be coy – Dr G Practitioner has heard it all before!)

- ✔ Whether your partner has ever had a vasectomy – and has it been successfully reversed

- ✔ If you've had a burst appendix or severe peritonitis in the past – possibly resulting in tubal or uterine problems

- ✔ How long your periods last and how long your cycles are from day one of one cycle to day one of the next

- ✔ The date of your last period

✔ Whether your periods are painful or heavy and how many sanitary towels or tampons you use a day

✔ Whether sisters or other close relatives have children

✔ Whether any known genetic factors exist in your family (check out Chapter 1 for more information on family genes)

✔ Whether you used ovulation predictor kits, and what they showed

If you haven't bought your first basal thermometer yet, you may also be told to start charting your daily temperature before getting up or going to the bathroom. Your doctor may also want to check your basal body temperature (BBT) charts (refer to Chapter 3 for more information about temperature charting) to see whether your temperature shows a pattern of ovulation. If your BBT chart indicates that you're not ovulating, take the charts to your next GP appointment and she may either prescribe infertility drugs for you or refer you to a specialist or clinic.

Dr G Practitioner may have a lot more questions aimed specifically at you. If you're overweight and have adult acne or facial hair, she may wonder if you have polycystic ovary syndrome (PCOS), because PCOS patients often don't ovulate. If you're very thin, she may be concerned about your not getting periods due to over-exercising, anorexia, poor nutrition, or a thyroid problem.

You may wonder why the doctor doesn't want to do loads of tests on your first visit to make sure that you don't have a problem that will require high-tech fertility treatments, such as IVF. The fact is, most patients who see a doctor because they're not pregnant have fairly simple problems, such as lack of *ovulation* (releasing an egg), or just bad timing of sex, and don't need the high-tech stuff. Despite the emphasis today on these methods, only a small percentage of infertility patients actually need IVF. Your doctor may check your blood to see whether your FSH (follicle-stimulating hormone) level is raised, which could indicate the perimenopause. But most doctors won't suggest any further investigations until they've tried some simple things first.

Carrying Out Tests on Your First Visit

Dr G Practitioner should listen to your story so far (your fertility diary will be useful here), ask questions about your general medical history, and give you (both) a physical examination. She will also check if you've had a recent smear test and that the results were okay.

Some initial tests

If your general medical history suggests no specific reason for you not being able to conceive, she may suggest a few initial tests. For you, these may include:

- A urine test for chlamydia (which in most infected women is totally symptomless but can cause blocked tubes).

- A blood test to check for immunity to German measles (rubella), which can harm your baby if you become infected in the first three months of pregnancy.

- A blood test to check you're ovulating by measuring progesterone levels, which start to rise just before ovulation, peaking about seven days after ovulation (that is, around about day 21 if you have a 28-day cycle, hence it's common name of the 'day-21 test') and which then fall quickly just before a period.

But not all the testing is reserved for you and so even the most reluctant male partner should also see the GP to allow the following tests:

- A urine test for chlamydia.

- A sperm test to check the quantity, shape, and 'swimming' ability of the sperm. This test may need to be repeated in a few weeks if the outcome is poor.

Hopefully, the test results will reveal why you're having problems getting pregnant. Sometimes the results may be good news, revealing no specific physical or hormonal problems – although frustratingly, this fact doesn't explain why you're still not pregnant. If this is the case and you've been trying for less than 18 months, Dr G Practitioner may simply recommend more sex and a few lifestyle or dietary changes (refer to Chapter 3). If she suspects you may have fertility problems, she'll discuss seeing a specialist either at a hospital, or even suggest that you 'do not pass go, do not collect £200' and go straight to a fertility clinic.

'Take two Clomid and call me in three months'

Clomiphene citrate, more commonly referred to by its brand name Clomid, is given to help you release an egg or to help you release a *better* egg; it may also help sustain a pregnancy with higher progesterone levels. Normally, you take Clomid for five days. Some GPs start you on it on day two of your cycle, and others start you on day three to five. The exact timing isn't important; the point is to start taking it before your ovaries begin to develop one dominant follicle.

Because taking Clomid significantly increases the risk of multiple (twin and triplet) pregnancies, 'best practice' in the UK recommends ultrasound monitoring for the first cycle of treatment.

Usually GPs give you one pill a day the first month or two and then move up to two or three tablets a day if you still don't seem to be ovulating regularly. Clomid comes in 50-milligramme tablets, so if your GP starts you at a higher dose, 100 to 150 milligrammes per day, you'll need to take more than one. After you stop taking the pills, you can check for ovulation by using your old friends, the basal thermometer and the ovulation predictor kits.

Clomid is an anti-oestrogen and works by fooling the body into thinking it's not making enough oestrogen. When your hypothalamus thinks that you're low on oestrogen, it releases GnRH (gonadotropin releasing hormone), which stimulates the release of FSH (follicle-stimulating hormone) into your blood. The FSH stimulates the ovary to recruit follicles that produce oestrogen. About 80 per cent of women taking Clomid ovulate in response to this stimulation, but only half of them will become pregnant with no other treatment.

Clomid works best for those whose ovaries are capable of functioning normally but need a little tune-up. If you're already ovulating a mature follicle regularly, Clomid probably won't help you get pregnant.

Your doctor may tell you to try Clomid and come back in three to six months if you're not pregnant. Most pregnancies from Clomid occur in the first three to six months, so if you're not pregnant by that time, your GP should refer you to a consultant or fertility specialist to investigate why not.

Clomid, which the Committee of Safety in Medicine recommends is used no more than a total of 12 months throughout a woman's entire life, has a few drawbacks:

✔ **Higher chance for multiple births:** Between 5 and 10 per cent of all Clomid pregnancies are twins and 1 in 400 is a triplet pregnancy. Multiples have a very high rate of premature delivery and significantly higher than normal maternal and infant complications. Multiples result from Clomid working too well and stimulating more than one follicle to grow, hence the need for ultrasound monitoring.

✔ **Ovarian hyperstimulations syndrome:** If you're making a large number of eggs, you may develop *ovarian hyperstimulation syndrome* (OHSS – see Chapter 12 for more), which can make hospitalisation necessary. If you're on Clomid and feel very ill, with a sudden weight gain, severe bloating in your abdomen, or abdominal pain, call your doctor immediately. This condition is a rare side effect of Clomid.

✔ **Visual disturbance:** Clomid can affect your vision. If you notice severe blurring, stop taking the Clomid at once and call your GP

✔ **Symptoms of menopause:** Clomid also has some less serious side effects. Because your body has been fooled into thinking that it doesn't have enough oestrogen, you may have some of the same symptoms women have when they enter menopause and their oestrogen drops and experience hot flushes, headaches, nausea, or blurred vision. Let your doctor know if you have any of these symptoms.

✔ **Effects on cervical mucus:** Clomid can also interfere with your production of cervical mucus, by making it more hostile to sperm. Therefore, if significant sperm problems exist, Clomid will not enable you to get pregnant.

✔ **Thinner uterine lining:** Because oestrogen also builds your uterine lining, some women on Clomid don't make a thick lining. If you have either of these side effects, you may need to take oestrogen after you start making a follicle.

Choosing Over-the-counter Remedies: Placeboes or Simple Solutions?

Some – but very few! – GPs who prefer the simple approach may suggest trying low-dose aspirin and cough syrup for a few months. Although no clinical evidence exists to suggest either can help you conceive, you may be aware of a 'friend of a friend' who swears by one, or both, and so they are worth discussing.

Low-dose aspirin

Low-dose aspirin (75 milligrammes) is prescribed for many middle-aged people because it decreases the normal clotting of the blood, allowing blood to flow more easily through the blood vessels. Some people believe that taking low-dose aspirin when you're trying to conceive may increase blood flow to the uterus, giving the embryo an improved lining in which to implant.

Low-dose aspirin can cause stomach upset or pain, in which case enteric-coated aspirin is a suitable alternative.

Don't take non-steroidal anti-inflammatories like normal dose aspirin (300 milligrammes) and ibuprofen (also known as Nurofen) mid-cycle, because they can prevent successful ovulation.

If you've had three or more miscarriages you may be tested for Anti-Phospholipid antibodies (sticky blood syndrome). The next time you conceive, your GP may recommend low-dose aspirin (in conjunction with heparin) to improve the blood flow to the placenta and reduce the risk of further miscarriage.

Cough syrup

The case for cough syrup is even less certain. Around ovulation, the cervical mucus should be thin and stretchy; in some women, the mucus doesn't thin enough for sperm to get through it. The theory is that pure cough syrup, or guaifenesin, thins all the mucus in the body, not just that in your chest, so the sperm can then get through the cervical mucus.

In addition to there being no evidence that pure cough syrup can help you conceive, many traditional cough remedies contain a sedative, so you may fall asleep before you actually get around to baby-making sex!

Chapter 5

Great Expectations . . . But: Early Pregnancy Loss

· ·

In This Chapter

▶ Understanding the meaning of 'a little bit' pregnant

▶ Dealing with a miscarriage or ectopic pregnancy

▶ Recovering after a loss

· ·

*N*ot getting pregnant is upsetting and frustrating, but getting pregnant and having the pregnancy end early in loss is even more devastating. Why do so many pregnancies end early, and what does it mean for future pregnancies? And how can you avoid personal feelings of failure when a loss occurs? In this chapter, we discuss how and why pregnancies are lost in the first 12 weeks, and we offer advice on how to pick yourself up and try again if this situation happens to you.

Getting 'a Little Bit' Pregnant – It's Possible

Most of you have heard that there's no such thing as 'a little bit' pregnant. This statement is true in one sense, but at times, you do feel that you're 'almost' pregnant . . . and you may be right.

More than 50 per cent of all embryos stop developing before they develop a heartbeat. Most of these, up to 30 per cent, are lost before the time when you would notice any signs of pregnancy. If this outcome happens, you may have no pregnancy symptoms at all, not even a missed period. Or you may have very early pregnancy signs, such as breast tenderness, which suddenly disappear. These signs may be followed by a slightly late, heavier-than-normal period, which is actually the passing of a very early pregnancy. You may pass more clots than normal (for you), or you may feel 'crampier' than usual.

You probably wouldn't even realise that you had been pregnant unless you did a sensitive early pregnancy test, such as a blood test. If you're having treatment with a fertility clinic, you may be asked to have a blood pregnancy test, to measure the amount of beta hCG (human chorionic gonadotrophin) about two weeks after ovulation or embryo transfer. This result may be positive (anything over 5 is considered positive but a 'good' result is at least 50) but very low when first tested, and it may be negative a few days later, at the second test. Your doctor may say that you had a *biochemical pregnancy* if this happens. What this term means is that the embryo started to implant and develop but stopped growing before the point at which even a very early ultrasound scan could be done; typically for one of the following reasons:

- **Abnormal embryo:** At least 50 per cent of the time, biochemical pregnancies are caused by the implantation of a chromosomally abnormal embryo, but other factors can also cause very early miscarriage.

- **Low progesterone levels:** ''In a normal pregnancy, the *corpus luteum,* or leftover 'shell' of the ovulated egg, produces a hormone called *progesterone.* Progesterone is necessary for the implantation and growth of the early embryo and it prevents the breakdown of the lining or endometrium in the womb. If your progesterone is lower than normal, the embryo may not be able to establish itself. We know how important progesterone is because the anti-progesterone called Mifipristone is used as an abortifacient to terminate an early pregnancy.

 A simple blood test can check your progesterone levels and if the blood sample shows less than normal progesterone, your doctor can recommend supplementing progesterone in the form of injections, pills, or vaginal suppositories. However, low progesterone levels are usually the sign of a failing embryo that does not have the potential to turn into a healthy baby. Increasing your progesterone levels may just delay the inevitable miscarriage rather than prevent it.

Even though people may say that you can't be a 'little bit' pregnant, the truth is that an embryo can start to implant and then stop developing before you even miss a period. You may not realise this event is happening to you without a very early blood pregnancy test. If your doctor suspects that you're having biochemical pregnancies, she will order further testing to see whether an easy fix, such as adding progesterone supplements, can help with the problem. However, because the vast majority of early pregnancy losses are due to embryos that are genetically abnormal, letting Mother Nature decide the outcome is often best. High-dose progesterone can stop the bleeding for a while, but it won't transform a faulty embryo into a healthy baby.

Suffering a Miscarriage

A *miscarriage* is a pregnancy loss that occurs after you know you're pregnant but before the fetus is *viable,* or able to survive on its own, usually before 24 weeks of gestation.

Miscarriages are very common: One in four women has a miscarriage during her reproductive years. In young women, one in six pregnancies will end in a miscarriage, by the mid-thirties the chance is one in four, at age 40, the risk increases to at least one in three and by 45, three-quarters of all positive pregnancy tests will not result in a healthy live birth. But knowing that miscarriages are common events and not likely to recur, doesn't make them any easier to deal with.

Eighty per cent of miscarriages occur in the first 12 weeks of pregnancy. Based on this fact, many couples decide not to shout the news to friends and relatives before this time has passed.

The terminology of miscarriage is difficult and upsetting. Gynaecologists may refer to a miscarriage as an 'abortion' even though that word is usually understood to mean the deliberate termination of pregnancy. It can be heartbreaking to hear the pregnancy that you have tried so hard to achieve, and now seem to have lost, described as an abortion. The doctor isn't being deliberately insensitive, she's just using the correct medical term. Here are some more medical terms:

✔ **Threatened miscarriage:** The first sign of possible miscarriage is usually spotting, although some women first report the loss of 'pregnancy' symptoms like breast tenderness or nausea. Sometimes bleeding can be quite heavy and yet the pregnancy can be fine, and sometimes you can have' only a slight loss of blood and yet the pregnancy has failed. After fertility treatment, up to 40 per cent of women report some bleeding in early pregnancy. Bleeding in early pregnancy tends to occur at around the time you would have been having a period. You usually experience only minimal pain, and if your doctor does a vaginal examination she will find that the cervix is tightly closed. Most doctors restrict sex and heavy exercise if some spotting has occurred.

Because spotting is common in pregnancy (occurring in one in five women), doctors don't always take it as a dire sign. Bleeding can be caused by implantation of the embryo or by the sloughing off of the lining around the area where implantation has occurred. If spotting and cramping stop quickly, the chances are excellent that the pregnancy will carry to term. If a scan has shown a beating heart in the womb then you have more than a 90 per cent chance of a good outcome.

✓ **Inevitable miscarriage:** An internal exam will show whether your cervix has started to open. An ultrasound done around six weeks will show whether a fetus is in the uterus and may show a heartbeat. A heartbeat *should* be seen by six and a half weeks. If your cervix has started to open, or *dilate,* and you're bleeding, you'll almost certainly miscarry.

Another type of inevitable miscarriage occurs when an ultrasound shows no fetal heartbeat. This occurrence is called a 'silent miscarriage' because the pregnancy has stopped growing but there have been no other signs such as bleeding or cramping. You will still 'feel pregnant' and without a scan you may not be aware that anything is wrong. In 80 per cent of these cases, a miscarriage will follow and you don't need to be hospitalised. Most doctors would advocate letting Nature take its course. Your doctor will want you to watch for signs of infection, such as a temperature over 39 degrees or a nasty vaginal discharge. Hospitalisation isn't necessary in most cases of miscarriage. If the bleeding becomes heavier than the heaviest day of a heavy period or you start to feel faint or dizzy or have severe pain, then call your GP or get a lift to the A & E Department of your nearest hospital. You'll probably continue bleeding for seven to ten days. Sometimes a 'silent miscarriage' may require a *dilation and curettage* (D&C), a minor surgical procedure to remove the tissue, because still 'feeling pregnant' and yet knowing it isn't a healthy pregnancy can be upsetting.

Don't be upset if your doctor calls your miscarriage a *spontaneous abortion.* This is the old medical term for a miscarriage.

Will you need a D&C?

You need a D&C, or *dilation and curettage,* if you don't pass all the pregnancy tissue on your own. This procedure involves gently dilating the cervix and scraping the uterus with a blunt instrument called a *curette,* or with a suction vacuum, to make sure that no tissue is left, because leftover tissue can cause an infection. This surgery is usually done under light general anaesthetic as a day case procedure. Your doctor may tell you not to take baths, swim, use hot tubs, douche, or have sex for a while. You may be asked to return for a follow-up visit to make sure that you're healing normally. You won't have any stitches to remove after a D&C.

Playing the blame game

Are you feeling guilty about your miscarriage because you once sneaked a cigarette, had a glass of champagne at a wedding, had sex, or went skydiving during your pregnancy? Maybe you've been depressed or had an abortion when you were 17. Whatever happened, now you blame yourself and your careless ways for the miscarriage. Don't. Although some of these actions may not have been the best decisions, the truth is that almost certainly *none* of them caused this miscarriage.

You should know, though, that regular cigarette smoking can increase the rate of miscarriage by 30 to 50 per cent, so cutting down drastically or stopping smoking is a good idea if you want a successful pregnancy.

More than 50 per cent of miscarriages are due to chromosomal abnormalities. In these cases, no amount of rest, or anything else that you do – or don't do – will prevent them. Other common causes of miscarriage, such as abnormalities of the uterus, lack of progesterone support after ovulation, or vaginal infection, can be evaluated before you try to get pregnant again. Having had one miscarriage doesn't mean that your next pregnancy is more likely to end the same way. Even after five miscarriages in a row you still have a better-than-evens chance of a live birth.

Gwyn and I (co-author Jill) saw two heartbeats at our six-week scan following IVF treatment with ICSI (intra cytoplasmic sperm injection – see Chapter 13) treatment and, over the coming weeks, delighted in the knowledge we were expecting twins. The queasiness was more than bearable, because we were expecting the babies we'd waited so long for. I moved on from the infertility books to the pregnancy books, and followed the embryos' growth and development from the week-by-week guides and was reassured that the sickness usually stops at the end of 12 weeks. Mine did; I was following the book exactly! Then I went for my eagerly awaited 13-week scan. And after being moved from one scan room into another 'with more sensitive equipment', followed by lots of silent scanning, the ultrasound technician gently told me 'I'm sorry, but you're not pregnant any more'. In seconds I had gone from the joy of expecting twins to being told there was nothing – not two babies, not even one baby, nothing. I sat up on the bed and wailed like a banshee. I looked down on myself, inconsolable, thinking of our babies who we would never know and that someone had played a huge and cruel trick on us. And how would – could – I tell Gwyn? . . . and my parents? And all the needles, the injections, the travelling, and all the other people involved in getting pregnant, and now nothing. But the ultrasound technician next words, eventually, did help: 'Mother Nature can be a bitch, but she does know best.' That time, our babies were just not meant to make it and had 'died' around ten weeks.

Playing the guessing game: Why did things start off so well?

Miscarriage has a number of causes, some of which may not be easy to pinpoint. More than 50 per cent are related to chromosomal abnormalities.

In trying to understand chromosomal abnormalities, you can compare a growing fetus to a house being built. If a builder orders a lot of bricks but no roofing materials, house walls can be built, but only up to the point where the roofing materials are needed. If the genes needed for the baby to develop are processed incorrectly at the time of conception, the baby will develop to the point where it needs those genes to keep growing. Without those genes, the fetus can't continue to develop. Its 'walls' will be built, but without the 'roof,' it can't continue to grow.

Blighted ovum

A blighted ovum is a variation of chromosomal error. *Blighted ovum* occurs when the placenta and amniotic sac develop and put out pregnancy hormones but the embryo itself doesn't develop. So you may test pregnant, but there's no fetus. You and your doctor may discover this fact when you start spotting and the doctor does a scan and finds no embryo.

Molar pregnancy

Another, somewhat rare type of chromosomal anomaly is called a molar pregnancy. Molar pregnancies occur in one in a thousand conceptions. *Hydatidiform mole* or *molar pregnancies* result when the embryo is abnormal; it has no chromosomal content to pass on, so you don't have any fetal development, only a placenta. The placenta usually grows very quickly; you may show signs of pregnancy very early and have unusually high pregnancy hormone levels. An ultrasound scan will show a swollen mass of vesicles in the womb that look like a bunch of grapes.

Molar pregnancies are treated with methotrexate, a chemotherapy drug, to stop the abnormally fast cell division. A D&C will probably be done as well; in fact, you may need more than one. Molar cells can spread very quickly into other areas, and you may need quite aggressive treatment to avoid serious complications. Very occasionally a molar pregnancy can develop into a *choriocarcinoma*. This condition is a highly malignant tumour but it's very rare, occurring in 1:40,000 pregnancies. The good news is that it's very responsive to combination chemotherapy based on methotrexate. You will be advised to avoid another pregnancy for 6 to 12 months after a molar pregnancy and to have regular blood tests to check that the pregnancy hormone levels fall and then remain undetectable to be sure that no abnormal cells remain in the body.

Playing the age game

As in most fertility issues, age is a definite factor in miscarriage rates. Consider these numbers:

- ✔ If you're under 35, the miscarriage rate is about 15 per cent.

- ✔ If you're pushing 40, the miscarriage rate increases to 25 per cent.

- ✔ If you're over 40, your chance of miscarriage is 35 per cent.

- ✔ If you're around 43, the rate goes up to nearly 50 per cent.

- ✔ After age 45, 87 per cent of all women are infertile, so pregnancy is rare, making miscarriage rates more difficult to gather. Also, periods are more irregular, so what appears to be a late period could be a miscarriage.

These statistics reflect the increased number of chromosomally abnormal eggs still left as you get older; your 'best eggs' have already been ovulated. We discuss age-related fertility issues more in Chapter 1.

Suffering the insensitive remarks of family and friends

What's worse after a miscarriage than friends who become pregnant? Or friends who continue to be pregnant when you're not? How about relatives who try to 'jolly' you out of depression with stories of how miscarriage was probably a blessing and that you should be thankful for the children you have? Or what about women who regale you with stories of their own miscarriages?

Everyone has her own way of dealing with people who can't be avoided. Some women politely ask that the matter is not discussed. Other women not so politely ask the offender to please shut up. Yet other women agree and pretend that they're feeling better. Try to remember that people are feeling awkward and don't know what to say, but they're trying to make you feel better because they care about you.

Remembering your partner's grieving, too

The good souls who are trying to comfort the woman who has physically experienced the loss are wonderful, but your partner often gets left out. After our (co-author Jill) miscarriage, Gwyn felt he had to be 'so strong' for me, and answer well-wishers' questions about how I was, that he never properly dealt with the loss of our twins – and certainly never grieved them. I didn't realise this fact until more than six months later at the time of the due date for the twins, when our heightened emotions enabled him to get angry and let me know just what he'd felt at the time, and ever since. When we started our next ICSI treatment I made sure that I was much more sensitive to his feelings and let my parents and close friends know, too – just in case we were to experience such a loss again.

Spouses may be having an equally difficult time, because few men discuss miscarriage with their friends; if they do, they may find little sympathy for an early loss. They may also feel out of the loop and uninformed about exactly what happened, and may not want to question you for fear of upsetting you more. If you can bring yourself to talk about things, a little conversation goes a long way toward making your partner feel more like a partner and less like a hindrance during this difficult time.

Ectopic Pregnancy: When the Embryo Is Developing in the Wrong Place

An ectopic pregnancy is a different type of miscarriage. In an *ectopic pregnancy,* the embryo may be developing normally, but it's growing in the wrong place, usually in the Fallopian tube. Like a miscarriage, an ectopic pregnancy ends your hopes for a baby *this time,* but it can cause other problems as well.

One out of 100 pregnancies is ectopic – and the percentage has been rising over the last 30 years. Ectopic pregnancies are much more common in women with tubal damage caused by infection, endometriosis or, sometimes, surgery. With an ectopic pregnancy, the fetus may be normal but attaches to tissue outside the uterus, usually in the Fallopian tube, and begins to grow there. (Figure 5-1 shows where ectopic pregnancies can occur.) The Fallopian tube is much smaller than the uterus, and the baby can't grow beyond a certain point, usually around seven weeks, before eroding into a blood vessel or rupturing the tube, causing severe complications. Ectopic pregnancy is the leading cause of maternal death in the first trimester of pregnancy.

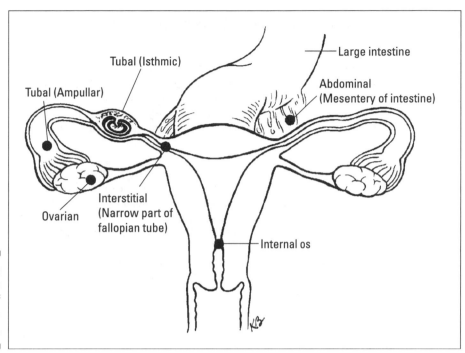

Figure 5-1:
Possible
sites of
ectopic
pregnancies.

What to do if you suspect an ectopic pregnancy

Although ectopic pregnancy is quite rare, women who know they're at extra risk (because they know their tubes are damaged or they have had a previous ectopic) must request an 'early scan' as soon as they know they are pregnant. This means booking a scan two or three weeks after the positive test.

An ectopic pregnancy can be a life-threatening event. If the fetus gets too big, the Fallopian tube will burst, and you could be in danger of bleeding to death. Any time you have severe one-sided pain, severe shoulder pain, or a feeling of light-headedness and weakness a few weeks after missing a period, you *must* go to hospital emergency to make sure that you don't have an ectopic pregnancy.

A positive pregnancy test and an ultrasound showing no fetus in the uterus can confirm an ectopic pregnancy. If you have no physical symptoms, an ectopic pregnancy may be suspected if the blood pregnancy test (beta hCG) is lower than it should be or isn't doubling every 48 hours; rarely, a urinary pregnancy test can also be negative. An ultrasound will show nothing in the uterus – no sac, placenta, or fetus.

Treating ectopic pregnancies

Treating an ectopic pregnancy involves either dissolving the developing pregnancy with a drug called methotrexate, the same drug used for molar pregnancies (see the section 'Molar pregnancy,' earlier in this chapter), or removing the pregnancy through surgery. Surgical removal of an ectopic pregnancy can also cause future infertility problems because the Fallopian tube may need to be removed, and adhesions or scar tissue may develop after the surgery.

Methotrexate causes the pregnancy to dissolve by stopping the rapid cell division necessary for a fetus to grow. Four per cent of women taking methotrexate have diarrhoea, mouth soreness, or stomach irritation because these cells are also fast-growing and affected by the disturbance in cell division. Serious side effects, such as liver toxicity or lung problems, are rare.

In the UK, the management of ectopic pregnancy usually involves laparoscopic surgery. If you are stable (no active bleeding, normal pulse and blood pressure, and ultrasound evidence of little or no internal bleeding) then laparoscopic 'keyhole surgery' may allow the surgeon to identify and remove the ectopic safely. But, if you do have bleeding, then this condition is a medical emergency and a *laparotomy* (a tummy cutting incision made just above the bikini-line) will be necessary.

I clearly remember (co-author Gill), as a very junior gynaecologist, the shiver of danger with which I would pick up a message on my pager that said 'Flat ectopic in casualty!' My first Professor of Obstetrics and Gynaecology, who was one of the kindest and wisest doctors I have ever had the privilege of working with, gave me a very useful piece of advice. He said, 'Gill, all women with tummy pain between the ages of 15 and 50 are pregnant with an ectopic until you prove otherwise!'

Methotrexate successfully dissolves an ectopic pregnancy 90 per cent of the time, but it must be used before the fetus grows larger than 3.5 centimetres (a little over an inch). After that, surgical removal is necessary. High levels of beta hCG, signs of bleeding, and some medical problems may mean that methotrexate therapy is not an option.

If surgery is required, your doctor may be able to save the Fallopian tube or reconstruct it if possible. Even if the Fallopian tube has to be removed, you can still get pregnant. An egg can even be released from the right ovary and find its way to the left tube if the right tube is gone.

Can the pregnancy be moved somehow from the Fallopian tube to the uterus? Unfortunately, no. Because the placenta and the tissues involved with growth are 'dug in' to the tube, removing the fetus from the tube and reattaching it to the uterus is not possible.

Understanding why ectopic pregnancies happen

Although anyone can have an ectopic pregnancy, ectopic pregnancies are more likely in women who have any of the following risk factors:

- ✔ If you have a swollen, dilated Fallopian tube, called a *hydrosalpinx,* you're six to ten times more likely to have an ectopic pregnancy. Hydrosalpinx is frequently caused by pelvic inflammatory disease (PID), often associated with a chlamydia infection. (Refer to Chapter 2 for more on chlamydia.)

- ✔ If you smoke, you're one and a half to four times more likely to have an ectopic pregnancy.

- ✔ If you've had a previous tubal ligation re-anastomosed (reverse sterilisation), you have a 15 per cent chance of an ectopic pregnancy.

- ✔ If you've previously used an IUD (coil), you have a slightly increased chance of an ectopic pregnancy.

- ✔ If you currently use progestin-only birth control pills, your chances of an ectopic pregnancy also increases.

- ✔ If you've had a previous ectopic pregnancy, your chance for another is 7 to 10 per cent.

- ✔ If you douche regularly, at least three times a week, you're more likely to have an ectopic pregnancy. Don't douche!

Some infertility treatments, such as in vitro fertilisation, are associated with a higher rate of ectopic pregnancies, often because they're being done for pre-existing tubal damage. Twin and triplet pregnancies are also associated with ectopic pregnancies; in some cases, one fetus may implant in the uterus and another in a tube, a condition called a *heterotopic pregnancy.*

Recurrent miscarriage: Why it happens

Recurrent miscarriage is defined as three or more consecutive miscarriages. By chance alone, one in 25 women will suffer two early miscarriages in a row and one in 125 will suffer three. If subfertility has been an associated feature, with long delays between failed conceptions, or if you have a family history of miscarriage then it's important that this problem isn't treated as 'Bad luck, try again!'

After three losses, the chance of a fourth loss increases to 40 per cent. But that still means a good chance of a healthy pregnancy.

What causes this repeated heartbreak?

- **Uterine problems,** such as fibroids that intrude into the uterine cavity, scar tissue in the uterine cavity (Asherman's syndrome), or malformations of the uterine cavity shape, can result in a miscarriage. If your mother took DES (diethyl stilbestrol, a drug to prevent miscarriage, in the 1950s and 1960s), you may have an unusually shaped uterine cavity. Between 15 and 20 per cent of recurrent miscarriages are caused by uterine problems. (We discuss this topic in depth in Chapter 7.)

- **An incompetent cervix** is responsible for 5 per cent of all recurrent miscarriages. An *incompetent cervix* is a cervix too weak to stay closed during pregnancy. The cervix dilates painlessly, resulting in the loss of the pregnancy; this event usually occurs after 12 weeks, when the growing fetus puts more weight on the cervix. An incompetent cervix can be diagnosed on ultrasound; the cervical length will measure less than 20 millimetres. An incompetent cervix can be caused by DES exposure before you were born, trauma to the cervix (such as a cone biopsy done to treat early cervical cancer), or congenital deformities. A multiple pregnancy increases the risk. Pregnancy loss can be prevented in most cases by placing a stitch, called a *cerclage*, through your cervix to keep it from opening too soon. This surgery is usually done after 12 weeks.

- **Chromosomal abnormalities** in either you or your partner cause 5 per cent of recurrent miscarriages. Chromosomal karyotyping, performed as a blood test on you and your partner, can be used to diagnose chromosomal abnormalities.

- **Immune problems,** including diseases such as lupus, may be a factor in a miscarriage. Antibodies called *antiphospholipid antibodies*, which cause clotting problems, and many other possible immune deficiencies are currently a hot topic in fertility workups. (See Chapter 7 for more information about immune issues.)

Pregnancy loss is an issue of biology, not morality. It's usually just genetic 'bad luck'. Fertility problems are not a punishment for anything; they're the result of biology gone awry.

Picking Yourself Up after a Loss

As if you haven't heard it enough, your body (and mind) needs to heal after a miscarriage. Your doctor may recommend that you wait up to three months before trying to conceive again. This time period gives your system time to completely recover from the stress of a miscarriage. If a D&C is required, remember that this treatment is a surgical procedure (albeit minor) that needs time to heal. Do *not* rush this process. However, some evidence suggests that women are 'extra fertile' in the period just after a miscarriage and many couples find it very upsetting to not even be allowed 'to try'. You are not risking anything by getting pregnant straight away after a miscarriage, so keep on making love as soon as you feel able to!

Time truly does heal, or at least dulls the pain. Each passing day will help to make your next pregnancy a joyous experience completely its own, not a shadow of the fear and doubt of your early pregnancy loss. You can never 'replace' a lost pregnancy but you may get a baby that otherwise wouldn't have existed!

Even the most optimistic of you will experience those times when your hope button is stuck on 'off.' This phase is a temporary, albeit painful, condition. Rebooting your emotions can go a long way toward resetting your physical condition as well.

What to do while you're waiting

Just like your body needs to repair itself, your spirit needs some help as well. As you count the days until you begin trying again, consider using this time to help your future child in another way. Here's your to-do list:

- ✔ **If you have already been blessed with a child or children, take a moment to appreciate them.** A hug from your precious one can right many of the world's wrongs.

- ✔ **Allow yourself the time to grieve.** Trying to pretend that you're back to normal when you're not may make you feel temporarily better. However, in the long run, covering up your grief rather than expressing your feelings and working through this period may cause the grief to resurface again, possibly during your next pregnancy, in the form of resentment or guilt. Take the time to heal.

- ✔ **Do something wonderful for yourself.** Whether it's a special purchase, a dinner out with your partner, or an ice cream sundae, indulge a whim.

- ✔ **Do consider professional help if your sadness is debilitating or lasts longer than three months.** A counsellor can help guide you through the minefield of emotions that you're facing.

You and your partner are allies, not enemies, no matter how differently you process the stress and grief of your loss. Helping your partner deal with his own emotions will help you come to terms with your own feelings as well. This experience can make you a stronger team if you work together.

What not to do

Taking care of yourself during this time and allowing others to care for you should be your first priority, if not your only one. Part of this task, which may seem daunting enough, is to keep in touch with your own feelings and stay in touch with those who care about you. To help accomplish this, here's our list of things to avoid:

- ✔ **Don't force yourself to do anything that you don't feel up to.** You may need to decline an invitation to a friend's maternity-leave party, a christening, or family gathering, and that's okay. This time is about getting better, emotionally and physically. Don't do anything to compromise your recovery.

- ✔ **Don't go into hiding.** You'll want to skip some events, but don't completely isolate yourself. Your community of friends and family can help you heal. Although pain is unavoidable, suffering, particularly alone, is optional.

- ✔ **Don't redecorate the nursery or wander through baby stores.** This type of behaviour is similar to picking at a scab. The temptation to do these things is great, and you can talk yourself into believing that these actions will be cathartic. In fact, they'll most likely cause you more pain and prolong your healing process.

An early pregnancy loss does have somewhat of a silver lining. It confirms that you can conceive, which often can be more than half the battle.

Part III
Tests and Investigations

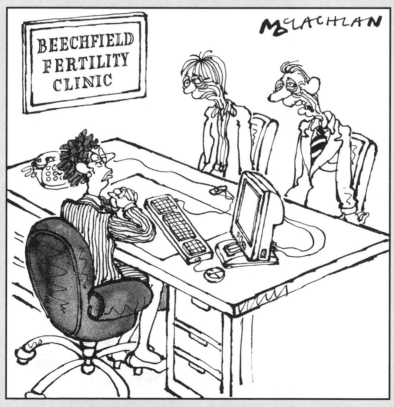

'I know we look too old to be starting
a family – we're just worn out trying.'

In this part . . .

When pregnancy doesn't happen easily, you may find yourself at the chemist's counter or in the doctor's surgery hoping that home-test kits or GP testing can reveal why. In this part, we explain the most common tests offered by a GP and the tests and surgical investigations a consultant may advise you to have. More importantly, we explain what the results mean. We also consider problems with sperm, because infertility can be a man thing too!

Chapter 6

Moving on Up: Seeing a Specialist

• •

In This Chapter

▶ Identifying a consultant

▶ Preparing for your first consultant appointment

▶ Undergoing investigations by a specialist

▶ Opting for IUI at your hospital

▶ Seeing a 'Man-Specialist'

▶ Understanding what you're told and what's happening

• •

*I*f after some GP blood and urine tests, a sperm test at your district general hospital (DGH), possibly a few courses of Clomid, and even more carefully timed (though possibly not quite so passionate love-making), you're still not pregnant, you have now completed the 'level one' fertility treatments, and you may, by now, have a better idea regarding the specifics of your fertility problems.

However, if your GP suspects *endometriosis* (where the cells from the lining of your uterus collect around the outside of the uterus and/or ovaries causing internal bleeding, pain, and reduced fertility) or *polycystic ovary syndrome* (PCOS; a hormonal imbalance that prevents egg containing follicles from developing properly – see Chapter 7 for more information on these conditions), or any similar condition, your GP will refer you to a specialist, because you may require surgery to alleviate the conditions and improve the chance of conceiving. Welcome to 'level two' fertility treatment.

A specialist is usually a consultant gynaecologist at a District General Hospital (DGH) with a specific interest in fertility, who assesses you for more tests, possibly corrective surgery, or even recommends 'high-tech' fertility treatment. Some DGHs are able to offer IUI (intrauterine insemination) with partner sperm to patients with a decent sperm count, who haven't been trying too long and where the woman's age is not a problem, before the need to consider moving onto the 'level three' fertility treatments. (These treatments are the high-tech options offered only by specialist clinics licensed by the Human Fertilisation and Embryology Authority (HFEA). See Part IV for more information on IUI, IVF, and ICSI.)

However, if your GP tests reveal abnormal hormone levels in you, or extremely few or sluggish sperm in your chap, he may suggest that you go straight to a fertility clinic, as further tests, investigative surgery, or even IUI at your DGH will not increase your chances of conceiving. (In which case proceed straight to Part IV and beyond.)

In this chapter, we help you identify your 'dream' consultant and discuss what type of specialists can help and what they *can't* do for you. We also give you some insight into how you make sure that a couple is treated as a couple, and what investigations and treatments you may have at your DGH. Finally, we help you decide if the time has come to try 'level three' assisted conception at a fertility clinic.

Seeking Dr Specialist

Your GP tells you he thinks 'you should see a specialist for some more tests'. A thousand questions fill your head, including:

- Which specialist?
- Are they at the local district general hospital or further afield?
- Can we choose who we go to see?
- How can we find out who is good at diagnosing the causes of infertility?
- Is this person the best one to see? Can they really help?
- How long will we have to wait for an appointment?
- Can we see someone faster if we 'go private'?
- Does our private health insurance cover investigations for infertility?
- Will the specialist be able to find out the exact reason for our infertility?
- Will the specialist be able to help us have a baby?
- Will my husband have to come to see the gynaecologist with me?

Of course, you can ask your doctor any (or all) of these questions, but, if your doctor names a consultant that you should see, ask him specifically why he recommends this particular person. He may choose them simply because they go back a long way or because the consultant is 'local'. GPs in the UK routinely refer their patients to the 'fertility clinic' at the local DGH. Remember to ask how long the waiting time for the first consultation is likely to be. If three months seems too long or you're impatient or worried (or rich) you may choose a 'one-stop-shop' fertility investigation package at a private clinic.

Talking to friends in your local area who have had similar advice can be useful. Find out who they saw and at which hospital. Did they see the specialist privately or on the NHS? Did they like him? Did they feel the specialist explained things clearly and helped either identify the cause of their infertility and, did he get them any closer to being able to have a baby?

Who are these specialists?

Both gynaecologists and obstetricians are qualified doctors who specialise in women's health. An *obstetrician* deals principally with the management of pregnancy and childbirth. A *gynaecologist* deals with disorders of the female reproductive system excluding matters relating to pregnancy. Whoever you see should have either of the following honours:

- ✔ **MRCOG:** In the UK a doctor wishing to pursue a career in obstetrics or gynaecology must demonstrate a high level of competence by passing the membership examinations of the Royal College of Obstetricians and Gynaecologists (RCOG). These qualifications are highly respected examinations and although it's not compulsory for them to do so, a large number of overseas doctors also choose to sit them.

   A doctor is admitted into the membership of the RCOG and may use the letters MRCOG after their name after they have passed both parts of the membership examination.

- ✔ **FRCOG:** After an obstetrician or gynaecologist has been a member of the RCOG for 12 years and has demonstrated a significant contribution to the field, they can apply to become a Fellow of the College. If the application is successful then the doctor may use the letters FRCOG after their name.

- ✔ Members of the RCOG who wish to specialise in fertility may choose to undertake 'sub-specialist' training in Reproductive Medicine; a further three years' study of all aspects of fertility. So now you know why Dr Specialist looks so worn out – he's been studying non-stop for 10+ years!

Choosing between a Ford and a Ferrari: NHS or Private?

After you identify which gynaecologist you need to see, your next big issue is, do you go with NHS or private? Which route you choose depends on a number of factors:

- ✔ **Time:** How long do you need to wait? Appointment waiting times vary around the UK from weeks to months. NHS treatment may be just as good as private, but private treatment may happen sooner. If, by this time, waiting months is unbearable to you, you may wish to by-pass waiting lists by going private.

  If you're happy to see your local hospital consultant, you may be able to get an earlier appointment if you go privately. Same doctor, but you'll see him at your local private hospital instead. (Incidentally, an NHS consultant post is usually a good yardstick for competence.)

- ✔ **Cost:** The NHS is free at the point of access. However, bear in mind that seeing a consultant privately may be more affordable than you think – sometimes around £150, plus the cost of hormone and sperm tests, for a single appointment, but certainly not thousands of pounds for most.

  Alternatively, you may want to see a consultant with a private practice elsewhere in the country, such as Harley Street in London, who is only available privately – but be prepared to pay big bucks for this!

Reassured by insurance

When Gwyn and I (co-author Jill) were told to see a specialist, we were both covered by my employer's private health insurance. This was a total revelation, because we thought that anything to do with infertility would be ineligible. In fact, all our tests were covered up to the point of diagnosis of the exact problem. Gwyn had another sperm analysis and I had my hormone tests again and was also advised to have a laparoscopy, which would have cost thousands of pounds with no insurance or placed me on a NHS waiting list for weeks or months, but which

was all covered by the insurance. I had the op within a couple of weeks, reducing the stress that was starting to build. More importantly, this time round the sperm test revealed Gwyn's sperm were swimming in circles and our consultant outlined how ICSI (a type of IVF where, in a laboratory, a single sperm is injected directly into an egg) could help. This opportunity meant we learned that we would need fertility treatment sooner than if we'd waited to see the very same consultant on the NHS.

Private health insurance may help – even if it's provided by your employer. Although it won't cover any fertility treatment, it may cover consultant fees and any tests for both you and/or your partner 'up to the point of diagnosis' of your infertility. This means you may get faster service and all your hormone and sperm tests (and even some investigative procedures, such as a *laparoscopy* – an examination of the pelvic organs with a fibre-optic telescope inserted surgically below the naval; or a *hysterocontrastsalpingography* (HyCoSy) – an X-ray of the Fallopian tubes through which dye is passed to see if they're obstructed) will be covered by your insurance. And all in the comfort of a private room, too! If you're covered, ask your doctor for a referral to a specialist who is registered with your health insurer.

Working with Dr Specialist

It's time to meet Dr Specialist. Your blood and urine tests have revealed no problems with your hormones and an initial sperm test reveals a sufficient quantity of 'swimmers', so you need more tests and/or investigations with the specialist, which we outline in this section.

Incredibly, some gynae outpatient departments are located close to the antenatal clinics of some NHS hospitals. You may find yourself surrounded by literature about pregnancy or termination and even be seated in a room full of pregnant women while you're waiting to see an infertility specialist. Take a deep breath, hold fast, and if necessary ask if you can wait elsewhere until you're called for your appointment.

What Dr Specialist will want to know

The specialist should have copies of your medical history and your test results from your GP, but be prepared to give him dates of any operations and last cervical smear test and pregnancies as well as any temperature charts and ovulation charts you have kept. In addition, be prepared to answer almost all the same questions your GP asked you (refer to Chapter 4). In addition, Dr Specialist may want to know:

- ✔ Details of your family's reproductive history – for example, parents, siblings, grandparents.

- ✔ Pertinent (or rather impertinent!) details about your sex life. A surprisingly high number of couples still think sex once or twice a month is enough to make a baby. Well it may be for some, but if you've got the Dr Specialist stage of your baby-making journey, that just isn't enough for you.

Investigations Dr Specialist may want to do

Generally, Dr Specialist may want to repeat some of the hormone tests, LH, FSH, and progesterone tests that the GP performed, but if all these have previously been normal, you may find yourself on your way for one or more of the following investigative procedures (check out Chapter 7 for full details of all the diagnostic tests and investigations Dr Specialist may consider for both you and your partner):

- **Hysterosalpingogram (HSG):** An X-ray of the uterus and Fallopian tubes that uses a dye to reveal any blockages that prevent an embryo from reaching the uterus or stop sperm swimming into a Fallopian tube and reaching the egg. This test is usually an outpatient procedure performed without sedation.

- **Hysterocontrastsalpingography (HyCoSy):** A procedure that uses a solution containing millions of microscopic bubbles instead of dye, and ultrasound instead of X-rays, to look for uterine abnormalities such as polyps and fibroids, and checks that the tubes are open and functioning normally. This test is useful for assessing your uterus, and it's less uncomfortable than an HSG and works in 'real time', to show how the Fallopian tubes are working. This method is an outpatient procedure performed without sedation.

- **Hysteroscopy:** Carried out under sedation and with pain relief or with general anaesthetic, this examination of the inside of the uterus uses a thin, fibre-optic telescope inserted through the vagina and cervix into the uterus. It can identify problems with the endometrium (lining of the womb) and to treat abnormalities such as polyps, small fibroids, or adhesions. This investigation is usually an outpatient procedure performed with little or no sedation, or may be carried out under general anaesthetic during a laparoscopy.

- **Laparoscopy:** Carried out under general anaesthetic, a thin, fibre-optic telescope is inserted through a small incision near a woman's belly button for a closer look at your uterus, Fallopian tubes, and ovaries. Gas is pumped into the abdominal cavity to let the surgeon get a better look at the internal organs, which may take a couple of days to disappear and sometimes causes pain behind the shoulder blade in the process. The procedure can identify cysts, adhesions (scar tissue), fibroids, and infections, some of which may be responsible for your infertility. It won't cure your infertility, but it may explain why you're not yet pregnant. A laparoscopy is usually a day case procedure but occasionally may require a stay overnight in hospital.

It takes two to tango, so if you're part of a couple, ensure that your gynaecologist treats you as a couple and doesn't just pursue female factor infertility possibilities. Although one or more of the above tests or the following surgical procedures may be perfectly valid to help diagnose the cause of your infertility, before you agree to treatment that requires sedation or general anaesthetic, ensure that your partner's sperm has been recently and thoroughly checked. This testing means more than just a count of the number of sperm, it involves an analysis of the shape (*morphology*) and swimming ability (*motility*) of the sample. A reduction in the quantity, morphology, and motility of the sperm may be the reason why you're not yet pregnant. If this is the case, you may not need to undergo invasive surgery before moving on to treatment at a fertility clinic. Go to the later section 'When to see Dr Man-Specialist' for info on what specialists deal specifically with male reproductive issues.

Dr Specialist and his amazing corrective surgery

If an HSG, HyCoSy, hysteroscopy, or laparoscopy reveals adhesions, scar tissue, polyps, fibroids, or endometriosis, Dr Specialist may advise one of the following surgical procedures to remove or correct the problem:

- **Adesiolysis:** A procedure that breaks down the fine filmy adhesions around the fimbriae at the end of the Fallopian tubes. If fimbriae aren't free to move, they're unable to 'catch' an egg as it's released from the follicle.

- **Myomectomy:** The removal of *fibroids* (non-cancerous tumours which sprout from the wall of the uterus). Myomectomy is the preferred treatment for fibroids in women who want to keep their uterus. Larger fibroids must be removed with an abdominal incision, but small fibroids can be taken out by laparoscopy or hysteroscopy.

- **Salpingostomy:** A surgical incision into a Fallopian tube to repair a damaged tube or to remove an ectopic pregnancy.

- **Polypectomy:** The removal of uterine polyps either by scraping or cutting away with an electric 'diathermy' loop or a laser. You'll probably need two to four visits to see Dr Specialist, by which time you will know the results of any tests and/or investigative surgery or corrective surgery. After this procedure you will be advised whether to continue trying to conceive naturally, or to consider fertility treatment as the possible solution to your infertility.

IUI at your DGH

Some large NHS district general hospitals (DGHs) are able to offer intrauterine insemination (IUI) to some couples. IUI is the putting of sorted and washed sperm directly into the uterus at the time of ovulation. It can be done in a natural cycle, that is, with no fertility drugs, or with a few drugs to help ovulation. In a DGH, IUI can only be done with partner sperm as donor sperm treatment is only permitted at HFEA-licensed fertility clinics. However, from April 2007, the EU Tissue Directive prevents many DGHs from continuing to offer IUI because of the high standards required for the laboratories.

If your partner has fairly good sperm, you haven't been trying to get pregnant for more than a year, your age is not an issue, and you have clear Fallopian tubes, IUI treatment may be suitable for you and available at your local DGH. If so, ask the following before agreeing to proceed:

- ✔ Will the IUI be a natural cycle (that is, with no drugs) or will stimulation drugs be required?
- ✔ Will you have to pay for your drugs, or will they be funded for you?
- ✔ Will it be carried out by a fertility specialist rather than a generalist gynaecologist?
- ✔ Can IUI be carried out at least five days per week, to allow treatment to coincide with when you ovulate? At smaller DGHs where IUI is available on only one or two days of the week, some patients have to wait for months before their ovulation coincides with when the IUI clinic is open. This practice is not recommended, particularly if you have had to pay for the drugs for a stimulated cycle.
- ✔ How many cycles are carried out at the DGH every year?
- ✔ What are the success rates for either natural or stimulated treatment?

For more information on IUI, head to Chapters 10 and 11.

When to see Dr Man-Specialist

If your GP's tests on your partner's sperm reveal a problem with the quantity or quality of his sperm and your hormone tests were normal, by-pass the gynaecologist and instead ask for a referral for your chap to an *andrologist* – a sperm specialist. The andrologist will perform a more detailed sperm assessment, check his hormones, check his chromosomes (karyotyping), and check that he isn't a 'carrier' of cystic fibrosis test his 'plumbing' with a vasogram and maybe biopsy (in which a tissue sample is taken) of the testes if no sperm are found in his semen sample. Many men hate hospitals and get confused between fertility and virility. You will need to be very supportive here!

If the reason for you not getting pregnant is because of penetration problems (problems achieving intercourse) or male impotence, your GP should refer you to an urologist, who is able to treat problems of the male reproductive system, including erectile dysfunction.

Facing the Stranger in Your Sex Life

Even at this pre-fertility treatment stage, you open the door to your private life – and especially your sex life – to a variety of strangers, otherwise known as medical staff. This loss of privacy is inevitable and takes some getting used to.

The frequency of intercourse, the quality and timing of your menstrual cycles, and your past history of pregnancies, whether by hit or miss, are crucial bits of information in piecing together your reproductive profile. Offer information willingly because doing so will help to give the specialist the full picture.

Your specialist (and his staff!) would rather discuss things other than your sex life (like last night's *Holby City*!) among themselves. They will not discuss your private life in their private lives. Their job, however, is to help you conceive a baby, and their questions are part of the process. Once again, consider this good training for possible fertility treatment, where the questions, prodding, and poking will become routine.

Understanding What Dr Specialist Says

Doctors and nurses aren't *really* trying to confuse you when they spew forth a list of initials or shortcut terms. But when your specialist says something like 'Get an HSG and scan, and then if your inhibin and FSH come back okay, we'll try some stim,' your immediate reaction may be 'Huh?'

You may find it important, even necessary, to take notes when your doctor is speaking. Some patients choose to tape record their conversations with their specialist, which may be helpful when relaying this information to your partner. Always ask your specialist if doing so is okay, particularly when it comes to taping your discussions. Most doctors are glad to accommodate you, but most *people* (including doctors) become a bit unhinged if they find out that they were being taped secretly.

Enlisting a second set of ears can also be helpful, which is the perfect spot for your partner to participate! Fertility is an emotional subject. Especially if the doctor is addressing problems that *you* have, you may be too close to the situation to hear and understand all the options that are available. Your partner or a friend may be a bit more detached and better able to comprehend and communicate the information to you. If English isn't your first language you may find it very helpful to take a close friend as an interpreter or the clinic may be able to provide an interpreter for you. Remember, doctors are much more concerned that you understand the tests, diagnosis, and treatment. They don't mind how many people are in the room!

Chapter 7

Finding the Female Problem: Testing, Testing, 1, 2, 3

*1*f you aren't pregnant after a year of trying, the time may have come to start doing some tests. Your doctor may suggest these tests to you, or you may suggest them to him, if you feel that time is slipping away and you want to find out why you're not yet pregnant, or why you can't stay pregnant.

In this chapter we give you a rundown of the tests that fertility doctors do most frequently, why they do them, and what you can expect to learn from the tests.

For about 30 per cent of couples trying to get pregnant, several problems contribute to infertility. This fact is especially important to remember if one of you has a known factor, such as previous tubal surgery or a known sperm problem. Many couples come to a clinic and tell the staff, 'I don't need to do any testing – we already know the problem is mine (or his).' You may think that you already know the problem, but keep in mind that for 30 per cent of you, tests will reveal another problem, and pregnancy won't occur until both problems are addressed. Mother Nature is quite good at letting you make babies (given enough time and opportunity!) as long as only one fertility factor is involved. But if more than one problem exists (even if all the problems are quite minor), then spontaneous pregnancy may prove elusive.

Cataloguing the Common Tests: ABCD HSG

Many factors can contribute to infertility, and determining what your fertility issue is can take some time and involve testing. Some tests, such as blood tests, are fairly simple, while others, such as laparoscopic surgery, are more invasive.

Your doctor may start with the most basic tests or go right to the more invasive tests if they suspect that your fertility problems involve uterine or tubal factors. The tests we list are the ones most likely to be suggested by your doctor, but you may not need all these tests.

Thirty per cent of infertility is related to sperm problems, so don't forget to have your partner tested, too!

Baseline blood tests

'Let's do some baseline blood tests,' your doctor may say when you first start looking for an answer to the 'why am I not pregnant?' question. This method is one of the simplest tests you can have done. You simply wait until your period starts, go to the practice nurse or hospital on day two or day three of your period, and have a blood sample taken. A follow up with the GP will give you quite a bit of information about your fertility. Here's what the tests reveal:

Try not to get hung up by numbers. If you're having a regular cycle then you're almost certainly ovulating (and the stress of going for blood tests can upset even the most well-behaved periods!).

- ✔ **Follicle-stimulating hormone (FSH):** FSH is probably the most important blood test. Your FSH level should be less than 8, depending on your lab, on day two or day three. A higher than normal FSH level may indicate that you're going into the *perimenopause* early – the period a few years before menopause; you may also not be releasing eggs every month. We discuss FSH in more detail in the section 'FSH, AMH, and inhibin B' later in this chapter.

You may wonder why normal ranges for FSH vary from lab to lab. The reason is that many labs establish their own norms based on their specific patient population. The instruments used in the lab can also cause variations from one lab to another.

✔ **Oestradiol:** Oestradiol on day two or three of your period is normally 25–50 pg/ml (picogrammes per millilitre). An oestradiol level that is very low, less than 10, may indicate that your ovaries are suppressed and may not respond well to stimulation to make a normal egg. An oestradiol level that is over 50 picogrammes per millilitre may indicate ovarian cysts or that your ovaries are likely to have a poor response to stimulation.

✔ **Progesterone:** On day two or three of your period, your progesterone levels should be low, less than 2. Progesterone levels go up in the second half of your cycle, after you ovulate, and should be measured on day 21 (if you have a regular 28-day cycle). The peak progesterone level is about seven days before your next period is due. A good result is over 30 nmol/l (nanomoles per litre) after you release an egg. Progesterone comes from the *corpus luteum*, the leftover shell of the follicle after you ovulate, and is necessary to help the embryo implant.

✔ **Luteinising hormone (LH):** The LH level is usually about 5 on day two or three; women with polycystic ovaries (we discuss this condition in the section 'Polycystic ovary syndrome (PCOS)' later in this chapter) may have an LH level that's significantly higher than their follicle-stimulating hormone level on day two. LH is the 'trigger' for ovulation so levels rise later in the cycle, usually going over 40 when you're almost ready to ovulate.

Your partner's hormone levels, especially LH, FSH, and testosterone, also need to be normal for good sperm production. Most doctors don't test the levels unless your partner's semen analysis is abnormal because a good semen analysis means his hormone levels are normal.

HSG (don't even try to spell out the word)

An HSG, or *hysterosalpingogram*, is an X-ray that outlines your uterus and Fallopian tubes to make it easy to see where abnormalities may be keeping you from getting pregnant (see Figure 7-1). Dye is injected through your cervix to make the uterus and tubes easy to see on an X-ray.

HSGs are a valuable tool in diagnosing fertility problems. Some of the problems that can be diagnosed with an HSG are fibroids in the uterus, large polyps in the uterus, an unusually shaped uterine cavity, a septum (a piece of tissue dividing your cavity), or adhesions (scar tissue) in the uterus. If you know that you have fibroids, an HSG can show whether they're intruding into the inside of the uterus, where they may prevent implantation of an embryo.

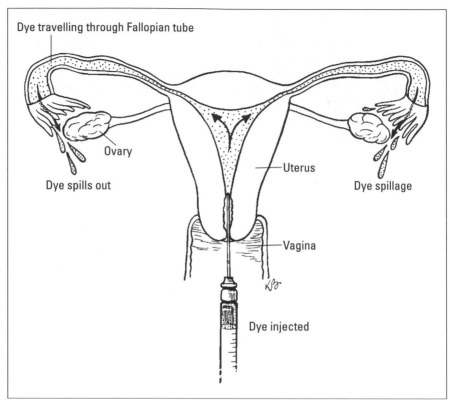

Dye travelling through Fallopian tube

Ovary

Dye spills out

Uterus

Dye spillage

Vagina

Dye injected

Figure 7-1:
Dye is
injected
when doing
a hystero-
salpingo-
gram.

The dye also outlines the Fallopian tubes, so your doctor can see whether your tubes are normally shaped and, most importantly, whether your tubes are open, which your doctor can tell by noticing whether the dye passes through the tubes and flows into the pelvis. The HSG is an important test because it lets you know whether your tubes are blocked in any way, or if they're very swollen, in which case an egg or embryo won't be able to get through to the uterus, or sperm to the egg. If dye does pass through easily, your HSG report will say that the Fallopian tubes 'filled and spilled,' meaning that the dye easily passed up from the uterus, all the way up the tubes, and out the end of the tube into the pelvis.

Here are some other things to know about HSGs:

✔ **They can be uncomfortable, causing mild to severe cramping.** How uncomfortable is an HSG? That depends on your own pain tolerance and whether your tubes are open. If the tubes are slightly blocked with debris, your doctor may need to push the dye more forcefully to clear the block, which may increase cramping. Most doctors tell you to take ibuprofen or a similar pain medication an hour or so before your test.

✔ **Both the dye and the pelvic X-rays can be harmful if you're pregnant.** Be sure to schedule your test for the early part of your menstrual cycle, usually before day 12 (before you ovulate).

✔ **Many doctors also do cervical cultures for gonorrhoea and chlamydia before doing an HSG.** If you have an infection, pushing dye through the uterus and Fallopian tubes can spread the infection and cause serious complications. Your doctor may also prescribe antibiotics (such as doxycycline) for you to take starting a few days before your HSG, because between 1 and 3 per cent of women experience some type of infection after the procedure.

✔ **If you're allergic to contrast dye or shellfish, you may not be able to have the test done.** Contrast dye and shellfish both contain iodine, and some doctors believe an allergy to shellfish means you've a higher chance of having an allergic reaction to the dye.

After the test, a small amount of bleeding is normal; you'll also leak a small amount of dye (which is clear, not coloured) over the next day or so. You may also have tummy cramps for a few hours after the procedure. Take someone with you so that you don't have to drive yourself home. On the positive side, the chance of conception appears to increase for a few cycles after an HSG as if the cobwebs in the tubes have been blown away.

Saline-enhanced ultrasound (sonohysterogram)

A *sonohysterogram* is very similar to an HSG, except that a saline solution, rather than a dye, is injected, and ultrasound, rather than an X-ray, is used to show uterine abnormalities such as polyps or fibroids. The test can be done in the clinic and requires no medication in most cases.

A sonohysterogram is very effective for evaluating your uterus but not as effective as an HSG for looking at the Fallopian tubes.

HyCoSy (hysterocontrastsalpingography): Don't even try to say it!

HyCoSy (also known as Echovist) is a new way of examining the inside of the uterus and the Fallopian tubes that doesn't require X-rays (like the HSG) or a general anaesthetic (like a laparoscopy and dye test). It involves injecting a starch solution containing millions of microscopic bubbles through the cervix under ultrasound vision and the outline of the uterine cavity can be clearly seen. The bubble mixture can be tracked in 'real time' on the ultra-sound screen flowing through the Fallopian tubes (if they're not blocked) and appearing in the pelvis. As with the HSG, discomfort, delay, or needing to use high pressures may indicate problems with the tubes.

Hysteroscopy

Sometimes smaller polyps and fibroids are hard to see on an HSG. For a close-up look at the inside of your uterus, your doctor may want to do a hysteroscopy.

A *hysteroscopy*, which can be done as an outpatient procedure, involves a small telescope with a fibre-optic light being guided through the cervix into the uterus. The uterus is distended, usually with carbon dioxide gas or some-times a neutral solution called Hartmann's, so that your doctor can clearly see the entire cavity including any small polyps, adhesions, or fibroids. You may be given local anaesthesia, such as a cervical block, or mild sedation, such as a benzodiazepine like Valium or Midazolam, for the procedure.

If the procedure detects polyps, scar tissue, or small fibroids in the uterus, your doctor may proceed to an *operative hysteroscopy*. In this procedure, the doctor inserts small instruments through the scope to remove the abnormal tissue. This op can be done in outpatients, or under may require an additional procedure under general anaesthetic if more extensive work needs to be done.

Laparoscopy

A *laparoscopy* involves inserting a thin telescope with a fibre-optic light at the end into the abdomen through a tiny cut made just below the navel, as shown in Figure 7-2. Other instruments can be inserted through cuts made in the pubic hairline. The incisions made are very small, about ½ inch or less, and the pro-cedure usually involves one to three incisions. Carbon dioxide gas is used to separate the organs inside the pelvic cavity making it easier to see the uterus, ovaries, and tubes. A special blue dye can be instilled through the cervix to check that the tubes are not blocked (the 'lap and dye' test). Apart from 'patent' or open tubes, the doctor is looking for signs of past or active infection, scar-ring, or endometriosis. Endometriosis and scar tissue can be removed during an operative laparoscopy using laser or *diathermy* (electric current).

A laparoscopy is usually done as an inpatient procedure in a hospital or sur-gical centre. It is a 'day case' so you can expect to go home the same day. The most common problems after the surgery are pain (usually minimal) from the incisions and pain at the shoulder tips from the carbon dioxide used to inflate the abdomen. Your abdomen may seem sore and bloated for a few days. The recovery period is usually short – less than a week.

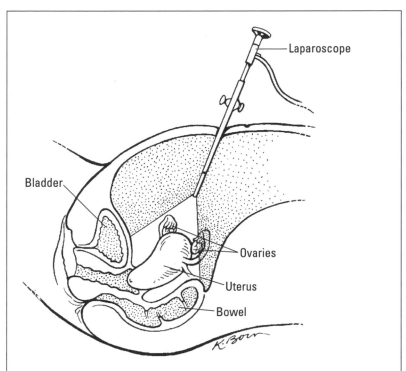

Laparoscope

Bladder

Ovaries

Uterus

Bowel

K. Bow

Figure 7-2:
A laparo-
scopy.

Post-coital tests

Post-coital testing (PCT) is, as its name implies, a test performed after sex. The test measures the sperms' ability to penetrate the cervical mucus. In addition to checking out 'the troops,' your doctor also examines the quality and quantity of the mucus itself.

Post-coital tests must be done around the time of ovulation. Timing of this test is very important to correctly evaluate the results. Your doctor will want you to have sex around the time of your LH surge (detected by ovulation predictor kits) and come into the clinic the next morning, anywhere from 4 to 12 hours later; different doctors seem to have different opinions on the exact timing.

The doctor or a nurse takes a sample of mucus from your cervix for the test, so don't take a bath, douche, or use lubricants, such as KY Jelly, for sex.

Generally, the post-coital test is time consuming, unreliable, and really, really embarrassing. However, some fertility doctors set great store by it and 'hostile mucus' is a diagnosis that can only be made after a PCT.

What you want to see in the semen

To evaluate the sperm's performance, the doctor puts the mucus on a slide and looks at it under a high-powered microscope. You hope that the doctor sees six to ten sperm moving forward per high-powered field. You *don't* want to see a few inert sluggards or a bunch of sperm seemingly stuck together; stuck-together sperm may mean that antisperm antibodies are present. *Antisperm antibodies* are immune cells that 'attack' the sperm and attach to their tails so they can't 'swim' to the target, which is your egg. (See the section 'Testing for immune disorders' later in this chapter, for more information about antisperm antibodies.)

Mucus matters

Your cervical mucus should be clear in colour; make a leaflike, fern pattern under the microscope; and be very stretchy, a quality known as *spinnbarkeit*. Good ovulation-time mucus can be stretched about 4 inches, but nobody will blame you if you don't want to check this fact out yourself! All these qualities are required for sperm to swim rapidly through the vagina without being mired down or destroyed.

Sometimes the mucus seen doesn't live up to all these great qualities; here are a few possible reasons why it may not:

- ✔ **You may not be ovulating.** If your predictor kit says that you're having a surge but your mucus is thick, your kit may be wrong. Your LH level may be high in conjunction with a high FSH level; this is common in premature ovarian failure, or in women with PCOS.

- ✔ **You may have a cervical infection.** With cervicitis, normal mucus producing cells in the cervix are replaced with 'squamous' or flat cells that don't make good cervical mucus.

- ✔ **If you're taking Clomid (a fertility drug), it may be affecting your mucus.** See the section 'CCCT (clomiphene citrate challenge test)' later in this chapter for more on Clomid.

- ✔ **If you've had any procedures done on your cervix for abnormal smears, your mucus-producing cells may have been destroyed.** Such procedures include *cone biopsy*, in which a wedge-shaped piece of cervix is cut out and sent to be tested for cancerous cells; *loop electrosurgical excision of the transformation zone* (LETZ), in which a layer of cervix is removed by using a fine wire; laser; or freezing (*cryocautery*).

Thyroid tests

The thyroid gland is the pacemaker that helps all the rest of your *endocrine* (hormone) system function. The best state to be in with your thyroid is *euthyroid*, which means that your thyroid is in balance. Thyroid problems are very common, with one out of eight women diagnosed with a thyroid problem at some point in their lives. Men can also have thyroid disorders, but women are five to eight times more likely to be affected.

Your thyroid can be either overactive (*hyper*) or underactive (*hypo*). Both hyper- and hypothyroid conditions can cause infertility problems in men and women:

- **Underactive thyroid (hypothyroidism):** A thyroid that is hypoactive usually causes fatigue, dry skin, cold intolerance, and weight gain. It can also cause a raised FSH level, so if your doctor says that you have a high FSH and it may mean you're heading for the menopause, get your thyroid checked out. Hypothyroidism can also be blamed for an increase in *prolactin*, the hormone responsible for maintaining breast milk production in pregnancy. High prolactin can cause a decrease in fertility.

- **Overactive thyroid (hyperthyroidism):** A hyperactive thyroid causes a rapid heart rate, anxiousness, sweating, and weight loss.

Both under- and overactive thyroid problems can be associated with infertility and miscarriage. Women seeking fertility treatment aren't routinely screened for thyroid disease but thyroid problems run in families, so if your mother, aunt, or granny had thyroid disease, mention it to your GP and ask for a TFT (thyroid function test).

In men, thyroid problems can cause a low sperm count and decreased sperm motility. Women may experience an increased rate of miscarriage, lack of ovulation, or irregular periods.

Thyroid imbalances can be treated by daily medication, radiation, or, in severe cases, surgery. Your thyroid medication will need to be adjusted when you become pregnant and your antenatal care will involve even more blood tests than usual.

FSH, AMH (anti-Müllerian hormone), and inhibin B

Follicle-stimulating hormone (FSH) is necessary for the production of an egg each month, but, like other things in life, sometimes too much of a good thing is a problem. FSH rises above normal levels when the ovaries stop producing enough oestrogen. The pituitary gland in the base of the brain produces more FSH to try to make the ovary recruit a follicle and produce more oestrogen. This change is reflected as a raised level of FSH in the blood. Your doctor may say that you're in *perimenopause*, which is the time from two to ten years before menopause.

Many doctors feel that a single, high FSH reading, meaning anything over 8–10 mIU/ml (milli-International Units per millilitre) – the exact number varies with your lab – means that you have diminished ovarian reserve, which can be defined as a reduced number of potentially viable eggs left within the ovaries. Many women have a raised FSH level and yet still have normal fertility, but a significantly raised FSH level can be a problem if you need fertility treatment that requires your ovaries to produce multiple eggs in a single cycle. If you're under 40 years of age and you have a very raised FSH level (>15 mIU/ml), you may be diagnosed with premature ovarian failure (POF). If you're over 40, your doctor may consider this rise in FSH to be a normal ageing response.

Because the level of FSH can fluctuate between months, a single 'good' result can offer false promise so if you're over 35, have any risk factors for poor ovarian reserve such as a family history of early menopause, or if your periods have become irregular or closer together, you should get another level checked before embarking on fertility treatment, such as IVF.

Two 'new' hormone tests, which involve measuring the levels of AMH (which stands for anti-Müllerian hormone) and inhibin B in the woman's blood, are proving very helpful in assessing 'ovarian reserve' prior to treatment. AMH can be measured on any day of the cycle and inhibin is best done on cycle day 4–6 if you've an average 28-day cycle.

A low level of inhibin B or AMH may indicate that your ovarian function is decreased and your response to stimulation during fertility treatment will be low. AMH and inhibin B testing are not widely available but some specialist labs in the UK will run the tests for you. Don't wait to find out that your ovarian reserve is very low *after* you've spent hundreds of pounds on medication that didn't work!

CCCT (clomiphene citrate challenge test)

The CCCT, often called the *clomiphene citrate challenge test*, is a measurement of oestradiol and FSH taken on day two or three of your period and then measured again after you take a medication called clomiphene citrate for five days. This drug has the brand name Clomid, and it's a fertility medication that stimulates egg production. Your oestradiol and FSH levels are checked with a further blood test after the five days of tablets. Your oestradiol level should rise by the fifth day, but if your FSH level is elevated on either day two, or after five days, you'll be told that you had a failed CCCT. Your doctor may feel that a failed CCCT means that you've a decreased ovarian reserve, which decreases your chance of getting pregnant with your own eggs.

Understanding Female Infertility Problems

Men's infertility issues seem simple at first because the problem all comes down to sperm: Are they produced, can they get out, and what do they do when they get where they need to be? Women's infertility issues can be more complex because so many different systems can be at fault. Is the problem uterine, tubal, hormonal, age related, or ovarian? Any one of these problems can cause enough trouble to prevent you from becoming and staying pregnant.

Looking in the uterus

Maybe you had an HSG to evaluate your Fallopian tubes and uterus, which we discuss in the section 'HSG (don't even try to spell out the word)', earlier in this chapter, or maybe you had a hysteroscopy for an even closer look into the uterus. Looking at the uterus is an integral part of any fertility workup because the uterus nourishes and holds a baby for nine months.

Fibroids, or benign tumours of smooth muscle, are commonly found inside or on the outside of the uterus. They're extremely common, with 40 per cent of women between the ages of 35 and 55 having at least one. Fibroids are even more common in black women, with 50 per cent having at least one.

Fibroids can cause bowel or bladder problems, very heavy bleeding, or pain. Fibroids can be either inside or outside the uterine cavity; their location determines whether they cause a problem with your ability to get or stay pregnant.

Fibroids include the following:

- ✒ *Pedunculated* fibroids are completely outside the uterus, but are attached to the uterus by a stem, and don't usually cause a problem with infertility.

- ✒ *Subserosal fibroids* are located in the outer wall of the uterus and generally don't impinge on the cavity. They don't have a negative effect on fertility but may undergo 'red degeneration' during pregnancy if they grow too rapidly and outstrip their blood supply.

- ✒ *Intramural fibroids*, those within the wall of the uterus, can disort the uterus in if they grow large enough.

- ✒ *Submucosal fibroids* grow through the lining of the inside wall and can make the cavity too small for a baby to gestate for nine months. A significant proportion of pregnancies miscarry if submucosal fibroids are present, and submucosal fibroids reduce the chance of IVF and ICSI working.

Fibroids can be surgically removed, a process called a *myomectomy*. You may need to deliver by caesarean section after a myomectomy.

Checking out the Fallopian tubes

Most women have two Fallopian tubes, one on each side of the uterus, next to the ovaries. Because these tubes are the only route from the ovary to the uterus, a problem with one or both tubes can have a big impact on your baby-making ability.

Sometimes a tube is surgically removed after an *ectopic* pregnancy, a pregnancy that starts to grow in the tube rather than in the uterus. If this pregnancy is found early enough, doctors may be able to dissolve the pregnancy with a chemotherapy agent called methotrexate. However, if the embryo grows large enough undetected in the tube, the tube can burst, causing life-threatening bleeding (we discuss this in Chapter 6). The only way to stop the bleeding is to remove the tube.

You can get pregnant with only one tube, but you must be aware that having one ectopic pregnancy leaves you at a higher risk to have another.

Women who have only the left ovary and the right Fallopian tube have got pregnant because the egg can 'float' to the remaining tube. Of course, this also applies to women who have the left tube and the right ovary.

Sometimes Fallopian tubes are seen to be enlarged on ultrasound or during an HSG. If the tubes are very swollen and dye doesn't flow through them, you may have a *hydrosalpinx*, the medical term for a chronically infected tube (see Figure 7-3). If both tubes are dilated, the condition is known as bilateral *hydrosalpinges*.

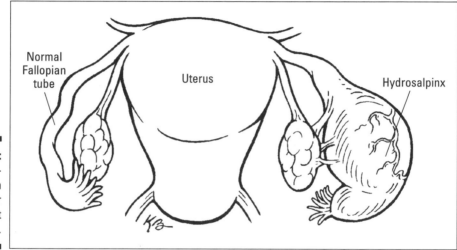

Figure 7-3:
A hydro-
salpinx can
affect your
ability to get
pregnant.

A hydrosalpinx interferes with pregnancy in two ways:

- ✔ The egg may not be able to find its way through the tube because the tube is so large and the passage may be blocked with infected debris.

- ✔ The embryo, if it makes it to the uterus, may not be able to survive because the infected material from the tube drips down into the uterus, making an inhospitable environment for the embryo to grow.

The treatment for a hydrosalpinx sounds drastic. The tube or tubes must be removed or at least be clipped or cauterised at the *cornua* (where the tube emerges from the uterus), and then you will need to have in vitro fertilisation (IVF) to get pregnant because your embryos can no longer be transported down to the uterus. This diagnosis is a hard thing for many women to accept because it definitely ends any chance that they'll be able to get pregnant on their own. However, overwhelming evidence exists that removing chronically swollen and infected tubes does improve the chance of IVF embryos implanting and reduces the chance of ectopic pregnancies occurring.

Women can be born without any Fallopian tubes; often the tubes are missing as part of a syndrome in which the external sex organs look normal, but the vagina, uterus, and Fallopian tubes are missing. Of course, if you've had two ectopic pregnancies, you may have had both tubes surgically removed also.

Sometimes Fallopian tubes look fine on an X-ray or ultrasound, but for some reason, don't 'work' properly so that the embryo can't get down to the uterus.

The tubes are lined by millions of tiny hairs called *cilia*, which beat synchronously, and waft a thin carpet of mucus along the tube carrying the egg and fertilised embryo towards the uterine cavity. If this 'ciliary carpet' is damaged then pregnancy is unlikely to occur. *Endometriosis*, a common condition in which the endometrium or lining of the womb grows outside the uterine cavity can grow in or around the Fallopian tubes and block them.

Because the Fallopian tubes play such a large role in getting pregnant, you'll probably need intervention, such as IVF, to get pregnant if a problem is discovered with them. Removal or absence of the tubes, or a blockage that can't be removed, makes IVF inevitable if you're trying to get pregnant.

The complications of scar tissue

Adhesions form when blood and plasma from trauma such as surgery form *fibrin deposits*, which are threadlike strands that can bind one organ to another (see Figure 7-4). Adhesions in the pelvis are common after surgery such as a caesarean section, an appendectomy, tubal removal for an ectopic pregnancy, or fibroid removal. Between 60 and 90 per cent of surgical procedures leave adhesions behind. Adhesions often cause pelvic pain; 30 to 40 per cent of women with chronic pelvic pain have adhesions, and one out of seven women has chronic pelvic pain.

Adhesions can be removed, but keep these points in mind:

- ✔ **Surgery to correct adhesions may result in – you guessed it – more adhesions.** The chance of adhesions forming can be reduced by careful surgical technique, handling the organs as little as possible, wearing starch-free surgical gloves, and using special tissues that cover 'raw' areas after surgery or a solution used to irrigate the pelvis.

    Your chances of getting pregnant after adhesion removal are highest in the first six months after surgery, before extensive adhesions form again.

- ✔ **Some adhesions can't be removed without damaging the tubes or ovaries.** If this is the case, you may need IVF to get pregnant.

In my years as an obstetrician, I (co-author Gill) saw at firsthand how scar tissue, or adhesions (as shown in Figure 7-4), can create problems in your reproductive system. Many women having a second or third caesarean section delivery had scar tissue throughout the pelvis that needed to be cut away before the delivery team was able to get to the uterus and deliver the baby.

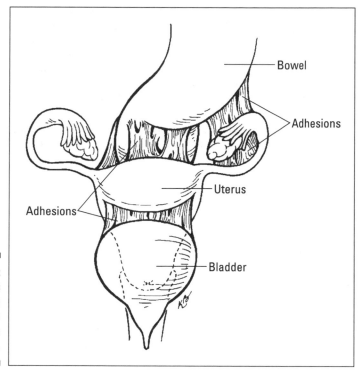

Figure 7-4:
Adhesions
in the
female
reproductive
system.

If you have adhesions within the uterus itself, you may be diagnosed with *Asherman's syndrome*, also called uterine synechiae. With Asherman's, the adhesions criss-cross the entire cavity and make it difficult, if not impossible, for a pregnancy to implant. Asherman's can follow a dilation and curettage (D&C), an abortion, or a uterine infection. It can be diagnosed during an HSG but is best diagnosed with a hysteroscopy, where the inside of the uterus can be seen. Asherman's also is suspected if you've scant or no menstrual flow or recurrent miscarriages following uterine trauma. If the mild-to-moderate adhesions are removed surgically, you've a good chance of becoming pregnant and carrying to term. Severe adhesions may destroy nearly all the normal uterine lining, and pregnancy may not be possible.

Testing for immune disorders

Immune testing in infertility, which in most cases simply requires a blood sample, is a highly contentious area. Different doctors have different opinions of the importance of immune testing in infertility. Some tests are widely done and the results almost universally accepted. Other tests are done only by doctors specialising in immune disorders, and not all doctors believe the results are important. In addition, the organisation of good clinical trials is hard. Randomised clinical trials, or RCTs, are the only effective way to tell conclusively if a particular treatment is effective and they involve allocating patients at random to different treatments or perhaps 'no-treatment' at all. Understandably, patients with a long history of miscarriages or infertility are not keen to risk being allocated to the 'dummy' pill or placebo arm of a trial.

The following sections discuss some of the most common immune tests, with information on what the tests mean and how you're treated if the tests are abnormal.

Antisperm antibody (ASA)

Many fertility centres do antisperm antibody (ASA) tests on all their patients. Both you and your partner may be positive for ASA. Women are tested through a blood test, and men are tested through a semen specimen.

Antisperm antibodies in either partner can cause problems with fertilisation. Males with ASA may need to do IVF with *ICSI* (intracytoplasmic sperm injection, or the injection of one sperm into an egg) if they have more than 20 per cent antibodies, because the antibodies cause the sperm to clump together instead of moving forward. (We discuss ICSI in more detail in Chapters 10 and 13.) About 70 per cent of men who have had a vasectomy reversal have antisperm antibodies; they're also common in men who have had injury to the testes. Ten per cent or so of infertile men have ASA.

Antisperm antibodies are less common in women; less than 5 per cent of infertile women have antisperm antibodies. They're found in the cervical mucus as well as the blood. The treatment is IVF with ICSI.

Antiphospholipid antibodies (APA)

Antiphospholipid antibodies can interfere with the embryo implanting or can cause miscarriage; they disrupt the normal clotting of blood and the implantation of the embryo into the uterus. You'll most likely be tested for antiphospholipid antibodies (APA or 'sticky blood' syndrome) if you've had multiple miscarriages or a history of clotting disorders, such as DVT (deep vein thrombosis) or PE (pulmonary embolus). The test for APA actually tests for a number of different antibodies including antiphospholipid and anticardiolipin antibodies; a moderate or high reaction to two or more antibodies is considered a positive reaction. Treatment is with low-dose aspirin and heparin (an *anticoagulant*, or blood thinner).

Antinuclear antibodies (ANA)

A high positive antinuclear antibodies (ANA) test can mean that you have a disease called systemic lupus erythematosus (SLE) – for more info, see the later section 'Lupus: Not just a rash'. At lower positive levels, especially if the pattern is speckled, ANA can increase your risk of miscarriage. A positive ANA level may be treated with low-dose steroids.

Antithyroglobulin (ATA)

Antithyroglobulin antibodies (ATA) can cause problems with your thyroid function. Because the thyroid is so important in maintaining your hormone levels, antibodies that interfere with the thyroid's functioning can cause problems with egg production. A high ATA level may be treated with steroids.

Antiovarian antibodies (AOA)

If you're in premature ovarian failure or early menopause, you may be tested for antiovarian antibodies (AOA).

Leukocyte antibody detection (LAD)

Foreign bodies are usually rejected because they're attacked by antibodies; the same would be true of a fetus if it didn't have the protection of *blocking antibodies*, which you make in response to the genetic material from your partner that's present in the embryo. If you and your partner have DNA that's too similar, those antibodies won't be activated, and the fetus will be recognised as 'foreign' and rejected. A positive leukocyte antibody detection (LAD) test is good; it means the antibodies are present. Previously if the test was negative, you may have been recommended to try leukocyte immunisation (LI) therapy, which injects white blood cells from your partner into you by using a small intradermal needle, similar to a tuberculin test. At present, LI therapy isn't widely used and most fertility specialists feel that the risks far outweigh any theoretical benefit.

A synthetic form of LIT using injections of a substance called Leukonorm showed promise in some early clinical trials.

Natural killer (NK) cells

Natural killer (NK) cells are part of white blood cells that attack and destroy anything they see as a foreign substance in the body. They're an important part of keeping cancer cells from spreading. A normal NK cell range is about 2 per cent; if the count is higher than 10 per cent, the cells may be too aggressive and attack a growing embryo. Treatment for high NK cells is intravenous immunoglobulin (IVIG) therapy or high dose steroids. IVIG is very expensive and highly controversial among infertility specialists.

Endometriosis: A 'bloody' pain

Up to 20 per cent of women have endometriosis, a common, complicated condition that affects 30–40 per cent of all infertility patients. Despite its prevalence, it's often under diagnosed and under treated.

Endometriosis is the presence of endometrial tissue, which should be restricted to lining the inside of your uterus, in places it has no business being. Endometriosis can be found throughout the pelvis – around the Fallopian tubes and ovaries – but it has also been found in the lungs, skin, and brain. What seems to happen is that every time you have a period, some of the *menstrual debris* (!), as gynaecologists refer to it, gets pushed back up the Fallopian tubes and settles around the back of the uterus and on the ovaries. Normally, the 'house-keeping' in the pelvis would clean it up before it had time to make the place look untidy, but in a proportion of women the debris (which contains tiny endometrial glands as well as blood) 'burrows' into the tissues and starts to grow. So whenever you have a period these tiny deposits bleed too and over time they form big cysts on the ovaries (*endometriomata* or chocolate cysts).

Because endometriosis is endometrial tissue, it reacts to hormone changes the same way your uterine lining does. So when you get your period or have mid-cycle spotting, the endometriosis tissue also bleeds. Because this blood can't escape to the outside world the way your uterine lining does, the blood stagnates, causing inflammation, irritation, and eventually scar tissue.

You may suspect that you have endometriosis if you have any of the following symptoms:

- ✔ Chronic or recurring pelvic pain
- ✔ History of ectopic pregnancy or miscarriage
- ✔ Backache or leg pain

- Nausea, vomiting, diarrhoea, or constipation
- Rectal bleeding or bloody stools
- Blood in urine
- Urinary urgency or frequency
- Chest pain or coughing up blood, especially at the time of your period
- Deep pain with intercourse (dyspareunia)

Because the symptoms are so broad and sometimes non-specific, endometriosis may be confused with the following conditions:

- Appendicitis
- Irritable bowel syndrome
- Bowel obstruction
- Ovarian cysts
- Pelvic inflammatory disease

Endometriosis affects fertility in many ways. It may cause adhesions, tubal blockage, and problems with ovulation. The problems may include luteinised, unruptured follicle (LUF) syndrome, in which a mature follicle develops but the egg inside doesn't release. Women with endometriosis may also have a lower oestradiol level at the time of ovulation, or a blunted LH surge, so that the follicle may not properly mature.

No complete cure is yet available for endometriosis, nor is there clear-cut evidence why some women develop endometriosis, although a familial link appears to be a possibility.

But effective treatments are available, of which one of the best is *diathermy* or laser treatment to the endometriotic deposits. Hormone treatment that mimics pregnancy by stopping your periods for a while (Depot GnRH analogues like Prostap SR or Zoladex) help the endometriosis settle down, but of, course you can't get pregnant while you're not having periods. Endometriosis is progressive but it can be kept in check to some extent by the oral contraceptive pill.

The amount of endometriosis present doesn't determine the degree of difficulty conceiving. You can have severe pain and infertility problems with a small amount of endometriosis, and less pain and fewer problems with a larger amount of endometriosis.

Amenorrhoea – not getting your period at all

Amenorrhea is the absence of menstrual periods. If you've never had a period, undoubtedly you've been examined sometime during your teenage years to see whether a structural problem, such as absence of the uterus, malformation of the vagina, or undeveloped ovaries, is the cause. However, many women have periods at one time, and then stop having them. This may happen if you develop Asherman's syndrome (discussed earlier in this chapter in the section 'The complications of scar tissue') because little normal tissue is left and the exit path from the uterus may be blocked with scar tissue, or maybe you aren't ovulating any longer.

Failing to ovulate

If you're not getting your period at all, or if you're having irregular periods, you may not be ovulating, a condition known as *anovulation*. Many factors, including emotional factors and stress, can cause anovulation.

Weight gain or loss

Of course, most women don't want to look at their weight. But even a slight deviation – about 15 per cent – either up or down may create menstrual irregularities and subtle infertility issues. After your weight falls into normal limits, your chance of getting pregnant without any other therapy may increase. A 10 per cent weight loss in overweight women (with a BMI of 30 or above) is enough to restart ovulation in the majority of cases.

In today's culture, where thin is in and 'you can't be too thin (or too rich!)' is a widely accepted standard, overweight women are far more likely to consider their weight a problem than the underweight. The fact is, however, that being underweight is equally as damaging as being overweight if you're having fertility problems.

Frequent, strenuous exercise

If your exercise regime causes your body fat percentage to drop to less than 22 per cent, the amount needed to keep menstruation occurring, your periods may stop.

Stress

Stress can alter your body functions, which can affect your menstrual cycle. The stress hormone is prolactin, which is the same hormone that suppresses ovulation in breastfeeding women (see the later section 'Hyperprolactinemia, or high prolactin' for more details on how prolactin itself can exacerbate fertility problems). If you have high stress levels this state may account for your irregular cycles. It's chill-out time!

Lowering stress levels is easier said than done, but if you're under severe stress, you may want to consider therapies such as biofeedback, acupuncture, or reflexology to decrease negative response to stress.

Polycystic ovary syndrome (PCOS)

Between 10 and 20 per cent of women have polycystic ovaries but only 5 per cent have the full blown syndrome (PCOS) – a hormonal imbalance that prevents egg containing follicles from developing properly. Many of these women have difficulty getting pregnant because many women with PCOS ovulate irregularly, or not at all.

Often your doctor will test for PCOS if you're overweight (50 per cent of all PCOS patients are obese) and are hairy where you shouldn't be, a condition that may be caused by an overabundance of male hormones called *androgens*.

If your doctor suspects that you have PCOS, they may do a pelvic ultrasound. Women with PCOS have lots of small follicles around the edge of their ovaries that are visible on ultrasound. Your doctor will probably check your hormone levels as well; PCOS patients often have a baseline blood LH level that is higher than normal. The high LH levels can cause abnormalities in eggs and also increase miscarriage rates. The syndrome is related to increased insulin resistance but these symptoms of the 'metabolic syndrome' can be treated by taking oral diabetic medications, such as Metformin. Obese PCOS patients have a higher chance of developing adult-onset diabetes and so it is vital for their general health, as well as their baby-making, that women with PCOS try hard to keep their BMI below 30.

Many women with PCOS respond well and begin ovulating if treated with Clomid or with injectable gonadotrophins to induce ovulation. In resistant cases of anovulation, your doctor may suggest *laparoscopic ovarian drilling*, a procedure in which your doctor makes small punctures in your ovary during laparoscopic surgery. Between 50 and 75 per cent of women start ovulating after this procedure, although the effect may be temporary. Risks of the surgery are principally related to scar tissue formation.

Hyperprolactinemia, or high prolactin

Although less than 1 per cent of women have high prolactin levels, high *prolactin* (the hormone responsible for maintaining breast milk production) levels are found in 10–40 per cent of premenopausal women who have stopped menstruating due to anovulation.

Women who are pregnant or breastfeeding should have high levels of prolactin. If your levels are elevated at any other time, ovulation may be suppressed. A tumour is found on the pituitary gland in about 30 per cent of women with very high prolactin levels; these tumours are almost always benign. Many drugs can cause high prolactin levels, including antidepressants and antihypertensives.

Tablets are available to lower your prolactin levels so that you'll start ovulating again.

Reversing Sterilisation

Nearly 25 per cent of UK women rely on sterilisation for contraception and 100,000 women, and 90,000 men, are sterilised annually in the UK. Unfortunately, at least 10 per cent regret their decision down the road and as divorce rates rocket and increasing numbers of couples are trying to conceive in second and subsequent relationships, the big question is 'Can surgical sterilisation be reversed?' The answer is 'yes, no, and maybe', depending on when the surgery was done and what kind of surgery it was.

A *tubal reanastomosis*, or tubal reversal, has several drawbacks. For one thing, it's expensive – about £5,000 – and the NHS, or insurance, usually doesn't cover the cost. For another, the success rate depends on how long ago your tubes were tied, and how they were tied.

Before you decide to have your tubal ligation reversed, consider these factors:

- ✔ **Your age:** Are you in your mid 30s or younger? If you're over 40, you may have other fertility problems related to age, and in vitro fertilisation (IVF) may be a better option for you.

- ✔ **Your partner:** If your partner has sperm problems, you may also be better off doing IVF rather than reversing your tubal ligation.

- ✔ **How your tubes were tied:** If your tubes were blocked off or clamped with clips or rings instead of being cauterised or having a large section removed, your chance of success is higher. Some doctors say that you need about an inch of healthy tube to successfully reconnect the tubes.

If you want a tubal reversal, look for a surgeon skilled in microsurgery. Depending on the surgeon and type of surgery done, your surgery can take up to six hours to perform and require several weeks of recovery.

Risks after surgery include scar tissue formation, infection, and increased risk of ectopic pregnancy. If the *fimbriated* end of the tube (the part that the egg enters from the ovary) is intact and your doctor believes that you've enough tube left to reconnect, your pregnancy chances after reanastomosis can be as high as IVF success rates. Because the risk of ectopic is high, arrange a scan as soon as possible after your positive pregnancy test (ideally two to three weeks later) to ensure that the pregnancy is in the right place.

Surgical sterilisation is very common and so is regret. Still, many women think that it is as quick, easy, and successful to undo as it was to do. It's not! So if you, or your little sister or your friend at work is contemplating a tubal ligation because you think that the 'pill' will make you fat or that the coil gives heavy periods, or that three perfect children is quite enough, think again!

Understanding Diseases That Affect Fertility

Just a few generations ago, systemic diseases such as diabetes or lupus ruled out the possibility of having a baby. Now, pregnancies in patients with systemic disease are commonplace, and obstetricians or perinatologists who specialise in high-risk patients guide women with a history of cancer, kidney problems, heart problems, or just about any other health condition through successful pregnancies. Discuss the potential problems of pregnancy with your doctor beforehand so that you can be prepared for the problems you may face in getting pregnant or carrying a pregnancy to term.

Diabetes: More than a sugar problem

Diabetes affects about 6 per cent of the population. There are actually several different types of diabetes, including the following:

- **Type 1 diabetes:** Used to be called juvenile diabetes. The condition usually develops before puberty but can develop at any age. Five to ten per cent of diabetics have Type 1 diabetes, which is an autoimmune disease. In Type 1 diabetes, the beta cells of the pancreas stop making insulin altogether, so people with this problem must take injections of insulin every day.

- **Type 2 diabetes:** Usually develops in people over 40, but it can develop earlier. The condition is often associated with being overweight; 80 per cent of Type 2 diabetics are overweight. It develops more slowly than Type 1 and possibly can be controlled with diet and pills rather than injections.

Men with diabetes often have problems with erection and ejaculation; about 40 per cent of male diabetics have *retrograde ejaculation* – a condition in which sperm back up into the bladder – or problems with erectile dysfunction.

Women with diabetes need to have well-controlled blood sugar during pregnancy. Even with good control, the rate of birth defects in women with diabetes is two to three times the normal rate. Overweight women with polycystic ovary syndrome are at increased risk of developing Type 2 diabetes later in life – yet another reason to keep that lock on the fridge! Pregnant women who are overweight are at risk of gestational diabetes and will need insulin in the latter stages of pregnancy. This type of diabetes usually gets better after the delivery.

Diabetics tend to have large babies, which can create problems at the time of delivery.

Lupus: Not just a rash

Systemic lupus erythematosus (SLE), commonly called *lupus*, is primarily a disease of women, although a small percentage of men also develop it. One of the outward symptoms of lupus is a facial rash, but lupus can affect every organ in your body. A few generations ago, women with lupus were advised not to have children, because it was felt that pregnancy worsened the disease. More recent studies have shown this belief not to be true, although a third of pregnant lupus patients have 'flares,' or increases in disease activity. About 10 per cent of pregnant lupus patients find that their symptoms actually improve.

Fifty per cent of women with lupus have normal pregnancies and normal deliveries; about 25 per cent deliver prematurely, and another 25 per cent experience miscarriage or stillbirth.

Miscarriage may be related to antibodies called antiphospholipid antibodies (discussed earlier in this chapter) found in some lupus patients. These antibodies cause clotting and interfere with the growth of the placenta. Baby aspirin and/or heparin may be given in pregnancy to help blood flow to the placenta.

About 20 per cent of lupus patients develop *toxaemia* (*PET or pre-eclamptic toxaemia*), a condition that results in high blood pressure, liver and kidney malfunctions, and premature delivery, and can lead to eclampsia, which can cause maternal seizures and death.

Men with lupus often have antisperm antibodies, so fertilisation may not occur without IVF and ICSI.

If you have lupus, you need to be followed carefully by an obstetrician who specialises in high-risk patients.

Cancer and female fertility: Good news?

Just a few years ago, having cancer meant that you would probably not be able to conceive and carry a child. Surgery, radiation, and chemotherapy, the mainstay treatments of most cancers, can destroy the egg cells within the ovaries and sperm cells as well as your hope of having a child.

Today, however, new advances have made it possible for cancer survivors to become parents, and the really good new is that more advances are being made all the time. The information of today may be obsolete soon, and the chances for parenthood will hopefully be better than ever.

Breast cancer survivors are now being told that pregnancy after treatment is possible, as long as their ovaries are intact and haven't been irradiated. Many doctors encourage patients to wait two years after treatment before trying to get pregnant. Pregnancy doesn't increase the chance of cancer recurrence, according to most recent studies, but doctors want to make sure that the cancer doesn't recur on its own.

If you do have a recurrence of cancer while pregnant and require chemotherapy, you need to be aware that chemo in the first trimester may cause fetal malformation, while waiting till the second or third trimester may result in pre-term labour or fetal loss. If you're taking tamoxifen, you may find that you're no longer ovulating, a side effect for some, but not all, women who are treated with the drug.

If you've been treated for ovarian cancer with radiation or ovarian ablation, your ovaries will not be functioning, and you'll need to use donor eggs to become pregnant. If you were treated with multiple-agent chemotherapy, there's a good chance you'll go into premature ovarian failure. A third of women under age 30 and two-thirds of those over 30 go into premature ovarian failure.

Your baby will not have a higher risk of birth defects or childhood cancer if you become pregnant after cancer treatment. For information about freezing embryos and sperm before chemotherapy, check out Chapter 14.

Chapter 8

It's a Man Thing: When Tests Reveal Sperm Problems

*A*lthough most men are happy to pursue treatment for infertility and show huge support and understanding while their female partner goes through tests and surgery to try to find out why they are not yet pregnant, things are a bit different when *he's* the one being poked and prodded. Even the most re-constructed man can feel his masculinity, personality, and whole being are being questioned when it's time to analyse his sperm – the commonly, but incorrectly held connection between virility and fertility suddenly becomes very important to him.

In this chapter we look at how sperm can be produced for analysis – either 'manually' or by a needle biopsy – and consider what the sperm specialists look for in a sperm sample. We also explain some of the illnesses and conditions that can affect sperm quality, as well as assessing the outlook for fatherhood after cancer. And because everyone going through fertility testing can use a bit of loving kindness, we offer advice on how to support your chap when he feels as if it's 'all his fault'.

Sounding Out Semen Analysis

Male factor infertility accounts for about 35 per cent of infertility. For that reason, semen analysis is a necessary first step. Yet you may find your partner acting a little funny when it's time to 'check out the troops'.

Collecting a sample

In order for the troops to be evaluated, your partner needs to produce a sperm sample that can be examined under a microscope. He'll be asked to pop into a small private room, usually equipped with some 'suitable' literature, to 'produce' his sample. (You can help him if you want, but no saliva or lubricants, please.)

To be valid, the sample has to be collected during a certain period of time – ideally, three to five days after his last ejaculation – which is rather coyly described as the 'period of abstinence'. If the period is too short or too long the result of the test may be misleading.

If you prefer, you can also bring a semen sample from home. If you decide to go this route, you must bring it in within a half hour of collecting it, and you must use a sterile cup or pot that the fertility centre supplies.

If you're bringing in a semen sample, keep it at next-to-body temperature – holding it under your armpit is ideal. Make sure that the lid's on tight!

Looking under the microscope

Sperm are extremely small, but under the microscope you can see how complicated they really are. A normal sperm (see Figure 8-1) has three sections: a head, a midpiece, and a tail. All three parts need to be normally formed for a sperm to be considered normal:

- ✔ **Head:** The head contains all the genetic material and is topped by a little cap called the *acrosome*, which contains some special enzymes that help the sperm to penetrate the egg 'shell'. A sperm with an abnormal head – such as a round head, pinhead, large head, or double head – isn't capable of fertilising an egg normally.

- ✔ **Midpiece:** This section is the 'outboard motor' for the sperm. It contains fructose, a sugar that supplies the energy the sperm needs to move rapidly.

- ✔ **Tail:** Needed for propulsion. Sperm with no tails, two tails, or coiled tails are all considered abnormal.

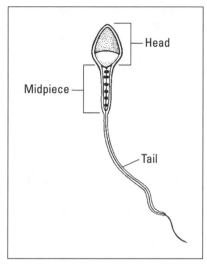

Figure 8-1:
A normal
sperm.

The World Health Organisation (WHO) has set standard parameters for a normal semen specimen, so your sperm sample must have the following in order to be graded A+:

- ✔ **Volume:** Needs to be 2 to 5 millilitres, or approximately a teaspoon.

- ✔ **Concentration:** Must be equal to or greater than 20 million sperm/ millilitres, or a total of greater than 40 million per ejaculate.

- ✔ **Motility:** More than 50 per cent of the sperm must be motile, or moving.

- ✔ **Morphology:** More than 15 per cent must be normally shaped.

- ✔ **Forward progression:** On a scale of 1 to 4, at least 2+ means a good number of sperm moving forward.

- ✔ **White blood cells:** To be no more than 0 to 5 per high-power field, or less than 1 million per millilitre. More may indicate infection.

- ✔ **Hyperviscosity:** Should gel promptly but liquefy within 30 minutes after ejaculation.

- ✔ **Ph:** Needs to be alkaline, to protect sperm from the acidic environment of the vagina.

- ✔ **HOS, or hypo-osmotic swelling:** Greater than 50 per cent of the sperm tails are likely to swell when exposed to a hypo-osmotic solution; this swelling is a sign of normal functioning. Where sperm are immotile then the HOS test can identify 'live' sperm suitable for ICSI injection.

✔ **Antisperm antibodies:** A normal semen sample contains no antisperm antibodies. Antibodies cause problems if they're attached to the sperm tail, because they interfere with movement, or to the head, where they may make conditions difficult for the sperm to penetrate the egg. For more on antisperm antibodies, refer to Chapter 7.

✔ **Acrosome reaction test:** The tip of the sperm is the acrosome. It contains enzymes that allow the sperm to penetrate the egg. If the proper enzymes aren't present, the sperm can't get through the egg's *zona*, or shell.

Interpreting Your Partner's Test Results

With some of the test results back, you may be even more confused than you were before. If your partner's semen analysis comes back with some results askew, he may be too embarrassed to ask what the results mean. Sometimes you may prefer to look up the problems in a book, so here you are!

Semen samples can vary from month to month, or even day to day. That's because the sperm takes about 70 days to develop. Unlike eggs, which are present from your embryonic days, sperm are replenished all the time. Because men are constantly producing new sperm, one 'bad' semen analysis needs to be followed up, to make sure that you're seeing the real picture. An illness, injury, or medication or drug used a few months before may make one sample seem sub-standard, but checking again a month later may show an improvement, revealing a much more promising picture. If the sample is unexpectedly poor with no or very few visible live sperm then the sample should be repeated much sooner because the result may be due to a 'technical' fault. If a sperm sample is kept above body temperature (37 degrees Celsius) for even a short time, then all the sperm will die.

Disappearing act: Where's the sperm?

Sometimes a semen analysis shows a very low number of sperm, less than 20 million, a condition called *oligospermia*. If no sperm are seen, this state is called *azoospermia*. Between 5 and 10 per cent of the male population have either azoospermia or oligospermia.

You can get pregnant without fertility treatments if your partner has oligospermia, but your chances of pregnancy are higher if you do one of the following:

✔ **Intrauterine insemination (IUI) or intracervical insemination (ICI):** The sperm is concentrated and 'washed' so that the best sperm are used for insemination.

✔ **In vitro fertilisation (IVF):** This treatment uses intracytoplasmic sperm injection (ICSI), the injection of a healthy sperm directly into an egg. The procedure is done by an embryologist under a high-powered microscope.

If your partner has azoospermia, you won't be able to get pregnant conventionally. Different factors can cause azoospermia; the production of the sperm, the 'plumbing', or the delivery of the sperm can be at fault.

Sperm production problems

Sperm production problems can be caused by the following:

✔ **Sertoli cell only syndrome:** In this condition, the germ cells that produce sperm in the testes are absent. No method is available for a person with this syndrome to father a child.

✔ **Anabolic steroids:** Their use may cause a possibly reversible shutdown of the sperm production.

✔ **Abnormal hormone levels:** Low levels of LH, FSH, or testosterone can cause low sperm production. This problem can be treated with hormone injections, pills, or transdermal patches.

✔ **Premature testicular failure:** This condition is diagnosed by finding very high levels of FSH (follicle-stimulating hormone). Just like a woman can have a 'premature menopause' so a man can have a 'premature andropause'.

✔ **'Recreational' drugs (especially cannabis):** Their use can seriously impair sperm production.

Plumbing problems

If the problem is obstruction (a plumbing problem), your partner may be referred to a urologist for assessment and possibly surgical correction, or he may need a testicular sperm aspiration (discussed in the sidebar 'If you need a sperm aspiration,' later in this chapter). This procedure must be done in conjunction with IVF with ICSI because the sperm need to be injected directly into the egg. Obstructive problems include the following:

✔ Absence of the *vas deferens*, the tube that delivers sperm to the urethra.

✔ Previous vasectomy.

Mechanical problems with getting the sperm where they need to be include the following:

- *Retrograde ejaculation*, in which the majority of the sperm go into the bladder.
- Spinal cord injury that prevents ejaculation.
- Previous injury from trauma.
- Previous injury from surgery, such as hernia surgery.
- A disease such as diabetes.

If you need a sperm aspiration

Sperm can be aspirated from the epididymis, which sits on top of the testes, or from the testes themselves. Four different types of procedures are carried out, each with advantages and disadvantages:

- **MESA (microsurgical epididymal sperm aspiration):** This procedure can be done only for obstructive azoospermia, because men with non-obstructive azoospermia rarely have sperm in the epididymis. A small incision is made in the scrotum, and then a dilated tubule in the epididymis is cut open and examined through a lighted microscope. Fluid is collected from the tubule and examined for sperm. MESA can be done as an outpatient procedure, but most require a general anaesthetic. If you're awake you are given a spermatic cord block and sedation during the procedure. You can generally return to work the following day.

- **PESA (percutaneous epididymal sperm aspiration):** This procedure is quite straightforward and is particularly suitable for men with unreversed vasectomies as the sperm pools up in the epididymis because the vas deferens has been blocked or tied off. A fine needle stuck into the epididymis is used to extract sperm-containing fluid. Local anaesthesia and sedation may be given.

- **TESE (testicular sperm extraction):** A small incision is made, and a tiny piece of testicular tissue is removed (a biopsy). Testicular sperm doesn't freeze or thaw as well as epididymal sperm because it's less mature, but may be the only sperm found in men with non-obstructive azoospermia.

- **TESA (testicular sperm aspiration):** This procedure is a needle biopsy done in the clinic using a special needle under local anaesthetic block. Because sperm production is 'focal', parts of the testis may still be producing sperm even if the rest has gone on strike.

All four techniques can cause bleeding, bruising, and *haematoma* (a collection of blood that can be painful). A biopsy usually requires only a one-day recovery and can be done under local anaesthesia or mild sedation.

Hormone tests are done before any sperm extraction procedure is attempted because (just like women) a very high FSH or a very low inhibin B means the treatment probably won't work, and even the bravest of chaps would rather have a blood test than a failed sperm aspiration.

Congenital bilateral absence of the vas deferens (CBAVD), the duct that leads to the urethra, is associated with cystic fibrosis (CF) in men. Genetic testing is likely to be suggested if this problem is found. Sometimes CBAVD is the only sign that a chap carries the cystic fibrosis gene but vitally, both he and his partner should have genetic testing. If she is a 'carrier' (that is, has one copy of the CF gene) any child they have together will have a high chance of being born with CF.

Judging sperm performance: Swimmers and non-swimmers

Sometimes plenty of sperm are seen in the ejaculate, but the sperm themselves are abnormal. Sperm are very complicated little creatures. Despite their small size, they contain three distinct sections (refer to Figure 8-1), and a problem with any section can cause infertility.

The head of the sperm contains the DNA, or genetic material. If the head is abnormally shaped, the sperm is probably incapable of fertilising an egg because its genetic material is abnormal. Sitting on the head is the cap (where else would a cap sit?) called the acrosome, which contains the enzymes that help the lucky sperm to penetrate the egg shell. If the sperm has no acrosome cap then this state is known as globospermia and ICSI is required.

The midpiece of the sperm contains the energy necessary to propel it to the egg. Sperm need a tremendous amount of energy to get to an egg. If they lack this energy, they're not going to make the whole distance. Think of swimming the English Channel.

The tail of the sperm makes the sperm move rapidly; if the sperm sample has a lot of coiled, rather than whip-like, tails, or no tails at all, those sperm may go in the wrong direction or may go nowhere at all – they may just twitch a bit. Again, these sperm aren't going to be able to get where they need to be.

Considering ejaculation issues: A sensitive topic

Abnormal sperm may be a problem you both can deal with. Problems with ejaculation, or the ability to sustain an erection, however, may be so difficult to address that you may have a hard time bringing the issue out into the open. Yet it's a common problem: Ten per cent of men between the ages of 18 and 59 have experienced erectile problems in the last year, and 10 per cent of men between the ages of 40 and 70 have complete erectile dysfunction (ED).

Plenty of medical-related conditions can cause problems with erection and ejaculation. Table 8-1 lists examples of what can cause such problems.

Table 8-1	**Possible Causes of Erection and Ejaculation Problems**	
Medications	*Diseases*	*Surgeries*
Antidepressants	Diabetes	Abdominal perineal resection
Antiulcer medications	Heart attack (myocardial infarction)	Proctocolectomy
Certain blood pressure medications	Hypertension or other vascular disease	Radical prostatectomy
Cholesterol-lowering medications	Hypothyroidism or hyperthyroidism	Transurethral resection of prostate
	Liver cirrhosis	
	Renal failure	
	Sickle-cell anaemia	

Radiation, trauma, heavy alcohol use, and neurological damage from surgery, stroke, epilepsy, or multiple sclerosis can all cause erectile dysfunction.

Erectile dysfunction (ED) may also result from psychosexual problems better addressed by therapy. The sheer stress of trying to 'perform' when required if you're having trouble making a baby can be enough to deflate a previously ardent chap. Your computer's spam box is probably full of unsolicited offers to supply Viagra and Cialis over the Internet. The fact is that these meds do work for many chaps. Don't buy from unreliable sources, though; see your GP. You may need to pay for a private prescription but the cost is worth every penny if it solves your ED problem. Whatever the reason, the first step in dealing with the problem is being able to discuss it, especially with an outsider, such as a doctor or nurse.

Two syndromes that affect male fertility

Klinefelter's syndrome and Kallmann's syndrome are two syndromes that affect male fertility.

✔ Klinefelter's syndrome is far more common than most people realise. One out of 500 to 1,000 males are affected. Symptoms of Klinefelter's are delayed puberty, decreased facial and body hair, small firm testes, and long legs. Blood tests show an increase in LH (luteinising hormone) and FSH (follicle-stimulating hormone) levels and a decrease in serum testosterone levels. Chromosome tests show a 47 XXY karyotype. Usually, no sperm is found in the ejaculation, and sperm retrieved from the testis may be genetically abnormal.

✔ Kallmann's syndrome is less common but may be familial. Symptoms can include absence of a sense of smell, delayed puberty, osteoporosis, red-green colour blindness, and possibly cleft palate and urogenital abnormalities. Treatment is with hormones, namely, pulsed GnRH (gonadotrophin-releasing hormone; the hormone that's 'missing' in Kallmann's) or FSH, LH, and testosterone injections.

Handling the emotional effect of male problems on both of you

A few decades ago, failure to produce a baby was always considered to be the woman's fault. In many cultures, a man was able to obtain a no-questions-asked divorce from any woman who didn't give him a child. With the advent of microscopes high powered enough to look closely at sperm, studies soon revealed that male factors are as important for reproduction as female factors.

Intellectually, which one of you has a problem shouldn't matter, but intellect and emotion are two different issues. For whatever reason, more men than women have an ego issue when it comes to their reproductive parts. Their sense of personal failure may be more pronounced than yours, and they may also be less willing to face the problem and do what's necessary to fix it.

If tests reveal that he's the problem, you may have to tread very gently around the issue, especially if you're the one more interested in having a child. He may consider the whole subject closed if he's the problem – no sperm, no child, okay, end of discussion. Not all men feel so closely tied to their semen analysis, but if your partner does, be prepared for some tense moments.

Reversing a Vasectomy

About 90,000 men are sterilised annually in the UK. Unfortunately, at least 10 per cent regret their decision down the road and as divorce rates rocket, increasing numbers of couples are trying to conceive in second and subsequent relationships. For that reason, many men decide to have the surgery reversed. Vasectomy reversal surgery is often successful in that sperm is found in the ejaculate in the majority of cases, but the number of sperm may be too small to make pregnancy likely, or antibodies attached to the sperm may make it nearly impossible for the sperm to swim properly or fertilise an egg.

Antibodies are found in 50 per cent of men after vasectomy reversal; men with antibodies generally need IVF (often plus ICSI) for their partner to become pregnant.

As with tubal ligation, vasectomy reversal success depends on what type of surgery was done. The reversal success rate is higher if the surgery was done on a straight section of the vas deferens, the pieces to be joined together are of equal size, and the reversal is done within ten years of the original surgery.

Your chance of pregnancy after sterilisation reversal depends on several factors. Consider carefully whether reversal is going to be more cost effective and offer a better chance of success than IVF, in which tied tubes can be bypassed or sperm can be removed directly from the testicles via sperm aspiration.

A recently reported study shows that less pain and less time is lost from work with sperm aspirations as opposed to vasectomy reversals.

My clinic (co-author Gill) pioneered a 'package' for improving vasectomy reversal outcomes. When a couple consider a vasectomy reversal, we do a 'fertility MOT' on the woman first. This involves checking her hormone levels and testing the Fallopian tubes. If she has tubal problems then IVF is a better option, and so we prepare for that eventuality, in case it's needed. Then, during the vasectomy reversal, one of our scientists attends the operating theatre and takes samples of sperm and testis when the surgeon is doing his 'micro-plumbing'. These samples are *cryopreserved* (frozen at the temperature of liquid nitrogen) in case the reversal operation fails. A few weeks later we do a series of semen analyses and freeze any sperm in the ejaculate (working with this type of sperm is always more successful). *If* the reversal is unsuccessful or if (as often happens) the vas 'blocks off' again before pregnancy is achieved, we have sperm all ready to use without having to do a new procedure such as PESA or TESA (read the section 'If you need a sperm aspiration' earlier in the chapter).

Overcoming Cancer and Male Fertility: The News Is Cautiously Optimistic

Over one in a thousand young adults are survivors of cancer. Modern oncology treatments, such as surgery, radiation, and chemotherapy, can offer the prospect of complete cure and a normal life expectancy. However, the treatments for most cancers can destroy the egg cells within the ovaries and sperm cells and reduce the chance of having a child.

Today, however, new advances have increased the possibility of cancer survivors becoming parents, and the really good news is that more advances are being made all the time. The information of today may be obsolete soon, and the chances for parenthood are hopefully going to be better than ever.

When diagnosed with cancer, a person's future fertility prospects are not usually uppermost in their, or even their doctors' minds. They naturally just want to have the surgery, start the chemo, and get better! But the opportunity to 'bank' sperm should be offered to all post-pubescent boys and men who are likely to have their fertility affected by cancer therapy. The equivalent treatment for young women is egg or oocyte freezing (flick to Chapter 14). This technique is a much newer and more complicated process, but one that is increasingly being seen as an option for young women undergoing cancer treatment.

Although testicular cancer is rare, making up only 1 per cent of all cancer, it's the most common cancer found in men between the ages of 20 and 34, and the incidence is increasing rapidly. It's four times more common among Caucasian men than black men. The good news on testicular cancer is that the disease is almost 100 per cent curable with modern chemotherapy. Young men need to be encouraged to freeze or 'bank' some sperm before they start their treatment, in the event that both testicles need to be removed.

If only one testicle is removed surgically, the remaining testicle produces enough sperm so that fertility won't be damaged. If both testicles need to be removed, several semen samples can be frozen before surgery and used for insemination later on. If only one testicle is affected, the man has a 2 to 5 per cent chance of developing cancer in the other testicle.

Some chemotherapy treatment causes temporary loss of fertility, but sperm counts may return to an acceptable level after two to three years. Radiation treatment is much more damaging to sperm production.

If certain lymph nodes are removed, the nerves that control ejaculation may be affected, although the sperm count may be normal. This condition may require sperm aspiration with ICSI and IVF to achieve a pregnancy.

Part IV
Eureka! Possible Solutions

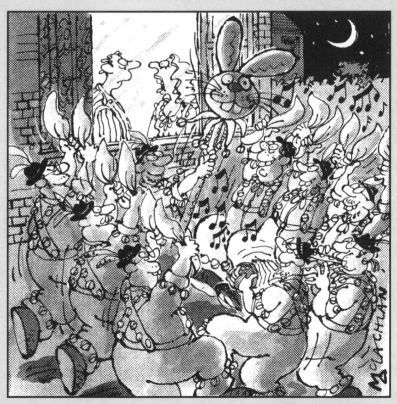

'I don't care if they are performing a
traditional fertility dance – just make
them go away!'

In this part . . .

*I*f you're still not pregnant after following diet and lifestyle changes, and having GP tests and consultant investigations, it may be time to find out what a fertility clinic can do for you. But where do you start, how do you pay for any treatment, and how do you get over the feelings of 'Why me/us?' In this part we explain how to research fertility clinics, decipher success rates, and use the Internet to get genuine patient testimonials. We look at the criteria and availability for NHS funding and take you through IUI, IVF, and ICSI cycles, as well as egg freezing and egg sharing treatments.

Chapter 9

Doing Your Homework: Researching Fertility Clinics and Funding Treatment

*I*VF – in vitro fertilisation – has become a catch-all term for tertiary level assisted conception, the top of the high-tech mountain of fertility treatment, which also includes IUI (intrauterine insemination) and ICSI (intra cytoplasmic sperm injection). Naturally, being told you 'need IVF' may make you a bit nervous about moving into invasive, expensive, no-guarantees treatment.

Despite IVF being used as a catch-all label, IVF, IUI, and ICSI are distinct treatment options. While IUI involves the fertilisation (the joining of egg and sperm) *in vivo* (in the body), for example, *in vitro fertilisation* means fertilisation that occurs 'in glass'; that's where the term 'test-tube baby' comes from. For an introduction to these procedures, head to Chapter 10. Chapters 11, 12, and 13 offer in-depth information.

Twenty years ago only a handful of clinics performed assisted conception. Now, more than 80 UK clinics offer IUI and most of these centres are also licensed for IVF and ICSI. In this chapter, we help you research different fertility clinics, decipher the statistics about success rates, and give you some help in deciding whether fertility treatment is the next step for you.

Dealing with First Reactions

So you're told by your GP or consultant that you need fertility treatment – and how do you feel? Nervous, daunted, 'why us'? But hopefully also excited and positive, too. All those months and years of negative pregnancy tests, being prodded and poked by various doctors and even having investigative surgery, and now you know what you have to do to have a chance of having a baby. But what else do you need to consider?

Here's the snapshot of assisted conception:

- ✔ Fertility treatment may be expensive.
- ✔ Fertility treatment is time consuming.
- ✔ Fertility treatment is unpredictable.
- ✔ Fertility treatment doesn't guarantee success.
- ✔ Fertility treatment has risks and side effects.
- ✔ Fertility treatment involves injections.
- ✔ Fertility treatment requires frequent ultrasound scans and blood tests.
- ✔ You may scream at the fertility nurses at least once during your treatment.
- ✔ You will scream at your partner at least once during your treatment.

Jill's reaction

I (co-author Jill) remember watching *John Craven's Newsround* in July 1978 about the birth of Louise Brown, the world's first 'test-tube' baby, when I was 12 years old. Fast-track 21 years and my husband Gwyn and I sit in the consultant's office as he tells us we need ICSI treatment to conceive. This followed marriage at 29, the successful reversal of my husband's 18-year-old vasectomy, not trying for a baby for two years (when career promotion and a larger home were our priorities), then joyful, spontaneous sex at any opportunity, which turned into carefully timed sex at the 'right' opportunity, following regular disappointment as my period started every month. Then, two laparoscopies, a tube-dye test and a hysteroscopy revealed I was fine, but a more detailed sperm analysis showed Gwyn's sperm were swimming in circles! ('Wouldn't you be if you'd been stitched up for so long?' he mused!) I was 33 and suddenly, getting pregnant wasn't me and him and a night of passion. The mention of fertility treatment meant we now had to consider, where, when, can we deal with it, can we afford it, will the NHS pay for it, who can we tell, who can we ask, will it ever work, will we *ever* have a baby? But our decision to opt for assisted conception also brought a feeling of empowerment. No more messing about, this treatment will be our best shot, let's do it!

That's all you really need to know at the beginning and you'll pick up the other vital info along the way.

Perhaps the most intimidating part of fertility treatment is the notion that high-end technology and lots of people you don't yet know are going to be involved in getting you pregnant. Although part of you may feel enormous excitement that you've finally found the 'magic' path, the other part may fear what will happen if treatment doesn't work. If it fails, you may have similar treatment again – but how many times? – or you may consider other means of creating a family, such as donor egg or adoption. Think of IUI, IVF, or ICSI as getting one step closer to your dream, however it may be attained.

Understanding that assisted conception may not work

Publicity for every celebrity IVF baby may also give you the impression that IVF is a sure-fire success method, when at best, the statistics for live births per IVF cycle are about 35 per cent – and that's for women under age 35. According to HFEA (Human Fertilisation and Embryology Authority) data (based on recent HFEA data), the statistics break down this way:

- ✔ **Under age 35:** A 28 per cent chance of a live birth per IVF cycle
- ✔ **Ages 35 to 37:** Approximately 24 per cent chance of taking home a baby per IVF cycle
- ✔ **Ages 38 to 39:** An 18 per cent chance of a live birth per cycle
- ✔ **Over age 40–42:** An 11 per cent chance of a live birth per cycle
- ✔ **Over age 45:** Virtually no chance of pregnancy unless you use donor eggs

Getting real: Managing your expectations

As the Romans said, 'caveat emptor' (let the buyer beware). When you're spending large amounts of money on fertility treatment, you have high expectations. Do your research on different clinics, listen to comments from family and friends – who will all know of someone who has had fertility treatment – and visit some of the clinics in your region. But always be aware that fertility treatment comes with no guarantees. You have a much greater chance of failure than success on your first attempt.

Researching Fertility Clinics

More than 80 UK clinics do IUI and over 70 offer IVF or ICSI. But these facilities range from the 'dabblers' that do maybe a dozen IUIs or egg retrievals a year to the large clinics that do more than 400–500 egg retrievals a year.

Bigger isn't always better, but when dealing with high-tech procedures such as IVF, success rates are highly dependent on the expertise of the doctors, nurses, and scientists. For that reason, a small clinic doing a dozen retrievals a year may not have the same clinical or laboratory expertise as a centre doing hundreds a year. So before you pick a clinic, you need to do a little (okay, actually quite a bit of) research. The following sections tell you how.

From April 2007, IUI, like IVF and ICSI, will only be available from clinics licensed by the HFEA, so you will probably need to go to a different unit within the hospital where you've seen your consultant, or to an entirely new clinic for your assisted conception treatment. Your consultant may steer you towards a particular clinic, especially if your treatment will be funded by the National Health Service (NHS), or you may be given a choice of clinics – particularly if you're self-funding. But such choice can be overwhelming, especially in the UK where we are not used to 'shopping around' for medical treatment.

First steps to finding a fertility clinic

Use the following steps to get a better idea of what each clinic offers and what its success rates are

- ✔ **Listen to word of mouth.** Most people know of someone who has had assisted conception. Do they rave about their clinic or do they consign the whole experience to the darkest recesses of their memories? Do they heap praise on individual members of the team and/or the clinic in general? Personal testimonials are powerful influencers.

- ✔ **Visit the Healthcare Commission (HCC) Web site www.healthcare commission.org.uk to review the inspection reports for clinics that offer fertility treatment.** Look in particular at how – and how often – the clinic didn't meet the required standards at the last inspection. The HCC assesses the performance of all UK private and NHS healthcare organisations, awards annual performance ratings for the NHS, and inspects all independent hospitals.

- ✔ **Request a copy of a clinic's patients' guide to services and annual report.** These documents should give an overview of the approach to treatment, admissions policy, list of fees, guidance to different treatments, and success rates – the most recent success should be no more than 2 years old. It should also describe the quality management system it adheres to and display any relevant 'kitemarks' as proof.

✔ **Visit online support group forums.** Check out www.infertility networkuk.com or www.fertilityfriends.co.uk, or www.midlandfertility.com. What do the patients say about their treatment and the clinics where they're getting it? Don't pay too much attention to individual high praise or grievances, but get a feel for what the majority write about each clinic.

✔ **Attend any open days or evenings offered by clinics.** These should be free to attend and offer no obligation to return!

✔ **Visit the Human Fertilisation and Embryology Authority's Web site at www.hfea.gov.uk and request a copy of the HFEA's annual guide to infertility and directory of clinics.** The HFEA is the organisation that regulates fertility treatment in the UK and all clinics are obliged to pass on information about the number and types of treatments it has started and the outcome of each treatment.

'Lies, damn lies, and statistics': Tapping into HFEA data

The HFEA's principal tasks are to license and monitor clinics that carry out IVF, donor insemination, and human embryo research and also to regulate the storage of sperm, eggs, and embryos. The HFEA also keeps a record of all registrations, treatments, and outcomes that result from assisted conception techniques at the UK's 85 licensed clinics. Every year, each clinic must advise the HFEA of:

✔ The number of cycles they do

✔ The types of infertility their patients have

✔ The outcome of their cycles

✔ Pregnancy rates

✔ Multiple-pregnancy rates

✔ Live birth rates

✔ Miscarriage rates

✔ Cancellation rates

In short, the clinics provide information on just about anything and everything concerning patients' treatment.

All UK clinics must provide a massive amount of information to the HFEA that can be audited and checked for data accuracy. UK clinics spend a huge amount of time compiling and reporting HFEA data to ensure that patients get an accurate impression of how well they perform. The HFEA confirms clinic-reported data by visiting clinics every year and auditing selected patients' records to make sure that the submitted information is accurate.

The HFEA publishes the statistics online at `www.hfea.gov.uk` for each clinic.

HFEA statistics may appear consistent across all clinics, but not all clinics treat all types of patients and so comparisons of results may not be an accurate comparison of the types of condition treated. For example, some clinics only treat women younger than 38 with a BMI of 20–26, with no history of endometriosis or PCOS. Such clinics have a higher pregnancy success rate than those clinics that don't discriminate against older patients with more complicated fertility problems. So don't be beguiled by the success rates of those clinics that carefully select their patients – they may decide not to select you!

Other considerations when looking for a clinic

Although statistics make interesting reading and may help you decide which clinic to use, they don't tell the whole story. You also need to check the following information:

✔ **Is the clinic located near you?** Although IVF can be done outside your home area, it's much simpler to do within a 100-mile radius of where you live. Monitoring needs to be done frequently, and having blood tests and ultrasound scans isn't that easy if your clinic is 300 miles away. But good reasons may exist to travel further afield for treatment, including:

- No IVF clinic is in your area.

- No clinic in your area will treat you.

- No clinic in your area does IVF cheaply enough for you.

- You qualify for NHS funding, but all the clinics in your area only treat private patients.

- You need extremely sophisticated testing or procedures that are done only at a handful of clinics in the UK.

✔ **Is the clinic currently accepting new patients?** Some clinics may not be able to offer a first appointment for a few months. Can you wait this long?

✔ **Does it treat NHS-funded patients, privately-funded patients, or both?** This answer is important to you, depending on who's paying for your treatment.

✔ **Will the clinic treat 'patients like you'?** An important consideration if you're over age 40 or have been turned down by another clinic. You also want to know how much experience the clinic has of treating men or women with your condition, such as PCOS, endometriosis, recurrent miscarriage, cystic fibrosis, and so on.

If you're looking at one of the big-name clinics, you're also being sized up as a candidate for treatment, and you could be turned down for treatment if you don't fit the clinic's criteria. Some centres don't want to give you false hope if they don't believe that they can help you, and others don't want to bring down their statistics.

✔ **What kind of feeling do you get from the clinic?** To answer this question, you probably need to make a consultation appointment with a doctor or nurse. The clinic usually charges for this appointment. Alternatively check if it offers any free, no-obligation open evenings.

You don't need to commit to treatment at your initial consultation. It never hurts to go home and think everything over before you go any further.

✔ **What are the treatment success rates for your age group?** Remember to compare like with like. That is, don't select a clinic because they have a 40 per cent success rate for women under the age of 35 having IVF if you're a 39-year-old who needs ICSI treatment because your husband has poor sperm quality.

Whether you need or want to know everything about a clinic before you go there depends on your personality. You may be happy to go where your best friend went or to go where your consultant tells you to go, or to the clinic around the corner. There's nothing wrong with trusting your instincts and other people's personal experiences. However, if you're already filling up infertility notebook number three, your GP's recommendation that you just go to his golfing partner probably isn't going to convince you.

Surfing fertility clinic Web sites

The best way to find a lot of information about fertility clinics is to check the Internet. The information will be much more up to date than what you find in books or the phone book; most clinics have Web sites that they update fairly often. However, typing 'UK IVF clinics' into Google currently brings up about 245,000 results, so you need to refine your search methods. The HFEA Web site, www.hfea.gov.uk, offers a Find a clinic button, with links to each clinic's Web site. This function may help you easily research the clinics either by reputation or location.

At the very least, a clinic's Web site should tell you the following information:

- ✔ How many egg retrievals the clinic does in a year
- ✔ How many embryo transfers the clinic does in a year
- ✔ Pregnancy rates for all age groups, broken down per egg retrieval and per embryo transfer
- ✔ Live birth rates per cycle and per embryo transfer
- ✔ Whether it freezes embryos
- ✔ Whether it does ICSI
- ✔ Whether it transfers three-day embryos or blastocysts
- ✔ Profiles of the clinical and scientific staff, listing their qualifications and experience
- ✔ Whether the clinic cycles patients through all the time or you have to wait for the next group
- ✔ Whether the clinic has a donor egg or embryo programme
- ✔ To what quality management system it operates

You may have other concerns relating to your own situation. If you can't find the answer on the Web site, call the clinic and ask to speak to a nurse. Usually they're happy to answer any questions you have about their services and you don't even need to register as a patient. (You needn't even give your real name if you prefer!)

Personality match or clash?

Fertility clinics have personalities just like people do. Finding one to suit you is as important as knowing about its success rates. You're going to spend a lot of time at this clinic over the coming months and you need to be sure that you like the place and the people who work there. The following sections give you a rundown of the most common types of clinics and what you may encounter when you enter their doors.

Dr Slick

You may already know Dr Slick's clinic by name and media status. But even if you're not aware of its national reputation when you walk in, you will be by the time you walk out. They're the best, they know it, and they capitalise on it.

Dr Slick's imprint is usually apparent the moment you pull into the car park, beside the doctors' convertible sports cars. The place is spotless, the staff's designer suits are immaculate, and the doctors wear theatre 'scrubs' to show how serious they are about their work. All kinds of achievement awards and recognition certificates line the walls, and 'discreet' and 'exclusive' shout out loud.

These places are selective and often expensive, and you'll probably feel like you're in first class, but only if they agree to treat you.

Dr Serious

Dr Serious is a technician first and a people-person second. Some doctors take everything about life much too seriously, including themselves. Nothing is funny here. Infertility is serious business, and none of the office staff ever seems to crack a smile. No one mentions babies – it's too big a taboo.

If you're very anxious about your treatment, you'll probably love Dr Serious, but if you're a little more relaxed, you'll never make it through your first visit because you'll start laughing and you won't be able to face going back for your baseline tests or your follow-up appointment.

Drs Doom and Gloom

Just as some doctors feed false expectations, others may choose to starve reasonable ones. Most patients would rather the doctor at least *appears* to be in their corner, fighting for fertility and family almost as hard as they are.

Drs Doom and Gloom are certainly realists. They recognise the innate difficulty associated with human reproduction, to say nothing of how hard the situation becomes when other factors are thrown in. Remember, however, that the statistics do have another side – the successful side, the side Drs Doom and Gloom don't acknowledge *until* you are successful.

Women who have spent time and money to consult with Drs Doom and Gloom often walk away with a heavy heart after being handed the possibility of just a tiny chance of success. Listen closely. If a doctor tells you that they've never had success with a patient with your condition, translate that into the fact that *the doctor personally* has no experience in making this happen. Other doctors may routinely work with patients like you and report better odds.

Dr Casual

Dr Casual's clinic is easy to spot. You open the front door and are amazed. All of life is here! The waiting room is busy, the phone rings non-stop, the receptionists are busy, busy, busy, and you wonder 'where's the hospital smell?' Staff don't wear uniforms but call you by your first name and know you instantly when taking phone calls from you. How do they do it? You may get to see Dr Casual, but more likely, most of your contact time will be with a nurse. Former patients return to the clinic with their babies and the doctors and nurses and lab staff alike, bill and coo over the beautiful babies you have made.

Casual and informal are great for many people. This environment can remove barriers during medical treatment, which is about as intimate as it gets. But Dr Casual's clinic should disguise robust systems and organisation beneath the surface. For example, during your appointments, a clinic should always have access to your notes and staff should constantly check your ID details at key stages of treatment. When Dr Casual becomes Dr Chaos, it's time to move on to a clinic in control of your treatment.

Footing the Bill: Who Will Pay?

So you've done your research, you've selected your preferred clinic, and you have an idea of the type of treatment you need. But how are you going to pay for it?

Options for self-funding may include your savings, a loan, or even 'The Bank of Mum and Dad!' Or maybe you're lucky enough to live in an area where NHS-funded treatment is available, as the NHS currently funds around 25 per cent (or almost 7,500) IVF cycles per year.

If you're not eligible for funded treatment or none is available in your area, you can always try asking your GP if the NHS will at least cover the cost of your drugs. This possibility can save around £300–£1,000 so may be worth exploring.

Never consider buying someone else's unused fertility drugs left over from their treatment cycle to reduce your costs – even if you know the person.

NHS-funded treatment

Although the recommendation is that every woman in England and Wales up to the age 40 who may benefit from fertility treatment should be entitled to at least one cycle, the reality is still quite different. NHS funding for fertility treatment still varies across the UK and where funding is available, criteria including the age of the woman, the length of relationship, and the number of existing children may differ from region to region.

You have various ways of finding out if you are eligible for NHS funding:

✔ Ask your GP.

✔ Ask your local clinic if it treats NHS-funded patients and if so, whether you can speak to the person with responsibility for NHS contracts.

> ✔ Visit www.nice.org.uk (for England and Wales only). This address is the Web site for the National Institute for Health and Clinical Excellence.
>
> ✔ Contact your Primary Care Trust (England), Local Health Board (Wales), Health Board (Scotland), or Health and Social Services Board (Northern Ireland) and ask for information on funding and the criteria for eligibility.

In England: The PCT and the postcode lottery

Each area in England has a Primary Care Trust (PCT), the organisation responsible for allocating funding for all health care, including fertility treatment, on behalf of the GP practices in that area.

Since April 2005, and after recommendation by both the National Institute for Clinical Excellence (NICE) and the then Secretary of State for Health, all women under 40 who need it, should be able to have funded treatment. But access to funded treatment continues to depend on where you live.

Some PCTs currently fund only a handful of treatment cycles in any year and others fund none at all. Sometimes only a few miles can determine whether you qualify for two fully funded cycles of IVF or ICSI, or get nothing at all.

But moving house is seldom a short-term option as PCTs require that you have lived at the new address and been registered with a new doctor for a minimum of six months or one year. Nor is this idea a long-term solution, as moving house is often vastly more expensive than the cost of going private.

Accessing NHS funding

Contact your PCT or Health Board for information on the availability and criteria for funded fertility treatment and be prepared to ask:

> ✔ Whether your PCT funds fertility treatment
>
> ✔ At which clinics it funds treatment
>
> ✔ The current length of the waiting list
>
> ✔ The criteria for eligibility
>
> ✔ The route for referral – GP, or consultant
>
> ✔ What types of treatment can be funded
>
> ✔ How many cycles each patient is offered
>
> ✔ The duration between each funded cycle
>
> ✔ Whether you make an application to the PCT or Health Board or directly to the clinic

Criteria for funding

All PCTs manage the list of patients waiting for treatment in different ways and each has different criteria for selecting patients for treatment, including:

- Clinical assessment should suggest that the woman has a good chance of responding positively to treatment
- Age of female patient
- Length of current relationship
- Duration of infertility
- Any previous sterilisation
- Any previous fertility treatment
- Existence of any children (from the woman or the man or the couple)
- The woman's BMI (her height-to-weight ratio)

  Evidence shows that if a woman's BMI is under 19 or over 30 she has a reduced chance of conceiving naturally or with assisted conception and an increased risk of miscarriage or premature delivery if she gets pregnant.

Your PCT can advise you of its specific criteria for receiving funded treatment.

Playing the waiting game

Waiting lists for NHS-funded fertility treatment can vary from just a few weeks to up to four years. If your PCT waiting list means you will have to wait for months or even years to begin treatment, make sure they can easily keep in contact with you. Keep in touch with the PCT and/or the clinic and let them know of any change to your circumstances including:

- Change of address
- Change of telephone number
- Change of GP
- Change of partner or living arrangements
- If you have a baby

It's amazing how many people forget to send that crucial 'change of address' card to the fertility clinic and then wonder why they never seem to move up the waiting list.

If you move to an area covered by another PCT you will no longer be entitled to funded treatment from the original PCT and will have to start any application process again with the new PCT.

While you're waiting, follow the usual common-sense advice about taking folic acid, keeping your weight to a BMI of 19–30, reducing alcohol, increasing the amount of fluid (not alcohol or caffeine!) you drink, quitting smoking, and getting a moderate amount of exercise.

If you decide to have privately funded treatment while waiting for PCT funding, contact the PCT or clinic in advance to check how it may affect your funding status. Your self-funding may affect your eligibility for funded treatment even if your treatment cycle was unsuccessful.

Getting the go-ahead

When your funding becomes available, it's time to celebrate. At last! Now's your chance! Your PCT or the clinic will contact you to:

✔ Advise you that the funding is now available

✔ Check that you still meet the criteria

✔ Confirm your BMI is acceptable

✔ Confirm the type of treatment being funded

✔ Confirm the number of treatment cycles

✔ Confirm a date for your next appointment

After you've got the go-ahead, try not to postpone treatment for any non-emergency reasons such as 'decorating the house', 'going on holiday', changing jobs, or promotions at work. After your name gets to the top of the list, seize the opportunity with both hands.

Appealing a 'No'

If your PCT won't agree to fund you and you think you have special circumstances not recognised by the criteria, you may appeal the decision. Contact your GP, who can advise you whether they will handle the appeal or if you need to go direct to the PCT.

You may be asked to write a letter, complete a form, or even attend an individual case panel to review the original decision. Remember to reinforce the recommendation by both NICE and the Secretary of State for Health that all women up to 40 should be allowed at least a single cycle of treatment. Make a noise, get yourself noticed. Many appeal panels then listen, take note, and award funding.

Funding your own treatment

Treatment won't necessarily be any better if you 'go private', but you may be able to start treatment sooner. For that reason, this section explains what you need to know if you choose this path.

Although some media coverage would lead you to believe that costs are prohibitive to all except the super-rich, paying for your fertility treatment – or 'going private' – doesn't always mean remortgaging your home or spending five-figure sums over a couple of years. In fact, IUI using partner sperm can cost as little as £300 to £500, and a cycle of IVF or ICSI can cost between £1,500 and £5,000 depending on the clinic.

For most people, funding private fertility treatment such as IVF or ICSI is a financial commitment that needs consideration and some belt tightening, but isn't impossible to achieve.

If you're self-funding, be sure that you know what the treatment fee covers. Some centres quote inclusive fees, which cover the procedure itself, all the drugs and all the initial consultations, baseline tests, follow-up appointments, post-transfer or insemination drugs, and pregnancy tests. Others may charge for all or some of these items separately. Clarify this breakdown at your visit appointment so you don't fall foul of any nasty surprises when you get the invoice.

When budgeting for your treatment at a particular clinic, consider *all* the following:

- **Cost of initial consultation and baseline tests:** This cost includes a review of your medical history, particularly any fertility tests or investigations, pregnancies, or children you may have already. Baseline tests usually include measuring your hormones, infection screening for both partners, a sperm analysis for your chap, and an ultrasound scan for you.

- **Cost per treatment cycle:** A treatment cycle usually includes treatment planning, ultrasound scans, and IUI procedure. For IVF and ICSI the cycle is usually egg collection, sperm preparation, fertilisation of the eggs, embryo transfer, pregnancy test, and pregnancy scan and/or a follow-up appointment to review the treatment cycle if it hasn't been successful.

- **Cost of drugs:** These costs vary depending on the type of treatment and the individual woman. For example, down-regulation and stimulation drugs for IVF may cost between £300 and £1,000, but the exact amount won't be clear until after your initial consultation and the results of your baseline tests.

    Ask your clinic if it can obtain the drugs for you from a supplier or pharmaceutical company, or whether you getting quotes from your local pharmacy and buying them with a private prescription from the clinic is worthwhile.

When I (co-author Jill) had to get my down-regulation and follicle stimulation drugs, I asked my clinic for two separate prescriptions after phoning an independent pharmacy, a supermarket pharmacy, and a national chemist for quotes and getting massively differing replies. In the end I saved about £300 by buying the drugs from two different places. But it still felt weird to hand over way more than the usual NHS standard prescription fee before I walked out of the pharmacies with my precious vials!

✔ **HFEA levies:** Also be aware of that your treatment will be subject to a levy from the HFEA of, currently, £104.50 if embryos are created in vitro, or if embryos are transferred back into the uterus, or of £52 for the use of donor sperm. All relevant treatments at UK clinics must include these levies, so they're unavoidable.

✔ **Distance prepared to travel:** While the ideal is going to the clinic that will give you the very best chance of having a baby, if that clinic is a hundred miles away and you and your husband work full-time, getting there may not be reasonable. Depending on your treatment, you may need appointments on three or four consecutive days. Is the travelling feasible? Don't add to your stress levels by clocking up miles on the motorway. Some clinics may be able to recommend somewhere closer to your home that can scan you and then you only need attend your chosen clinic for critical parts of the treatment, such as IUI insemination or egg collection and embryo transfer.

Although cost is important, fees don't automatically reflect the quality of the service or the success rates of a clinic. The most expensive clinics don't necessarily have the best results – especially in your age group and for women or men with your particular reasons for infertility – but may simply be located in the most expensive building!

Getting creative when you're out of other options

If you can't get NHS funding, don't have savings, and don't want to borrow the money to fund your treatment, you may be able to get help from the clinic.

Egg sharing to reduce costs

If you need IVF or ICSI, some clinics have egg-share programmes that let you donate half your eggs to another couple in return for greatly subsidised treatment. The recipient of your eggs pays for your drugs, your egg retrieval, and embryo transfer. Circumstances vary, but some clinics may still require you to pay for the initial consultation, baseline tests, and the storage of any embryos that may be frozen.

Always ask the clinic in advance if it has an egg-share programme and again, check the live birth rates of IVF and ICSI cycles using donor eggs, before committing to having your treatment at that clinic.

See Chapter 15, for more information on egg sharing for donors and recipients.

Joining a drug study

Joining a drug study is a rare, but not impossible, route to partly or fully funding your treatment. Ask the clinic if it works with any drug companies that are carrying out clinical trials in IVF.

Some studies have very specific requirements for age, weight, and infertility problems. Others are less strict with their requirements and let the clinic select the patients they feel are suitable.

In most studies, patients trial a new drug that is not yet licensed for use in the UK. If you sign up for the study, you need to understand that you may get fewer eggs or embryos than you would from proven drugs. Most studies require that you sign a document stating this fact. You may also have to keep a diary of all the side effects and have frequent interviews with the person running the study. However, the rules about clinical trials in the UK are very strict and the drugs are tested for effectiveness and safety in smaller studies before they're made available for a clinical trial.

Shopping for money-back guarantees

Some clinics try to overcome resistance to the high cost of IVF by promoting 'special offers'. These offers are rare, and while they may sound good, they often have many catches.

The specifics vary, but usually you pay an upfront fee, for say, four IVF cycles. If you get pregnant in any one of the cycles, the clinic keeps all the money. If you don't get pregnant at the end of the last cycle, you get your money back. You must pay extra charges for ICSI or using an egg or sperm donor or a surrogate.

Patients must meet certain requirements for acceptance to the programme; usually you must be under a certain age and have a normal uterine cavity, and normal baseline blood test results.

Are these 'shared-risk' offers a good deal? Well, if the clinic has poor success rates, probably not. If it has good results and you get pregnant on the fourth cycle, you'll have had a good price for each cycle. If you have a baby from the first try, you'll have spent a great deal for just one cycle, far more than you needed. But if you have a baby from just one cycle, will you care about the cost? If not, such a programme may be for you.

Whether a clinic offers a 'shared-risk' three- or four-cycle programme or even a BOGOF – buy one get one free – deal, it's only a good deal if the centre is reputable and has good success rates. If the clinic doesn't have a proven track record or good success rates, you won't get a good deal no matter how many free cycles it gives.

Why fertility treatment costs so much

Fertility treatment all seems very expensive, with no guarantee of a baby at the end, or even a free gift along the way. But put it into perspective – the average cost of IVF is:

A luxury summer holiday for two

Half the cost of a second-hand car

1,200 glasses of wine or pints of beer in a pub

200 takeaway meals for two

66 meals in an average restaurant for two

While the cost isn't small potatoes, nor is it 'the moon on a stick' for many couples.

But why is treatment so expensive? Although supply and demand may have a bearing on costs – in other words, clinics charge what they can – the fact is that fertility treatments are usually high-tech procedures and 'high-tech' costs money. A fertility clinic costs over a million pounds to set up. In addition, your clinic has many other expenses:

✔ **Salaries:** Employees include doctors, nurses, nurse assistants, andrologists, embryologists, semenologists, lab assistants, biomedical scientists, secretaries, business managers, admin assistants, receptionists, finance staff, medical assistants, maintenance engineers, and housekeepers.

✔ **Supplies:** The clinic where we (co-authors Gill and Jill) work uses the following disposable supplies in a month for 80 egg retrievals: 100 retrieval needles, 600 pairs of sterile gloves, 200 speculums, 1,000 swabs, 100 IV cannulae, and 500 syringes.

✔ **Maintenance of equipment:** Clinics need such things as oximeters (to measure oxygen levels in the blood), automatic blood pressure cuffs, a complete crash trolley of medications, and ultrasound machines.

✔ **Embryologists' equipment:** These specialists use expensive culture media to grow and nurture embryos, micromanipulation tools for ICSI and assisted hatching, and expensive microscopes, plus liquid nitrogen tanks to store sperm and embryos.

✔ **Basic office expenses:** These costs include rent, utility bills, the phone bill (which can be enormous), postage costs, copiers, paper, computers, and so on.

A good fertility clinic is an expensive practice to run and although the tabloids may be full of stories about fertility treatment millionaires, most fertility doctors, nurses, and scientists are ordinary people who are passionate about their work and just want to help you become a parent.

A word about health insurance

First the bad news: Health insurance that covers the cost of fertility treatment isn't available in the UK. However, some policies cover the cost of private consultant fees and tests up to the point of diagnosis that you require fertility treatment. This fact means that your policy may cover the cost of blood tests, sperm analysis, and even investigative surgery, such as a laparoscopy or hysteroscopy, and so allow you to bypass any NHS waiting lists for these procedures. If you're already in your mid-30s where age can become an issue, this option may enable you to start your treatment sooner.

Chapter 10

All The 'I's: Introducing IUI, IVF, and ICSI

After tests with your GP, more tests at the hospital, possibly a little exploratory surgery to check your Fallopian tubes and uterus for evidence of cysts, endometriosis, fibroids, scarring, or polyps, and after your partner has had his sperm analysed, you're told those important four words: 'You need fertility treatment.'

You may have expected this outcome all along and you may actually be thankful that the GP and hospital testing can now stop and the treatment can start. Or, you may be devastated and view your options with fear and dread.

In this chapter we outline the tests that every clinic does before deciding which treatment is best for you and introduce all the 'I's – IUI (intrauterine insemination), IVF (in vitro fertilisation), and ICSI (intra cytoplasmic sperm injection) – the three main treatments given to the majority of patients who have assisted conception.

Doing the Groundwork

The clinic needs to identify and understand the reasons why you've not been able to get pregnant naturally before it can plan the best way for you to conceive with assisted conception.

Initial consultation

At your first visit the doctor or nurse talks to you and your partner about your lifestyle, your medical histories, and any fertility investigations, tests, or treatment you may have already had. You need to give a detailed medical and sexual history, and it's best to be honest and matter of fact, even when the issues are difficult or sensitive. The woman needs to give details of:

   ✔ Length of her menstrual cycle

   ✔ Any known fertility problems – for example endometriosis, PCOS, and so on

   ✔ Pains during ovulation or intercourse

   ✔ Any previous pregnancies, miscarriages, stillbirths, or children

The man needs to give details of any vasectomy or vasectomy reversal he may have had and also discuss any problems with erectile dysfunction or ejaculation.

They will discuss your lifestyle, including exercise, diet, smoking, and alcohol consumption, as well as your work, stress levels, any medications or conditions such as anorexia, epilepsy, high blood pressure, or genetic disorders in either partner's family. The fertility expert also explains the legal framework that the clinic operates within, including the issues of 'welfare of the child' and 'informed consent'.

Every UK clinic is required by the Human Fertilisation and Embryology Authority (HFEA) to consider the welfare of any existing child or any baby born as a result of treatment, including the need for a father. This may seem intrusive and unfair to couples who are having trouble conceiving, because the same considerations are not applied to women and couples who conceive naturally, but this procedure is something the clinic is currently obliged to follow by law.

Patients' written consent is required at key stages of all types of assisted conception. Consent, which must be given in writing with a signature, rules out phone consent and email messages, and may require the consent of both partners before treatment can progress.

Consent must be 'informed', meaning that the issues are clearly explained to you and the clinic must offer you counselling to discuss any concerns you have about the treatment or storage that requires your consent. Currently the HFEA requires patients to give written consent on three occasions:

   ✔ **Consent to the use and storage of eggs, sperm, and/or embryos:** You and your partner must give written consent to the use of eggs and sperm throughout your treatment and to the use or storage of any embryos created from them.

✔ **Consent to treatment:** For example, if you're having IVF treatment you need to give consent to the egg retrieval and transfer of any embryos to your uterus. If your treatment includes donor eggs or sperm, you have to give consent to treatment using these, and to an embryo transfer.

✔ **Consent to disclosure of information:** Before a clinic can tell your GP or anyone else about your treatment, you must have given your written consent. You're able to decide and limit the information you allow to be disclosed, so this needs to be discussed in detail with the fertility specialist you meet at your first consultation.

The nurse or doctor also explains that, with your permission, they need to contact your GP before your treatment can begin, to confirm your medical and personal histories.

Baseline tests

Baseline tests of hormone levels and sperm samples are vital for effective treatment planning. For the woman, the baseline tests need to be done on days two to five of your cycle, where day one is the first day of your period.

You've probably already had many blood tests to check your oestradiol, progesterone, LH, and FSH hormone levels. Very occasionally the results of these tests can be used by the clinic to help plan your treatment, but usually the clinic prefers to repeat the test from a current blood sample for analysis in their own labs. Here's what the tests reveal:

✔ **Follicle-stimulating hormone (FSH):** Your FSH level should be less than 8, on day two or day three. A higher than normal FSH level may indicate that you're going into *perimenopause*, the period a few years before menopause.

✔ **Luteinising hormone (LH):** The LH level is usually about 5 on day two or three; women with polycystic ovaries (we discuss PCOS in Chapter 7) may have an LH level that is significantly higher than their follicle-stimulating hormone level on day two. LH levels rise later in the cycle, usually going over 40 when you're almost ready to ovulate.

✔ **Oestradiol:** Oestradiol on day two or three of your period is normally greater than 10 but less than 50. An oestradiol level that is very low, less than 10, may indicate that your ovaries are suppressed and may not respond well to stimulation to make a normal egg. An oestradiol level that is over 50 picgrammes per millimetre may indicate ovarian cysts.

✔ **Progesterone:** On day two or three of your period, your progesterone levels should be low, less than 2. Progesterone levels go up in the second half of your cycle, after you ovulate, and should be over 12 after you release an egg. Progesterone comes from the *corpus luteum*, the left-over shell of the follicle after you ovulate, and is necessary to help the embryo implant.

But the clinic also needs to test your partner, too – even if GPs and consultants have overlooked the importance of this action in the past. He'll have to produce the sperm sample at the clinic, or be able to keep it at body temperature and get it to the lab within one hour of producing it at home. The SFA – seminal fluid analysis – analyses the quantity, quality, *motility* (movement), and *morphology* (shape) of the sperm. These can vary from week to week and so the clinic usually prefers a fresh sample to analyse. (For more information on sperm tests, see Chapter 8.)

 Your partner's hormone levels, especially LH, FSH, and testosterone, also need to be normal for good sperm production. Most clinics don't test the levels unless your partner's semen analysis is abnormal because a good semen analysis means his hormone levels are normal.

You also need to have an ultrasound scan to check your cervix, uterus, Fallopian tubes, and ovaries and look for evidence of fibroids, polyps, or endometriosis. This scan is done by an ultra-sonographer, a nurse, or a doctor, with either of the two following types of ultrasound scan:

✔ **Transvaginal ultrasound:** This procedure uses a long, wand-like probe which is inserted into the vagina. It can be embarrassing if you're very modest – but get used to it, because much more is to come, and the staff do it countless times every day! The moving probe may cause pressure, but it's not usually even as uncomfortable as a smear test. This method, which can be done with an empty bladder, gives better images than abdominal ultrasound scanning in most cases.

✔ **Abdominal ultrasound:** This procedure requires a full bladder. The images aren't usually as clear as the trans-vaginal ultrasound. You pull your pants down to the pubic hair line. Jelly is placed directly on your stomach, and the technician then moves the *transducer* (a small hand-held device about the size of your hand) over it. Be aware that, because you've a full bladder, this pressure can be uncomfortable.

 Why is a full bladder needed for an abdominal ultrasound scan? The uterus and ovaries normally lie behind the intestines, but a full bladder moves the uterus back and pushes the intestine up, so the uterus and ovaries can be seen more clearly. The bladder also provides a fluid contrast that makes the uterus easier to identify.

The ultrasound causes no known side effects. When your ultrasound is finished, you can go home with no special instructions.

Calculating your fertility age

A few UK clinics offer an ovarian reserve test to calculate your fertility age, rather than your chronological age. This test is especially useful if you're 34 or over as it can give an indication of your chances of conceiving spontaneously or with assisted conception. Measuring inhibin B – and the newer test to measure anti-Müllerian hormone (AMH) – may provide vital information about whether you can 'safely' postpone trying to conceive for a few years, or whether your 'ovarian reserve' is so low that any delay is going to further limit any chance of pregnancy. In the worst case, the test may confirm that you've little or no chance of either conceiving naturally, or with assisted conception using your own eggs.

Resist the temptation to do an 'over-the-counter' ovarian reserve test. They are very expensive and don't include the pelvic ultrasound scan and one-to-one consultation with a fertility expert that good clinics offer.

Routine infection screening

Clinics have to carry out routine infection screening on blood samples from both partners who are to be treated. It is a requirement of the HFEA to screen each patient for HIV – the virus that causes AIDS – hepatitis B, and hepatitis C in order to reduce the risk of cross infection during the storage of sperm, eggs, or embryos in liquid nitrogen. Some clinics require all patients to be infection screened before any treatment begins.

The results of the blood tests are confidential and are not passed on to anyone else without your consent. If any of the tests return a positive result, the clinic advises you if it's able to continue with your treatment, or alternatively, refers you for specialist help to continue your treatment.

Both partners are also screened for sexually transmitted diseases including syphyllis, gonorrhoea, and chlamydia and the woman is checked for immunity to rubella (German measles).

Genetic screening

If a history of any genetic condition exists in the family of either partner, such as cystic fibrosis, muscular dystrophy, or fragile 'X' syndrome, a blood test can indicate whether an increased chance exists of any child born to that couple of having a genetic disorder. The couple will either be reassured with the outcome or offered counselling and advice about their options.

Follow-up appointment and treatment planning

About one week after your baseline tests, the results of all the tests and scans can be discussed at your follow-up appointment. Your fertility specialist is in a position to identify or confirm the reasons for your subfertility – even, frustratingly, if this continues to be 'unexplained' – and recommends a suitable treatment or treatment alternatives, or whether you're offered counselling about coming to terms living without a child.

Now is the time to ensure that you're told about possible risks and the success rates for people of your age and with your condition(s) at that particular clinic. If the time is right for you, funding is available, and the fertility specialist confirms you don't need any more advanced tests, investigations, or counselling, you can begin to plan your treatment at this appointment.

Occasionally, the clinic may suggest you talk to a counsellor before treatment begins or progresses. The outcome of the counselling is not shared with the clinic unless the clinic specifically requests a counselling assessment. This happens rarely and only in complicated or unusual circumstances, but the outcome can determine whether or not the clinic will continue treatment.

Tailor-made treatment

Your follow-up appointment is the time to discuss the very best treatment options for *you*. This stage is when 'off the peg' protocols may be adapted to fit your hormone profile and the specific challenges of your sub- or infertility.

The best clinics vary drug protocols to get the best chance of a positive result for individual patients. This lateral thinking can sometimes lead to more 'creative' approaches.

For example, a woman with a poor or thin womb lining will seldom get pregnant even with the very best quality embryos. As part of her fertility treatment, before her egg collection, her fertility expert may prescribe controlled doses of Viagra to stimulate her blood supply and thicken the womb lining ready for her embryo transfer. Following this tailor-made approach to treatment, babies have been born in the UK to women who may otherwise never have even had a positive pregnancy test.

If your circumstances are unusual or particularly complicated, always ask how a clinic has approached similar cases, and whether any patient has got pregnant or had a baby from such an approach.

Deciding How Much Treatment You Need

The results of your baseline tests may be fairly conclusive and indicate a specific type of treatment. If the results suggest the frustrating and, unfortunately, still quite common 'unexplained' infertility with 'normal' sperm, the clinic may recommend artificial insemination with the husband's or partner's sperm (AIH), in the first instance. Alternatively, the tests will suggest that you need IVF or even ICSI as a recommended first course of treatment and that AIH is a waste of time, money and emotional investment.

Some clinics operate a 'try three times' rule before moving 'up' to the next type of treatment, but this decision depends on many factors including your age, your bank account, and your ability to deal with the emotional turmoil fertility treatment brings to some couples.

And then there's always the 'just one more and I know it'll work!' positive thinking. But, in the worse cases, for how long can you remain that positive if each cycle brings a negative pregnancy test? Deciding both what kind of treatment, and how much treatment, you need is a moveable feast that changes with your response to, and the outcome of, any treatment cycle. Ultimately, the decision is a personal choice you need to make with informed clinical advice and, if preferred, with the help of a fertility counsellor.

Discovering IUI, IVF, and ICSI – the Basics

Tests by your GP are the first stage of assisted conception treatment, and more tests, possible corrective surgery, or even partner IUI by a gynaecologist is the second stage. This section gives an overview of the third level of assisted conception treatment – IUI, IVF, and ICSI, which are the three most commonly used types of assisted conception at a fertility clinic.

ICI and IUI

AIH, which is another term for both intracervical insemination (or ICI) or intrauterine insemination (or IUI), means simply that sperm is placed into the cervix or the uterus to give it a 'leg up' on getting where it needs to go, which is to your egg.

A first single cycle of ICI or IUI normally takes an average of four to five weeks from the beginning of the treatment cycle to pregnancy test. Subsequent cycles may be slightly shorter.

If your partner's sperm is fine, you may just be monitored with blood tests and ultrasounds to be sure that you're making an adequate follicle and releasing an egg every month. In which case, the clinic may advise you to have an *intracervical insemination* (ICI), a procedure in which the fresh sperm is inserted into the cervix.

If the problem is diagnosed as *mild male factor* (a slightly lower than normal sperm count or motility), the fertility specialist will probably suggest doing an IUI, where the sperm can be 'washed' and concentrated, and then placed directly into the uterus.

If you're not producing an egg or not releasing an egg, you may be prescribed stimulating drugs to increase egg production. If you have a period less than two weeks after you ovulate, your doctor may prescribe progesterone for a suspected luteal phase defect (Chapter 11 has more information about this).

If you try all these individually and don't have a positive pregnancy test, you may end up doing all three: IUI, *gonadotrophins* (stimulating drugs), and progesterone. If this method brings no success, the fertility specialist may recommend you move up to IVF, where the insemination process can be more carefully controlled outside of the body.

Many fertility specialists say that AIH will not increase your chances over timed intercourse if you have a normal semen analysis and normal postcoital test (see Chapter 7 for more about both). Neither ICI nor IUI will be effective if the problem is *severe male factor* (a very low sperm count or antisperm antibodies) or caused by blocked Fallopian tubes.

Although statistics reported for IUI seem to vary widely, most clinics claim about a 10 to 15 per cent per month success rate for women under age 35, with decreasing success as your age goes up. Producing more than one follicle a month by using Clomid or gonadotrophins also increases your chances of pregnancy per month. Many experts believe that your chance of getting pregnant with further IUI after six failed IUIs is slim and would recommend 'moving up' to IVF.

In vitro fertilisation (IVF)

In vitro fertilisation, more commonly referred to as IVF, has been available since 1978 and more than 1 million babies have been born as a result. Unlike IUI, where fertilisation occurs in the body as with natural conception, with IVF the eggs and sperm are collected outside the body and the fertilisation takes place in a sterile plastic dish – but no longer the glass tube of the original 'test-tube' babies!

Women with blocked Fallopian tubes, men with mild sperm problems such as reduced, but not poor, motility, and both men and women with 'unexplained' infertility, may benefit from IVF. But be prepared for many injections, lots of transvaginal scanning, possible mood swings and temper tantrums, an egg retrieval under sedation, and an approximate one in three chance of having a baby as a result.

IVF requires the woman to take injected drugs to down-regulate her body to a temporary 'menopausal' state and also to inject gonadatrophins to stimulate the growth of the follicles on the ovaries that will contain the eggs. IVF requires the man to provide a sperm sample that will contain sufficient good quality sperm for embryologists to place about 150,000 with each of the retrieved eggs. The procedure also requires both partners to give huge and constant support to each other. A single cycle of IVF can take from 5 to about 11 weeks from initial consultation to pregnancy test, depending on your drug protocol.

Intra cytoplasmic sperm injection (ICSI)

Intra cytoplasmic sperm injection (ICSI) was a very happy accident! In 1990 Belgian scientists tried to assist insemination and fertilisation by injecting four or five sperm between the zona pellucida 'egg shell' and the softer, jelly-like centre of an egg. Well, the needle 'slipped' and the sperm went right into the egg, and although it was monitored overnight, they believed that the process would damage the egg making it unviable. Surprise and delight followed as the egg developed into a healthy embryo suitable for transfer.

Available in the UK since 1992, ICSI has revolutionised the success of fertility treatment where the main cause of infertility is male factor, as it requires only a single healthy sperm for the insemination of each egg, rather than about 150,000.

Like 'standard' IVF, ICSI requires the two to three weeks of down-regulation drugs and one to two weeks of gonadotrophins injections, lots of transvaginal scans and an egg collection under sedation for the woman, and the production of a sperm sample into a sterile pot for the man!

After the sperm is washed, sorted, and prepared, embryologists catch and inject a single sperm into the centre of each collected egg under a high-powered microscope, using a needle $\frac{1}{10}$th the width of a human hair. As with standard IVF, these inseminated eggs are left to incubate overnight and checked regularly for signs of development the next day. Forty-eight hours after egg collection, the embryologists will know how many eggs have been successfully inseminated to become viable embryos suitable for either transferring back to the woman's uterus, or freezing in liquid nitrogen for possible future transfer.

Deciding How Long to Keep Trying

You may find that a lot of data is available regarding IVF, but much less data is available for some of the medium-tech methods, such as IUI. You may also notice that every doctor has a different take on your odds for success. Although most doctors quote you numbers that reflect their *own* success with any given process, they may also alter them a bit to better reflect your age, or your response to treatment so far.

Growing sick of getting stuck

Perhaps you grew sick of waiting when the first home pregnancy test read negative. But even if you're more patient, what if a month, or two, or three, of nightly injections of hormones is just about all you can handle?

First, be assured that your impatience and irritability aren't a reflection of your winning personality, but more likely the side effects of the drugs you're taking. Most women find that acknowledging that their moods or mood swings are largely chemical in nature does lessen the burden. If you haven't confided in a friend about your fertility struggles, perhaps now is as good a time as any.

Being sensitive to your partner's feelings

Just as you may find the fertility rituals to be all consuming, your partner may be sharing your views – more than you know. The partner being treated may feel that she is undergoing the lion's share of discomfort and disappointment. But remember, even if your partner isn't experiencing every needle stick or test result, that person is watching you go through it. 'Big deal!' you scoff. Well, it can be.

Watching another person experience pain or sadness can be as difficult as going through it yourself. The silent partner also must suffer with feelings of inadequacy and powerlessness in being unable to relieve your discomfort. Partners of terminally ill patients often need their own support networks as well. And, as a recent study reveals, fertility patients, due to the sometimes long nature of their treatment, share some of the same issues faced by the chronically and terminally ill.

Encourage your partner to share his or her feeling with friends, family, or a professional. Although you may feel as though you're losing your sanity, your partner may feel as though they're losing you.

Share the shots! Get your partner to help you prepare your drugs by mixing the powders and diluents and drawing them into the syringe. If they – and you – are up for it, get them to give you the injections too. It'll involve them right from the start in the whole high-tech baby-making process, and emphasise that this is treatment you are *both* receiving (even if the needle is actually going into *your* leg or tummy!).

Coping when you're both sick of everything, including each other

Many say that the rigours of fertility treatment are an opportunity for couples to grow closer. But this scenario is generally *not* the case. With chemically induced moods raging, money being spent at high speed, and disappointment doled out in monthly doses, it takes a lot for couples to remain civil and calm with one another.

If you and your partner are unable to deal with anything, including each other, you may want to consider counselling and/or a break from your fertility treatment. Don't forget the importance of your relationship. Couples who do, may find themselves miles apart, whether or not they conceive. Remember, your goal is to make a family, not break one up.

Thinking Ahead: Health Effects of Fertility Treatment

Fertility drugs, or *gonadotrophins,* are powerful stuff. Anyone who takes them through even one cycle can attest to the physical and emotional effects of having one's hormones surging at a much higher level than nature ever intended. Do people suffer long-term effects 2 or 20 years down the road? No one knows for sure, but here are the most recent conclusions on the safety of taking gonadotrophins.

Effects on the mother

At this time, experts have no evidence that taking gonadotrophins has *any* long-term effect on women. Some studies have shown a possible link to fertility medications like Clomid and ovarian cancer, but other studies have not supported these findings.

One thing most studies have agreed upon is that the risk of ovarian cancer is higher in all women who've never become pregnant, regardless of whether or not they've taken fertility medications. So if you've taken fertility drugs for any amount of time and never had a child, make sure that you have an annual gynaecological check-up. This precaution is especially important if other women in your family have had ovarian cancer, because doctors have established a genetic link for this type of cancer, among others.

Effects on the baby

No one is sure whether fertility drugs will have a long-term effect on the children conceived through their use – many of the children born through high-tech methods such as IVF aren't old enough yet for this risk to be determined. However, the first IVF baby, Louise Brown, who was born in 1978, was pregnant with her first (naturally conceived) child in 2006. Her younger sister, Natalie – also conceived through IVF – had given birth to two children by 2006. Their babies reassure clinicians, scientists, and the public about some of the long-term effects of assisted conception on the babies conceived through such treatment.

Research into the possible long-term impact on assisted conception babies is ongoing. Some studies have indicated that assisted conception babies have lower birth weight and mild developmental delays, but this may be explained by other factors, and not directly as a result of the drugs or laboratory processes involved in creating the embryos. For example, more twins and triplets are born to mums using fertility drugs, and *all* multiple births more commonly have low birth weight and developmental delays. Also, more babies are born to older mothers through assisted conception treatment, and older women tend to have more complicated pregnancies than women under age 35.

Recent studies have shown that couples with mild subfertility – that is, those who take longer than one year to conceive naturally – also have babies with lower birth weights. Therefore, the subfertility, rather than the treatment, is the cause of such lower birth weights.

Because some men who need ICSI to conceive have part of their 'Y' chromosome missing, which results in their infertility, some of their sons may have the same chromosomal abnormality and may also need to do ICSI (or whatever high-tech methods are available in 30 years) to have children.

Chapter 11

Giving Mother Nature a Helping Hand: Intrauterine Insemination (IUI)

*S*tarting an IUI (intrauterine insemination) cycle or a stimulated medication cycle is a big step up from just trying to figure out when you're ovulating and planning to have sex accordingly. IUI cycles involve monitoring blood and ultrasound results, and often involve injecting potent hormones called gonadotrophins.

In this chapter, we explain how IUI and stimulated cycles work, and discuss some of the testing involved and the medications you may be taking. We also help you find those expensive gonadotrophins as cheaply as possible, and we give you tips on how to inject yourself with them safely and painlessly!

Deciding How Much Treatment You Need

You have several routes available to you when seeing a fertility doctor, and the one that Dr Special sends you down on depends on your reason for infertility:

✔ If your partner's sperm is fine, you may just be monitored with blood tests and ultrasounds to be sure that you're making an adequate follicle and releasing an egg every month.

✔ If the problem is diagnosed as *mild male factor* (a slightly lower than normal sperm count or motility), your doctor may suggest doing an IUI so that the sperm can be 'washed' and concentrated, and then placed directly into the uterus at exactly the right time.

✔ If you're not producing an egg, or not releasing an egg, you may be prescribed stimulating medications to increase egg production.

✔ If you're getting your period less than two weeks after you ovulate, your doctor may prescribe progesterone for a suspected luteal phase defect, which we explain in the next section.

✔ If you've gone several months without a positive pregnancy test, you may end up doing all three: IUI, gonadotrophins (stimulating medications), and progesterone (luteal phase support).

Treating Luteal Phase Defects

Luteal phase, in fertility circles, means the two weeks after you ovulate and before your period starts. You may be diagnosed with *luteal phase defect* (LPD) if your period starts ten or so days after you ovulate, rather than the normal two-week period. If you've been monitoring your BBT (basal body temperature) you may see an early drop in your temperature as well. LPD can be caused by problems with the corpus luteum, or with the uterine lining.

After you ovulate, the leftover shell of your follicle, now called the *corpus luteum*, starts to produce progesterone. Progesterone stimulates the uterine lining to produce extra blood vessels so that the embryo has a good supply to support its growth if it attaches.

If you get your period less than two weeks after you ovulate, some fertility doctors may suggest you have a biopsy done to check your progesterone. An *endometrial biopsy* involves scraping a little of your uterine lining with a small curette. The scraping is then checked to see whether the lining received the proper amount of progesterone. A biopsy is an outpatient procedure and can be done on the day of a negative pregnancy test before your period starts.

Treatment for luteal phase defects depends on what's happening:

✔ A poorly developed follicle, or one that releases an abnormal egg, won't put out enough progesterone to develop the lining properly. In this case, the treatment isn't more progesterone after you ovulate, but stimulating medications to produce a better-quality follicle.

✔ Sometimes you have a follicle that doesn't release the egg inside. This follicle may produce some progesterone, and you may think you've ovulated, but you won't get pregnant, because the egg was never released. An ultrasound before and after your LH (luteinising hormone) surge can help diagnose this syndrome, which is called *luteinised unruptured follicle syndrome* (LUFS). If LUFS is suspected then your doctor may prescribe an injection of hCG (human chorionic gonadotrophin) at around the time of ovulation to help ensure that the egg is released. Ovulation is an 'inflammatory' process so taking high doses of anti-inflammatory medications may interfere with ovulation.

Acquiring Help through AI

Artificial insemination (or AI, another term for intrauterine insemination) means simply placing the sperm into the uterus to help it get where it needs to go, which is to your egg. At the time of ovulation (either spontaneous or triggered by an hCG injection) your partner produces a sperm sample that's washed and prepared in order to select a high concentration of good quality sperm. This sample of gold medal swimming sperm is loaded into a *catheter* (a fine plastic tube) and injected through your cervix towards the top of the uterus where the Fallopian tubes join (see Figure 11-1). This method has the effect of doing half the journey for the sperm, by-passing any possible problems at the cervix and flooding the Fallopian tubes with good sperm at exactly the right time.

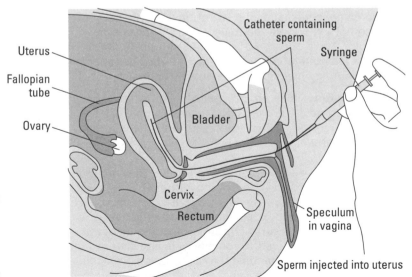

Figure 11-1:
Sperm is
injected into
the uterus.

You may or may not be taking stimulating medications to create more eggs during an IUI cycle. Some doctors start with Clomid, a pill given to increase your egg output, and move up after a few months to stimulation with gonadotrophins. Others may simply monitor your normal cycle and inseminate, hoping to fertilise the one or possibly two follicles you produce each month.

Measuring your chance for success

Unstimulated IUI may have relatively little to offer with a normal semen analysis and normal postcoital test (refer to Chapter 7 for more about both). IUI will be ineffective if the problem is very severe male factor (a very low sperm count or antisperm antibodies) or blocked tubes.

Although statistics reported for IUI seem to vary widely, this variable may reflect the length of time that a couple have been trying before they start IUI. Most clinics claim about a 10 to 15 per cent per month success rate for women under age 35, with decreasing success as your age goes up. Producing more than one follicle a month by using Clomid or gonadotrophins also increases your chances of pregnancy per month. Many experts believe that your chance of getting pregnant after four to six failed IUIs is very low and you should consider in vitro fertilisation.

Collecting sperm

Semen collection and concentration are a big part of IUI. Several methods are used both to collect and to concentrate the sperm:

- ✔ **Clean container collection:** A sterile container is used to collect the sample obtained through masturbation.

- ✔ **Condom collection:** A special condom containing no lubricants or spermicides is used if the semen sample has to be collected during intercourse. This method is useful for those whose religious beliefs prohibit masturbation.

When your partner is directed to produce a semen sample by the clinic he may have several reactions. I (co-author Gill) have seen strong, confident men faint, giggle, or just run away when confronted by the little plastic pot! Because timing is crucial, your mate can't get away with saying that he 'Doesn't feel like it today' or he has just remembered a phone call he must make! For some men, the concept of masturbating, let alone collecting the result in a pot and handing it to a stranger who's going to analyse and process it, is way beyond what he had in mind when he agreed to come to the clinic with you. No easy solution exists for this problem other than lots of support and encouragement. Get him to practise at home or let you help!

Don't be insulted if the *andrologist* (the person who deals with sperm) asks if there was any spillage. This comment isn't a jibe on your general clumsiness or the look of your sample! The first part of the semen has the highest concentration of sperm, so if any was lost, your semen sample may not be as good as it can be.

Sperm need to be 'washed' before they're ready for IUI. Washing must be done because unwashed sperm contain large amounts of *prostaglandins*, chemicals that cause smooth muscle contractions. If a large amount of 'raw' semen – more than 0.2 millilitres – is injected unwashed into the uterus, the prostaglandins can cause severe cramping at the least, and a shocklike, life-threatening reaction at worst.

If you're picturing the washing process being done in a little machine with a spin cycle, you're partially right! Sperm are spun down into a little pellet in a centrifuge before being placed in the uterus. One method spins the sperm in a centrifuge, and another puts the sperm on the bottom of a test tube and allows the best sperm to swim up. Another common method puts the sperm on top of several layers of washing media; the tube is spun down, and the pellet on the bottom will contain the largest amount of motile, healthy sperm. The sperm pellet is then placed, via catheter, into the uterus.

The main risks of doing IUI are the risk of infection (tiny) and risk of multiple births (considerable) if you're taking medication to stimulate growth of more than one follicle. This reason is why all gonadotrophin-stimulated cycles must be monitored by ultrasound, and abandoned if more than three follicles develop.

Checking out your egg

IUI, and timed intercourse (timed for your ovulation) works only if the sperm is placed in the right place at the right time – when you have a mature egg. To increase your chances of pregnancy, make sure that you're making a follicle and checking it for maturity before an IUI.

Monitoring your hormone level

One way to be sure that you're making a good egg is to monitor your hormone levels. As you start to make a mature egg, your oestradiol starts to rise. A good egg can produce an oestradiol of 150 to 300 picogrammes per millilitre. About 30 hours before your egg releases, your LH also starts to rise; a good LH surge is usually over 40.

Thar she blows: Ultrasounds before and after ovulation

Many fertility doctors use pelvic ultrasound to monitor the growth of ovarian follicles. Ultrasound works by bouncing high-frequency sound waves off internal organs. Unlike X-rays, ultrasounds don't expose you to radiation. Two types of pelvic ultrasound exist: *transvaginal*, in which a long, wand-like probe is inserted into your vagina; and *abdominal*, in which jelly is placed on your tummy and a handheld device is moved over it.

If your doctor does ultrasounds during the first two weeks of your cycle, you'll see your follicle growing as your estradiol rises and your LH surges; usually the follicle is about 22 to 25 millimeters at the time of ovulation. Many centres do an ultrasound the day of IUI and the day after, to make sure that the egg has released from the follicle; when this happens, the follicle shrinks on ultrasound. Even if you're not having a 'natural' cycle with no stimulation, you may be given an injection of hCG to ensure that you ovulate and release the egg. Pregnancy can't occur unless the egg releases.

Moving Up to Controlled Ovarian Hyperstimulation

Clomid is usually the first drug given to start your follicles growing because it can be given orally and has fewer side effects than injections, including a lower risk of multiple pregnancy. If Clomid isn't working for you after a few months, your doctor may suggest moving up to the big time: injecting gonadotrophins, a technique called *controlled ovarian hyperstimulation*, or COH for short. We talk about gonadotrophins in the section 'Defining gonadotrophins' later in this chapter.

With COH, the goal is to make more than one or two follicles. The reasoning is that if you make a few more follicles, you've a better chance of getting pregnant each month. The chance of pregnancy with one egg each month is between 5 and 20 per cent, depending on your age.

Clomid works by increasing the amount of FSH (follicle-stimulating hormone) you make. The alternative is to give you more FSH directly, but this substance has to be done by injection because the hormone would be broken in your digestive tract and your liver. So the logical next step, if you're not making follicles on Clomid, is to move up to injections.

Getting injections

Obviously, taking injections is a big step. Not only do you have a possibility of making too many follicles when taking injectable stimulating medications and having to paying out for the cost of the medication (typically £15 a day for 10 days if you're having private treatment), but you also have to deal with the logistics of COH, including going in for frequent blood tests and ultrasounds, and finding someone to give you your injections. The best person to do that is yourself! Stimulating injections are mainly given sub-cut (subcutaneously) and they're really easy. Some medications even come ready mixed with a cute little pen so you can alter the dose easily. You may want your partner or someone else to come in to give the injections.

Giving yourself the injections

Most of the time, you give yourself the injections. This way is easy, convenient, safe, and allows you to take control. If you know that you'll be doing your own injections, ask your doctor if he can give you subcutaneous gonadotrophins. These are injected with a very tiny needle – like a diabetic needle – and can be used in the top of your leg, or in your stomach. Subcutaneous gonadotrophins are *recombinant* – meaning that they're made in the lab from animal, not human, proteins – or urinary-based gonadotrophins, so they can be injected subcutaneously without causing a rash.

If you end up taking intramuscular injections made from human urinary proteins, standing in front of a mirror when you give them may be helpful. Or ask your clinic if you can inject them into the top of your leg.

Your doctor may recommend that you take all medication intramuscularly if your body mass index (BMI) is over 30, so that the medications are absorbed better.

Getting injections from your partner

Believe it or not, most partners do very well giving injections – after the first few times, that is. Especially if they're good at darts! Giving injections is a learning experience, and unfortunately, *you* are the learning tool in this experience.

Your clinic will probably show you and your partner how to give injections, and it may send you home with a video and an information sheet that you'll refer to frequently in the first few days.

Is it really safe to put a needle in the hand of a totally untrained person and tell them to go for it? Statistically speaking, yes. Millions of diabetics inject themselves every day, or have someone else do it. The biggest risks are from infection and hitting a nerve. You can prevent infection with a careful sterile technique, and hitting a nerve can happen to anyone, even a professional, because your anatomy may not look like the textbook picture.

If at all possible, insist on doing your first injection in front of someone at your clinic, so a person skilled in this procedure can advise and give pointers. Also, after you and your partner have done it once, your partner is less likely to pass out when you do an injection at home.

Defining gonadotrophins

Gonadotrophins are *stimulating medications*, meaning that they make follicles grow. Each follicle should contain an egg, so making three follicles each month, rather than one or two, gives you a better chance of getting pregnant.

The gonadotrophins your doctor prescribes are made from pure follicle-stimulating hormone (FSH) or a combination of FSH and luteinising hormone (LH):

- ✔ Pure FSH (also called recombinant FSH) is manufactured in the lab by several manufacturers and is the most expensive. FSH can also be purified from human menopausal urine (urinary FSH) and this version is generally less expensive. The clinical effect is the same.

- ✔ Some doctors prefer that you have a little LH because they feel it aids stimulation, although others prefer a pure FSH product. The combined product usually contains a 50/50 mix of FSH and LH and is called hMG (human menopausal gonadotrophin). Combination products are cheaper and some need to be injected intramuscularly.

Because these drugs contain hormones, you can expect to be more hormonal when taking them. The most common side effects are headache, bloating, weight gain, and mood swings. Obviously, the hormone changes are going to be a big part of making a stressful situation worse for some people.

Deciding which medication to use

The choice between recombinant, pure FSH, and LH/FSH combination medications depends on several things:

✔ **Doctor preference:** Which medication does your doctor feel most comfortable working with? If your doctor has a preference, ask them why. The doctor may have done or read studies that have influenced their opinion that one is better than the other.

✔ **Cost:** If you're paying for your medication then cost is important and you may want to go with the least expensive. Little evidence shows that one 'brand' is better than another and if you require higher than average doses then cost is a consideration.

✔ **Convenience:** Urinary gonadotrophins come as a powder that needs to be mixed up into a solution before each injection.

✔ **Pain tolerance:** Subcutaneous injections can be given with a very fine needle and may sting less than intramuscular (IM) injections.

Apart from the convenience factor and comfort, no evidence is available to suggest that one is better than another at making babies with COH for IUI. They're like brands of washing powder – they all get your socks clean and your shirts white!

✔ **How needlephobic are you?** If you're extremely needle-phobic, you need to go with subcutaneous medications (see the section 'Giving yourself the injection' earlier in this chapter) or risk being a wreck for two weeks, dreading each injection.

✔ **Do you have someone to give you your injections?** If you'll be doing most of your shots yourself, you'll probably want to do subcutaneous injections.

✔ **Have you taken one or the other in the past?** How did you respond? If you've taken stimulating medications before, you have some kind of track record. Did you do well on that medication? If not, you'll probably want to try something different. If you did well, you may want to do the same, because changing to something else may change your results.

Recombinant medications are more expensive – about a third more – because they're produced in the lab. But they're all given subcutaneously.

LH/FSH products are less expensive, but they may need to be injected intramuscularly because the proteins in them can cause skin rashes. New, highly purified FSH products can be given subcutaneously and are a little cheaper than recombinant products.

Injecting hCG to mature your eggs

The last injection you'll take when doing COH is called hCG, or *human chorionic gonadotrophin*, a luteinising hormone substitute given to mature your eggs and help them release from their follicles. You're usually given this injection a day or two before your IUI.

Not all doctors give hCG. Some doctors prefer to see whether you release your egg on your own. Taking gonadotrophins sometimes affects your follicle release. Your LH may rise but not enough to mature and rupture the follicle and release the egg. If this happens, you'll probably be given hCG. If you have an adequate LH surge on your own, you won't need to take hCG.

hCG helps the eggs in the follicles to mature and complete the cell division needed before they can be fertilised. hCG is made by several companies (see Chapter 21) and is usually given intramuscularly; a newer recombinant hCG called Ovidrel can be given subcutaneously.

Don't take non-steroidal anti-inflammatories such as aspirin or ibuprofen during the middle part of your cycle. They may inhibit prostaglandin production, which may keep you from ovulating.

Ensuring proper monitoring throughout your cycle

If you're taking stimulating medications of any kind – injectables or Clomid – your clinic may want to monitor you to make sure that you're not making too many eggs. Some centres may cancel your IUI, or insist that you do in vitro fertilisation if you're making a lot of eggs, because the risk of hyperstimulation and getting pregnant with triplets – or more – is increased.

Ovarian hyperstimulation syndrome (OHSS) is a serious complication that can land you in hospital. The risk starts when you take injectable, stimulating medications and make a lot of follicles. If your oestradiol rises too high and you go on and get pregnant, OHSS may occur; it's more common with IVF but can also occur with IUI cycles. Some symptoms of OHSS are the following:

- ✔ Difficulty urinating
- ✔ Difficulty breathing
- ✔ Sudden weight gain of 10 pounds or more

If you have OHSS, your clinic may want to monitor your blood count, liver function, weight, and urine output. OHSS may not resolve itself for several days or weeks, and symptoms may worsen if you're pregnant.

OHSS isn't the only complication of taking gonadotrophins or Clomid; multiple pregnancies of three or more babies are usually the result of stimulating medications. These high-order multiples are more often the result of IUI or timed intercourse than IVF because IVF can control the number of embryos put back into the uterus, whereas IUI can't. The number of follicles you have is the number of babies you may end up with!

Boosting Progesterone

Because progesterone is essential to maintain pregnancy, many doctors give progesterone supplements in pill, suppository, or injection form to their infertility patients on an 'it can't hurt and may help' basis. Most doctors want to see a progesterone blood level of at least 10 and preferably 15 nanogrammes per millilitre after ovulation.

Another way to raise progesterone levels is to give hCG 'boosters,' usually a 2,500 IU injection of hCG every few days. hCG stimulates the corpus luteum so that it puts out more progesterone. The disadvantage to boosters is that your pregnancy test is positive, even if you're not pregnant, for up to ten days after the last hCG injection.

If you've taken gonadotrophins, you may be given both progesterone and oestrogen supplements after you ovulate. Your doctor may prescribe them because gonadotrophins can affect embryo implantation in several ways.

Because gonadotrophins can shorten the luteal phase, progesterone is given to make sure that the two-week wait actually *is* two weeks, so the embryo has time to implant before the lining starts to break down.

Stimulated cycles usually result in higher-than-normal oestrogen levels. Higher oestrogen may cause the lining of your uterus, where the embryo implants, to develop too quickly. When the embryo arrives in the uterus, the lining may have developed past the point where an embryo can attach to it.

Higher oestrogen levels can also affect the movement of the embryo through the Fallopian tubes. If the embryo moves too quickly or too slowly through the tubes, the lining won't be ready for it to implant when it arrives in the uterus.

A few recent studies show that the ratio of progesterone to oestrogen is as important as the actual values of each. Some doctors are now giving both oestrogen and progesterone after ovulation to patients who've taken stimulating medications, to keep the oestrogen and progesterone in proper balance during the luteal phase.

Chapter 12

Making Test-Tube Babies: IVF

*I*n vitro fertilisation (IVF) is the highest-tech method of getting pregnant. During an IVF cycle, you take powerful stimulating hormone drugs called gonadotrophins so that you'll make lots of eggs. Then you go through an *egg retrieval*, a minor surgical procedure to take the eggs out of the follicles they grow in. After that, the eggs are fertilised in the lab and then the resulting embryos are put back into your uterus so they can grow.

In this chapter, we discuss how to get through an IVF cycle with the least amount of frustration, explore what egg retrieval involves, and explain how your best friend's cycle may be completely different from yours, and why you needn't worry about it. (For information on what happens after the IVF cycle – creating an embryo and what to expect during implantation – skip to Chapter 16.)

Starting an IVF Cycle: A Roller Coaster Ride of Emotions

In vitro fertilisation is a complicated process. It involves you injecting powerful medications with potentially serious side effects for several weeks, taking time away from work to have blood tests and ultrasounds, and undergoing surgery, albeit minor, to retrieve your eggs. And that's just the beginning! Every step of the way through IVF is crucial, and every day brings news that will potentially thrill you or bring you to your knees in despair. Is it any wonder that you're feeling scared? And if it works, it will change your life forever!

Aggravation is a 'given' in IVF. You're late for work too often because the ultrasound scanning machine was on a 'go-slow'. Just how often will your boss believe you had a dental appointment, couldn't find the cat, lost your car keys? Your partner isn't giving you the injections properly. Your follicles aren't growing, or are growing too fast! Be prepared for all this aggravation, and you won't be quite so upset when it occurs.

Try to reframe your anxiety as excitement. You *are* in the big time and probably closer to your dream of having your baby than ever before. IVF will also give you answers that will help your doctors understand exactly what's going on. For the first time, your medical team will see your eggs, determine their quality, see firsthand whether fertilisation is occurring, and figure out what kind of embryo you make. You'll know a lot more when all is said and done.

From the emotional side, rely on that support network that you've been building. Many women on chat room sites, in self-help support group meetings, and in mind-and-body classes find 'cycle buddies,' literally other women going through IVF (or any of the lower-tech measures) at the same time. You may find comfort in sharing your experiences, good and bad, with someone else who is going through the same thing at the same time. Remember, though, to share and not compare! You're not in competition with anyone. You're trying to have *your* baby.

Looking at your drugs protocol

When you first meet your in vitro fertilisation specialist, you may come to think of him as Dr Magic. He'll probably give you a stack of totally incomprehensible paperwork that you will be tempted just to file. One of those undecipherable papers is probably your protocol. A *protocol* is nothing more than a blueprint or schedule of how your cycle will be done. It includes the medications you'll be taking, instructions on how to take them, and the procedures you need to follow throughout the cycle.

Dr Magic may review your protocol with you, or he may mumble something about the IVF nurses going over the protocol with you. If he reviews it that day, you'll probably be too excited, nervous, or scared to remember exactly what he says. Ask your favourite nurse to go over the protocol with you – it really does matter!

So it's time to take out your protocol. Step Number 1: Read the protocol. You would think this would go without saying, but it doesn't. Read the protocol! Chaps, remember the saying 'when all else fails, read the instructions' – with IVF you 'read the instructions first'!

Doctors rely on a few standard IVF protocols (we list them in Table 12-1), and most doctors prefer to use one over the others:

- ✔ **Long protocol GnRH (gonadotrophin-releasing hormone) agonist (generic names buserelin or nafarelin):** If you're under 38 and your baseline hormone levels are normal, your doctor may choose to start you on a 'long' down-regulation cycle, starting GnRH agonist a few days after you ovulate (typically on cycle day 21). This drug, which can be sniffed or injected, shuts down your normal hormone production and encourages the growth of many follicles instead of one or two. The drug also keeps you from ovulating before egg retrieval. You then start your hormone-stimulating drugs a little while after your period starts. Some centres call this a 'long' cycle, and others call it a 'down-regulation' cycle.

    GnRH agonist is an amazing drug that prevents the normal growth of one dominant follicle by suppressing your pituitary gland. Instead of stimulating a single 'dominant' follicle, as happens in a natural cycle, it allows multiple follicles to develop at the same time when you start the stimulating drugs.

- ✔ **'Short protocol' GnRH antagonist (ganerelix or cetrorelix):** Your doctor may prefer to use a newer drug called ganirelix, a GnRH antagonist (with the brand name Orgalutron), or cetrorelix (with the brand name Cetrotide), in conjunction with follicle-stimulating medications. This drug suppresses your LH surge so you won't ovulate before your egg retrieval, which makes for a shorter treatment time, but you may not get so many eggs. Pregnancy rates are similar whether you are on a 'long' or 'short' protocol, but some doctors have very strong preferences for one or the other.

- ✔ **Flare-up cycle:** If you're over 38 or have reduced ovarian reserve many IVF centres prefer to use a modified protocol, sometimes called a 'short' cycle because you take GnRH agonist for just a few days and then stop when you are ready to take your hCG. This protocol is designed to decrease the suppressing effects of the agonist that can be detrimental to those over 38 or women who are known to produce fewer eggs.

- ✔ **'Natural cycle' or minimal stimulation protocol:** You can also do a 'natural' protocol, with no, or very little, medication. This protocol isn't common, but it's used in women who don't respond to even large doses of stimulating medication due to age or previous very poor response to the stimulating drugs. In this type of cycle, your natural follicle recruitment is tracked with ultrasound and then the GnRH antagonist injections are started (along with some FSH) to stop you ovulating before egg retrieval. Because only one or two follicles grow in a 'natural cycle', success rates are very low (only 5–7 per cent per cycle started) and only half of all women having 'natural cycle' IVF get as far as embryo transfer (ET).

Your doctor will prescribe the protocol and medications he feels most comfortable to use for *your* particular case. Try not to compare what you're getting to what anyone else is using.

Table 12-1	Common IVF Protocols at a Glance		
Protocol	*Used For*	*Average Days on Medication*	*Vials of Medication Needed*
Long GnRH agonist (buserelin or nafarelin)	Women under 38; good responders	21–28 days total, including 14–21 on GnRH agonist alone	24–36 × 75 IU vials
Short GnRH antagonist (ganerelix or cetrorelix)	Poor responders on a 'long' protocol	10 days on stimulating medications; start ganirelix/ cetrorelix on day 6 of stimulating medications	About 30 to 40 vials of stimulating medications plus 5 to 6 prefilled syringes of Orgalutron or Cetrotide
'Flare-up' cycle	Poor responders; women over 38	10 to 12 days of GnRH agonist and stimulating medications	30–60 vials of stimulating medications; one bottle of GnRH agonist

Make sure that you understand your protocol before you leave the clinic. It's much better to ask questions at this stage than worry all night that you've done something wrong. You may be a brilliant tax accountant, teacher, chef, or cellist but nobody expects you to know how to give injections without being shown! Having your partner inject medications is one of the scariest parts of IVF – for you *and* for your partner. Make sure that you get very clear instructions on how to do this. (Refer to Chapter 11 for more discussion on both subcutaneous and intramuscular injections.)

Working with the staff at your IVF centre

If your IVF centre is large, nurses probably take care of only IVF patients. If your programme is smaller, the nursing staff may take care of both non-IVF and IVF patients. Some programmes have only one IVF nurse with whom you deal throughout your cycle; others have so many nurses you can't tell who's who without a checklist. Remember that, however many or few there are, they all want you to get pregnant first time!

Try to understand how your IVF unit works and to whom you need to talk about your cycle. In many centres, the IVF nurses do blood tests and also do your ultrasounds; some centres have a separate staff that take blood, and ultrasonographers who do the ultrasounds. Some centres are 'nurse led' and you may have the same nurse looking after you all the way through your IVF journey. Make sure that you talk to the right person when you have a problem, or need help.

Also, be aware that you're going to be talking to the nurses a *lot.* You'll phone to ask questions. They'll supply you with information. You'll phone again to ask yet more questions. At a certain point, you may begin to *feel* it – you've become an annoyance to the nurses. You picture the nurses throwing the phone to each other when you call, in a version of patient hot potato. You feel terrible about this. Everyone wants to be liked, and every patient also wants her questions answered without feeling like a pest.

If you're getting bad vibes, you may want to try and clear the air with the staff. Politely explain (not when everyone is busy) why you feel things are strained, and encourage some open communication about how you can best work together. Everyone benefits if the communication between you and the staff is good, and unfortunately you're the one who'll suffer the most if you don't get along with the rest of the team. Every clinic in the UK has a 'complaints procedure', and maybe a quick chat with the complaints officer will clear the air in time to salvage your cycle. Remember, needing and having IVF is very stressful. The team just want it to work for you, too, and are well aware how hormones can turn perfectly reasonable, intelligent, caring pillars of the community into wild-eyed banshees with a death wish!

Dealing with a disappearing doctor

After your initial consultation you may wonder where your doctor went. In smaller centres, doctors may do follow-ups with your blood results; some also do their own ultrasounds. In larger centres, you may feel as though your doctor has vanished from the face of the earth because all your instructions come from the nurses. This system of patient communication can be upsetting if you came to a centre specifically to deal with a particular doctor. Rest assured that your doctor *is* reviewing your progress and instructing the nurses on what you need to do next. If your centre has more than one doctor doing IVF procedures, you may also feel as if you've lost the doctor you came to see. Many centres rotate doctors through IVF on a one- or two-week cycle; you may never see the doctor you had your consultation with again! Sometimes you can request that a certain doctor does your procedure, but granting that request may not always be possible. Your doctor may be operating in another hospital or seeing patients for new appointments in the week of your retrieval.

The doctor you saw on your initial visit to the clinic may not be the doctor who is managing your IVF procedure. Try to find out what your centre's policy is for scheduling doctors and whether you can request a doctor of your choice.

Taking your medications without having a nervous breakdown

Suppose that you attended your 'taking your injection' class a week ago, and on this beautiful bright Sunday morning, you're ready to begin taking your medications. Your partner, with shaking hands, opens the first vial to mix your first injection. 'No, no!' you scream, as he proceeds to draw up the liquid. 'That's not how she said to mix it!' He stops, and both of you stare dumbfounded at the boxes, the needles, and each other. In one week you've forgotten every word the nurse said. You look at the video or DVD you were handed on giving injections again, read the instruction leaflets that tell you how to mix and inject, and still feel confused, scared, and totally out of control. And it's a Sunday. What on earth are you going to do?

Being confused: Par for the course

First, take a deep breath. Of course, giving yourself injections is hard to do. Do you think doctors and nurses were born knowing how to mix and inject medications? Most people are scared the first time they give an injection or mix a medication. Your reaction is normal.

Second, call your clinic. Some centres do IVF procedures at weekends, and if yours does, you may be able to talk to someone who can talk you through the mixing and injection. All clinics in the UK must have an emergency help line number that patients can call 24/7.

 The doctor on call won't be annoyed (unless you're ringing at 2 a.m. to say you think you left your medication on the bus!), and can at least give you some guidance. Some centres also have nurses who carry beepers so they can answer questions when the clinic is closed. If you got your medications from a large mail-order pharmacy, it may have a nurse on call who can give you instructions also. Call the main number and ask. Never got to know the doctor or nurse who lives next door? Now is as good a time as any to strike up an acquaintance! Such a person is likely to be more adept than you and can help with that vital first injection.

If you can't get anyone, take a little break, compose yourself, and then go back and try again. The procedure probably won't look quite as overwhelming the second time.

Annoying the nurses: A small price to pay

Yes, you may hear a bit of strain in the nurse's voice when she tells you, for the third time in one day, how to mix your medication. No matter. That's what she's there for, and *every* nurse would rather hear from you three times than get a phone call three days later that says you've been taking your medication wrong, wasted your very expensive medications, and probably messed up your very expensive IVF cycle. Every nurse has stories of couples who took too much, too little, or the wrong medication and had to have their cycles cancelled. You'll feel angry and stupid, the nurse will feel guilty, and you may have wasted a lot of money. So call the nurse – and don't bother to disguise your voice. She knows who you are!

Monitoring your progress (more poking and prodding)

After a few days of injections, you'll start to feel like a pro, your partner will have his injection techniques perfected, and your protocol will start to make sense to you. It's time to find out how well this process is working. It's time to have a blood test and an ultrasound.

Most centres monitor you every few days to see how you're responding to the medication. If your follicles are growing nicely and your oestradiol is rising, your medications will probably not be changed. If you're stimulating too well, or not stimulating well enough, your medications may be decreased or increased.

As a rough guide, you'll probably be on stimulating hormones ten days before you're given hCG to mature the follicle for your retrieval. During those ten days, you'll probably have blood tests and ultrasounds done four times, or maybe more or less, depending on your circumstances. Some centres insist that all your ultrasounds are done at their facility; others allow patients to be monitored at outside facilities closer to their homes. You need to find a place capable of doing same-day reports and willing to fax results to your clinic.

Some clinics operate 'satellite' IVF where your stimulation and monitoring is done at your local hospital or clinic, and you only go to the IVF centre for the egg retrieval and embryo transfer.

Getting to the point of injections

I (co-author Jill) really worried about the injections; I was always the one at school to faint after rubella and TB vaccinations, and giving blood has always got me hot, bothered, and fuzzyheaded. I discussed taking naferelin – the sniffing down-regulation drug – with my nurse, but combining working and sniffing twice a day was not practical. Asking Gwyn to inject me was no option either, as he was regularly away from home overnight or in the early morning – and anyway he has the biggest hands I have ever seen! So I bit my lip and 're-framed' self-injecting as a challenge I could overcome. I used an auto-injector so as not to see the needle going into my leg, and sometimes didn't feel it either. I'd count to five to 'release' the drug, but then try to take myself by surprise (!) I'd press the button around three or four! The red dot on my leg was usually the only telltale sign I'd done it properly and each pinprick brought us one step closer to getting pregnant!

Table 12-2 A Typical 'Long Protocol' IVF Cycle – Yours May Vary

Day of IVF Cycle	Monitoring	Medication (you have been taking GnRH for 2 to 3 weeks and continue until your hCG injection)	Time Taken
1–5	'Down-regulation' scan	FSH or HMG	150 IU once a day
6	Ultrasound and blood test	Adjust according to monitoring results	Change if clinic tells you to
8	Ultrasound and blood test		
10	Ultrasound and blood test		
	Take morning medications	Take hCG at exact time clinic tells you	
12	Egg retrieval		

The dangers of over stimulating: OHSS

Stimulating too well can be another example of too much of a good thing. The goal of IVF is to have a number of follicles grow so that plenty of eggs can be retrieved. This result hopefully prevents you from having to do multiple cycles of IVF to get pregnant, because your extra embryos may possibly be frozen and used later if you don't get pregnant on your first try. With some women, especially those who have polycystic ovaries (Chapter 7 has more on this condition), hyperstimulation can get way out of hand very quickly.

If your oestradiol rises too fast, or if you make too many follicles – 20 or more – you run a risk of developing OHSS, or ovarian hyperstimulation syndrome. Patients with OHSS can be very ill after egg retrieval, with swollen ovaries and fluid in the pelvis and around the lungs. Some women become sick enough to require hospitalisation, and a few patients have died from severe OHSS, which causes fluid volume shifts through your whole body and can make your blood very thick, and prone to clotting.

Because OHSS is potentially so serious, IVF centres watch patients on stimulating medications very closely, monitoring their blood and ultrasound results every few days. If your clinic thinks that you're in danger of severe OHSS, you may have to freeze all your embryos after retrieval and not do an embryo transfer. OHSS becomes worse if you become pregnant, due to the rising hormone levels from the pregnancy. Some centres may not do egg retrieval at all, because the hCG trigger given before retrieval also makes OHSS worse.

The downside of under stimulating

If you're not stimulating well, your clinic may increase your medication to see whether you can do better. This situation also requires closer monitoring because your medications may require frequent adjustment. See Table 12-2 for a typical IVF stimulation cycle, but remember that your cycle may vary.

Waiting for the phone to ring . . . again and again

The phone rings at 4 p.m., and you grab it off the hook. 'Hi, this is Nancy Nurse,' chirps the voice on the other end. Your whole world stops for a second, as you try to decipher from the tone of her voice whether she has good news or bad news.

Waiting for the phone to ring is just a part of IVF. Do you remember what is was like when you sat waiting for the phone to ring because you were sure that the nice boy you met at the pizza house really had asked your friend for your phone number? IVF is a bit like that. You find yourself leaving whole volumes of information on how to reach you that day (mobile phone, home phone, don't leave a message with the babysitter, partner's number, don't call before 6 p.m., don't call after 6 p.m., don't leave a message, I really need to talk to you) on the message pad because this call, whether good or bad news, is the highlight of your day.

If your clinic has a lot of staff, try to cultivate a good relationship with one or two nurses you feel comfortable with. It doesn't hurt to ask to speak to that nurse when you call. Most nurses are happy to call you if you personally ask for them. Also, if you get to know one or two people well, you hopefully won't have to explain all the ins and outs of your case every time you call in.

Feeling as if everyone in the waiting room is doing better than you

You're sitting in the waiting room, listening to the person ahead of you brag about how well her cycle is going, how she's got 20 beautiful follicles, how good her partner is at giving the injections, how she loves the nurses so much she's baking cakes for them to say thank you, how great her veins are, and how happy she is to be alive. You look at your poor black and blue arms and think about how you've only seven follicles on ultrasound, how your partner seems to hit a nerve every other day, how much you hate all the nurses, and how much you hate this whole process.

In some centres, the waiting room is like group therapy in a psychiatrist's office: All the patients pull their chairs together while waiting for their ultrasound appointments and talk about IVF and life in general. This kind of place can provide you with new friends who know exactly what you're going through, but it can also turn into a sort of golf course with chairs – she got pregnant on the first try, she has the most follicles, she's doing better than she did last cycle, she's having twins . . .

Stay out of the comparison contests, if you can. Everyone responds differently to medications, and in the end, the person with three follicles may get pregnant, and the person with twenty follicles may not. Remember that the only statistics that matter are your own.

If talking to other people about your problems makes you feel worse, don't join in. Bring a book and headphones and put an unapproachable expression on your face. Arrive as close to the time of your appointment as you can, get engrossed in the TV, or hide in the ladies!

On the other hand, if you can listen to other women's tales and not compare yourself to them, the waiting room can be a great source of camaraderie and a place to make lasting friendships.

Feeling as if you've been on gonadotrophins your whole life

Are you setting some sort of record for the most days ever spent taking gonadotrophins? It probably feels like it. Gonadotrophins can cause mood swings, headaches, and bloating, all side effects that make you anxious to discontinue these drugs as soon as possible. You'll probably be on medications for at least ten days if you're doing a standard protocol; slow starters may spend nearly twice that amount of time on medications before their follicles are big enough to go to retrieval (usually about 18 to 20 millimetres). Although some doctors believe that staying on these medications too long negatively affects your egg quality, other doctors don't see a problem with continuing these medications for 15 or 16 days as long as your follicles are growing.

Recognising when your oestradiol level is too high

Your oestradiol level (the active oestrogen hormone produced by the granulosa cells in the follicles, shortened to E2) is usually directly related to the number of follicles you have. Each follicle produces an oestradiol of 100 to 200 units, so if you've ten follicles, your E2 (oestradiol) will be between 1,000 and 2,000 units when the follicles are mature.

When the skinny little blonde in the waiting room says proudly, 'My oestradiol's over 3,000', you wonder – even though you know not to make comparisons – 'Isn't that too high?' How high is too high? Most programmes consider you to be moderately hyperstimulated when your oestradiol is over 2,000, and classify you as severely hyperstimulated when the level reaches 4,000 or 5,000.

If your E2 is too high, you won't be able to do a fresh embryo transfer, so most centres try to keep your E2 and follicle count to a reasonable number. In an ideal world, every patient would have 10 to 15 follicles and an E2 of between 2,000 and 2,500.

Ovarian hyperstimulation syndrome (OHSS) is a potentially life-threatening complication of taking infertility medications; it's more common in IVF patients because they usually take high doses of stimulating hormones. OHSS causes severe fluid shifts in your circulatory system, with fluid from your blood vessels leaking into your surrounding tissues. Sudden large weight gain, difficulty urinating, and shortness of breath are some signs of OHSS that your centre will want you to know about and report to them as soon as possible.

Feeling blue is normal

We can't stress enough that mood swings are normal with high hormone levels. You also may experience a let-down feeling when doing an IVF cycle. You've planned for it and fantasised about how things would go, and now it's almost over. It's like Christmas: Sometimes the anticipation surpasses the reality. When you're almost ready for egg retrieval, you can't change things. It's too late to say, 'We should have waited another month' or, 'I ought to have taken more meds, less meds, or different meds.'

Taking a Shot in the Dark: Time for hCG

It's Nancy Nurse on the phone again, and this time you can tell that she's got *really* big news. 'It's time for your late night injection of hCG!' she says, and because she sounds so excited, you feel excited too. If you've read your protocol, you know what hCG (human chorionic gonadotrophin) is; if you haven't, here's a refresher course.

hCG is a crucial part of your IVF cycle. hCG is given about 35 hours before your egg retrieval; its job is to mature your eggs and prepare them to be fertilised. Giving hCG allows the IVF staff to plan egg retrievals for a reasonable time during the day, instead of waiting for your natural LH surge to occur. That's why the timing of your hCG is very important.

The hCG instructions include a specific time to take your injection, and following the directions is absolutely critical because timing really is everything. Your injection may be scheduled for midnight, or even a few hours later, if your centre has a lot of egg retrievals to do on one day.

If your injection is scheduled for, say, 2 a.m., you can mix the medication a little ahead of time and put it on your bedside table; then set your alarm for the time you need to take the hCG. Giving the injection at an odd hour is easier if you don't need to fumble around mixing medications when you're half asleep. If you normally have a close friend or neighbour to do your injections, you may have a problem getting them to give hCG in the middle of the night. Be aware ahead of time that you need to find someone willing to do this when the time comes.

Going for the Gold: The Egg Retrieval

Almost before you know it, it's time for your egg retrieval. Some IVF centres do egg retrievals every day of the week. Others do retrievals only Monday through Friday and start their patients' medications all at the same time to avoid the weekends. Still others cycle patients through in batches, doing retrievals only every other week. You probably won't have much say in what day or what time your retrieval is done.

Reducing the anxiety with medication

All kinds of emotions are probably churning around inside you and your partner. This is the culmination of several weeks of injections, emotions, and worries. It's your big day! How do you feel?

Surgery is always a little scary, even when it's surgery for something you want very badly. You may be having a general anaesthetic or (preferably) just sedation, but either way you will get medication to make you comfortable during the retrieval, and some centres give medications before the retrieval to relax you.

Signing here . . . and here . . . and here . . .

Informed consent is a very important part of an IVF cycle and all these forms need to be taken very seriously. Some centres ask you to sign consent forms ahead of time for your egg retrieval, but you may be asked to sign the day of the retrieval. Usually a nurse reviews the consent forms with you. Keep in mind that your anxiety level will be through the roof, and the chances that you'll be able to read and comprehend the pages of legal jargon on the morning of your retrieval are slim. If possible, ask for the consent forms ahead of time so that you have time to read and understand what you'll be signing.

The HFEA (Human Fertilisation and Embryology Authority) has official consent forms that are centrally registered, and the clinic has its own forms relating to the procedure itself and any additional bells and whistles you may be having, such as ICSI or assisted hatching. You will be given a copy of all the consents that you sign, which you need to keep them in a safe place!

Here are the most common concerns that people have with IVF consent forms:

- ✔ Having pictures taken of themselves, their eggs, sperm, or embryos, for use in any type of publication. Many people have no objection to this, but some do.

- ✔ Allowing medical, nursing, or other students in the room to watch the procedure.

- ✔ Using any sperm, eggs, embryos, or tissue for research. 'Tissue' can mean fluid from follicles, endometrial tissue, or anything else removed at the time of retrieval or transfer.

- ✔ Freezing of any embryos not transferred on a fresh transfer. Some people have religious objections to embryo freezing, and they want to inseminate only a few eggs so that they can use up all their embryos and not have any left to freeze. Discuss this step ahead of time with the embryology staff to make sure that everyone understands exactly what will be done.

Rescheduling the retrieval

You can count on Murphy's Law occurring at retrieval time. If you have a big event coming up around the time of your egg retrieval, the day of the big event will be the same day your retrieval is scheduled. In most cases, your doctor may be able to do your egg retrieval a day earlier or later to get you through a big occasion. Sometimes, however, due to your blood levels indicating that you may ovulate if you wait, your centre may not be able to schedule around your event.

If you know ahead of time about an event that may conflict with your egg retrieval, tell your doctor about it *before* you start taking your stimulating hormones. Sometimes the time of an egg retrieval can be held off for a few days if you take the GnRH agonist a few extra days before starting your stimulating medications. After you start stimulating medications, influencing the day of your retrieval is harder.

Your IVF cycle is the most important thing in your life at the moment so don't arrange it during the firm's annual sales conference, your stepdaughter's A levels, or your great granny's 100th birthday party!

If you have objections to anything in the consent forms, address them before the morning of your egg retrieval. If your clinic has a problem with your requests, it may delay or cancel your retrieval.

Meeting the retrieval team

You'll probably have met all or some of the people who will be with you for the egg retrieval; that's great. During the egg retrieval, a nurse or a medical assistant may be in the room helping the doctor and the embryologist will be very nearby. Hopefully, you'll know the nurse. With any luck, you'll also know the doctor, too, although, the doctor you had your initial consultation with may not do your egg retrieval.

Undergoing the egg retrieval procedure

Different centres do things different ways, but in most centres, you're taken to the IVF suite, a part of the building that you may never have seen before and had no idea existed. You may change into a gown, hat, and shoe covers because the IVF suite is a sterile area where an attempt is made to keep outside germs from entering. IVF centres vary about how 'clinically' they do things. There is no evidence that scrubbing everyone and everything with Dettol makes any difference to the pregnancy rates!

An intravenous (IV) infusion is started. The purpose of the IV is mainly to have access for giving you medication, but it's also there in case any complications require you to be given large amounts of fluid quickly. If you know that certain of your veins are better than others for the IV, don't be shy about informing the person starting your IV!

The embryologist usually comes in to see you before the procedure starts to ask you to verify your name, clinic number, and information about your partner. The purpose of checking this information is to prevent any type of mix-up with eggs, sperm, or embryos.

The doctor generally comes into the room at the last minute, hopefully introduces himself if you don't already know him, and instructs the person giving you medications to start giving them. The doctor inserts a speculum and wipes the vagina and cervix gently, trying to keep the area as clean as possible and may give a local anaesthetic injection either side of the cervix.

You won't remember the rest, so we explain what happens next. The doctor inserts the vaginal ultrasound probe into your vagina. On the top of the probe is a needle guide along which a long metal needle slides. The doctor locates your follicles on ultrasound with the probe and then punctures the back of the vagina with the needle, entering each follicle and sucking out the fluid. The follicular fluid is given to the embryologist, who examines it under a microscope and says, hopefully, 'Egg one, egg two' and so on. When the follicles are all emptied, you'll wake up and be taken to a nearby bed for a short time to recover. An egg retrieval (see Figure 12-1) usually takes about 15 to 20 minutes from start to finish, and you'll be asleep the whole time or so drowsy that you may just as well be asleep.

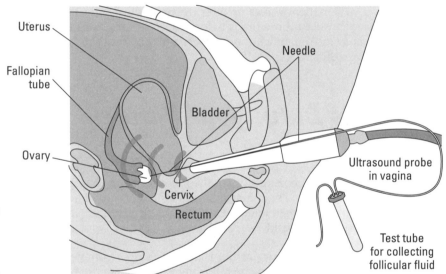

Figure 12-1: IVF egg collection.

Knocking you out: Anaesthesia choices for the retrieval

IVF centres vary considerably in their methods of anaesthesia for egg retrievals. Some centres do all their retrievals in a hospital operating suite, so an anaesthetist gives your medications. Smaller centres may have only an assistant or the nurse giving medication under the guidance of your doctor. Still others offer you a choice between conscious sedation and general anaesthetic. With conscious sedation, you receive some version of medication in the valium family, possibly Valium or Midazolam, and also some type of narcotic, such as Fentanyl, or Pethidine. The degree to which you're awake during your procedure varies quite a bit among individuals. If you've taken narcotics frequently in the past, you may develop a tolerance to them, and they may not make you comfortable. Some women are much more sensitive to all drugs and need very little medication to put them to sleep. Your vital signs, including your heart rate, blood pressure, and respirations, are carefully monitored during your procedure.

Certain medications, such as Midazolam, have amnesiac properties, which is a fancy way of saying that you won't remember what went on during the retrieval. This effect lasts for a short time after the procedure as well. Nearly every IVF patient wakes up after the procedure and asks, 'How many eggs did I have?' at least three times before she's actually awake enough to remember the answer! You may not remember walking from the table to a bed, either, but you did!

Doing His Duty: Your Partner Is Busy, Too

While you're snoozing away in the recovery suite, your partner may be flicking through the 'top shelf' magazines helpfully provided for him to masturbate to produce a semen specimen. This can be a tricky issue for some men and downright impossible for others.

If you think that your partner is going to suffer from performance anxiety on retrieval day, consider the following ways to take the pressure off:

✔ **You can have him freeze a specimen ahead of time.** Most centres prefer to use fresh sperm, but if your partner knows a frozen backup is available, he may have an easier time in the producing room.

✔ **He can go to a nearby hotel, or home, if you live close enough** – within 15 to 20 minutes away – use a sterile pot the andrologist will give him, and produce there.

✔ **You can help him produce.** You may feel uncomfortable going in with him, but believe me, it's no big deal – people do it all the time. But andrologists enforce two rules: no saliva and no lubricants. Either one can mess up the semen specimen. If you're going to help him, then do so before your egg retrieval . . . you may not be much use afterwards if your tummy hurts and you keep falling asleep!

Answering Common Egg Retrieval Questions

Almost everybody asks these questions about their egg retrieval:

- ✔ **Can I see my eggs before I go home?** You can't see your eggs because they can be seen only under a microscope, and no embryologist in the world is going to let a patient still lurching around in an anaesthetic daze mess around with an extremely expensive microscope or those precious eggs!

- ✔ **Can my partner be with me in the retrieval room?** In some centres, partners are allowed to be present at the egg retrieval. Other centres don't allow anyone else to be in the room for the retrieval, although they're often allowed in for the embryo transfer. Usually the rooms are too small to allow extra people, and no one wants partners feeling woozy in the retrieval room and knocking over the ultrasound equipment if they fall.

- ✔ **Do I have to have an intravenous access (IV)?** Yes, it's a little plastic tube inserted in a vein in your hand, through which you will receive the drugs required for the egg retrieval.

- ✔ **Are you *sure* that you won't mix up my eggs (or sperm or embryos) with someone else's?** Yes.

  With several mix-up cases in the news recently, most centres are anxious to reassure patients on this topic. Mix-ups with sperm, embryos, or eggs happen only when someone is extremely careless, and all centres are very aware of the recent cases in the news and are being extremely careful to avoid such an incidence.

  Most centres label all dishes, collection pots, and so on with the patient's name, clinic number, date of birth, and sometimes a colour code. Egg retrievals and embryo transfers are done one at a time – never two at the same time. Catheters used for embryo transfer are never reused, so someone else's embryo won't be stuck in your catheter!

  After an embryo transfer, the catheter used is examined again to make sure that none of your embryos decided to stay behind. All those little guys should be in the uterus, where they belong!

  In the UK we have a system of *double witnessing*, which means that at every step of the way, whenever eggs or sperm are prepared or moved or used then a second witness, as well as the embryologist doing the procedure, has to confirm all the details are correct!

- ✔ **Where do you keep the eggs?** Eggs are kept overnight with the specially prepared sperm in a petri dish (shallow plastic dish) in an incubator and then checked in the morning for fertilisation.

✔ **Where do you keep the frozen embryos?** Frozen embryos are kept in little colour-coded straws in a liquid nitrogen tank.

✔ **What happens if your power goes out? How do the embryos survive?** Nitrogen tanks don't use electricity. For everything else, centres have backup generator power. In the UK, all liquid nitrogen tanks must be fitted with automatic temperature alarms that activate if the temperature changes even a fraction of a degree. If this happens out of hours, the sensors then automatically dial all the scientists on the rota until someone answers and comes in to sort the problem out. Don't worry!

✔ **How many eggs did you say I have?** Sigh.

Chapter 13

ICSI: It Only Takes One Good Sperm!

*E*ven though standard IVF, covered in Chapter 12, is quite useful for moderately poor sperm (low counts of less than one million, or sperm that can only doggy paddle rather than swim 1,000 metres free-style, or sperm that are really, really funny shapes), some sperm wouldn't recognise an egg or know what to do with it if they bumped into one. Fortunately, ICSI (intracytoplasmic sperm injection), which Belgian embryologists discovered by accident, means that such sperm have the chance to fertilise an egg.

A happy accident

Many good things happen by accident in medicine, and ICSI is the new technique that has transformed the chances of parenthood for infertile men. By 1992, realising that some sperm can't penetrate the outer 'shell' of the egg (the *zona pellucida*), some talented embryologists in Belgium started to introduce a few sperm through the outer layer into the 'gap' between the zona pellucida and the actual egg (the *ooplasm*) in the hope that the sperm would be able to do the last bit of the journey. This method was called SUZI (subzonal insertion), and was very difficult to carry out and not very successful!

What everybody knew (or thought they knew!) was that you can't inject a sperm directly into an egg, because if you did, the egg would die. Well, it turns out that everyone was wrong. The embryologist doing SUZI accidentally injected sperm directly into a few eggs. Not only did the eggs not die, but they fertilised beautifully and went on to make fine young embryos. ICSI was born and was soon being performed all over the world.

So now we have two things to thank Belgium for: Tin-Tin and ICSI! If you get a chance, do see ICSI happening (most IVF units have tapes or training videos you can watch).

In this chapter, we explain who can benefit from ICSI, how it works, and what you need to know before you pursue this treatment option.

Understanding How ICSI Works

In ICSI (intracytoplasmic sperm injection), a sperm is injected directly into an egg. To accomplish this technique, the embryologist has to prepare the egg and then the sperm for the eventual meeting.

Here's the process in a nutshell:

1. **The sperm are washed in special solution to clean off the debris.**

2. **The sperm are placed in a warm incubator that encourages the good sperm to start swimming.**

3. **The embryologist removes the cumulus and the coronal layers from the egg, which helps prepare the egg for injection.**

4. **A tiny amount of the washed sperm is put in a very thick solution (called PVP) to slow them down and allow them to be 'caught'.** ICSI is done under a high-powered microscope, subject to the most sterile conditions possible. Because there's no room for wobble when injecting an egg invisible to the naked eye, micromanipulators are necessary. They 'gear down' the embryologist's movements, enabling her to work with precision.

5. **The 'naked' eggs are placed into droplets in the same little dishes as the sperm.** The embryologist takes the dish to the microscope equipped with micromanipulators. It's time to go on a sperm hunt.

6. **The embryologist patiently stalks and then catches a sperm.**

7. **The embryologist breaks the sperm's tail.** Breaking the tail stops the sperm from thrashing around inside the egg and disrupting the delicate structures in the *ooplasm* (the 'jelly' in the egg).

8. **Using a tiny glass needle about ¹⁄₁₀th the thickness of a human hair, the embryologist picks the sperm up and injects it into the egg.** During the injection, the egg is held steady at the correct orientation so that the spindle isn't damaged.

9. **The embryologist finally withdraws the needle and sets of in pursuit of another lucky sperm.**

Knowing Who Can Benefit from ICSI

ICSI is the fertility treatment of choice for men who have these fertility issues:

- ✔ Very low sperm count (*oligospermia*).

- ✔ Abnormally shaped sperm (poor *morphology*) and/or sperm that are poor swimmers (poor *motility*).

- ✔ Sperm that can't penetrate their partner's eggs (*egg-sperm interaction failure*) or absence of the *acrosome* (*globospermia*).

- ✔ Tubes carrying sperm from the testes to the penis (vas deferens) are damaged or blocked (by infection, trauma, or vasectomy) or missing (congenital bilateral absence of the vas deferens, or CBAVD for short, as in cystic fibrosis).

- ✔ Immune system reacts to the sperm they produce (antisperm antibodies).

- ✔ Problems with erection or ejaculation (spinal cord injuries, Hodgkin's disease, diabetes, and prostate surgery).

A clinic may also sometimes recommend ICSI if previous egg collections for IVF have produced only a few eggs or unexpected failure of fertilisation occurs.

Recognising a Good Sperm When You See One

Embryologists recognise that they have a big responsibility to pick the best sperm for ICSI. This task can be very time consuming if the sperm count is very low. Sperm that are moving are probably healthy, and if moving, active sperm aren't available, the embryologist tries to pick out sperm for fertilisation that are at least 'twitching.' If the sperm are all lying motionless at the bottom of the dish then a technique called HOST (hypo-osmotic swelling test) will identify the live sperm that are suitable for injection.

Thinking Ahead: Things to Know about ICSI

Some studies have shown that ICSI embryos have a higher than normal rate of *aneuploidy*, or abnormal chromosomes. This higher rate may occur because men with severe male factor (very low sperm count) have more chromosomal abnormalities, such as Klinefelter's syndrome.

A low sperm count caused by genetic problems can be passed on to a child, so you may be advised to take a blood test to check your chromosomes before going ahead with ICSI. Remember these tests can show that you carry a gene for a serious genetic or inherited disease so you may want to talk to a genetic counsellor or the clinic's counsellor before having the tests. Because ICSI is a fairly new technique, doctors don't yet know whether injecting the sperm into the egg to achieve fertilisation may have possible long-term consequences for the child. Although some studies suggest that ICSI is associated with certain genetic and developmental defects in a very small number of children born using this treatment, this possibility may be caused by the underlying infertility problem rather than by the technique itself.

You also run the risk that if your ICSI-conceived child is a boy, he may inherit his father's infertility problems along with his blue eyes and blond hair (or Daddy's other characteristics!). This consequence is because the genes for making sperm are all found on the Y chromosome. It's too early to know if this is the case, because the oldest boys born from ICSI are still only in their early teens. By the time they want to be fathers, we'll be even better at IVF!

Chapter 14

'Babies on Ice': Egg Freezing and Fertility Treatment

*M*en with cancer who need chemotherapy, radiotherapy, or surgery have been able to freeze their sperm for the last 50 years. Recently, a baby was born in the UK from sperm that had been frozen for over 20 years. Fish fingers may need to be eaten after three months in the freezer but, at the ultra-low temperatures of liquid nitrogen, sperm will last forever.

Until recently, however, little was on offer for young women facing a choice between the chemotherapy that could save their lives, and the certainty of premature menopause and sterility.

Early attempts proved that freezing eggs was more problematic than freezing sperm. Oocytes (eggs) are large (well, about the size of the point of a pin!), delicate structures, which when frozen are very susceptible to 'ice crystals' that form in the egg and shatter the spindle apparatus that controls the genetic machinery.

The first human live births resulting from previously frozen eggs were in 1986 when the world's first 'test-tube baby', Louise Brown, was still only 8 years old. The technique wasn't widely adopted due to the extremely low success rates: Few of the eggs survived the thaw, the fertilisation rates were very poor, and anxieties existed about damage to the cells. At that time doctors estimated that 100 healthy eggs were required to get just one live birth.

Fortunately, the problems that plagued early efforts have been solved, and egg freezing and fertility treatment is now a possible option for women.

Freezing Eggs: Coming In from the Cold

The most successful egg-freezing recipes depend upon a 'slow freeze, rapid thaw' method using high concentrations of glucose (sugar) as a dehydrating agent and a special 'antifreeze' to stop ice crystals forming. (But don't offer to do a deal with your local garage next time they top up your radiator; you need a very, very special antifreeze!) The freeze–thaw cycle causes hardening of the egg shell (zona pellucida) and fertilisation requires the ICSI technique (refer to Chapter 13) in which an individual sperm is injected into a mature egg; see Figure 14-1.

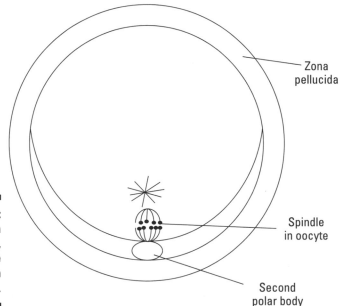

Figure 14-1:
The human
egg,
showing the
'spindle' in
the nucleus.

Zona
pellucida

Spindle
in oocyte

Second
polar body

The even newer technique of *vitrification* (flash freezing) now offers egg survival rates of 70 per cent, and pregnancy rates per embryo transfer that compare well with those of frozen embryos (more than 25 per cent per transfer). Fertilisation rates with ICSI are equivalent with fresh and frozen eggs. Strawberries go all squishy in the freezer, but eggs don't!

Eggs for freezing are collected in just the same way as eggs for IVF (refer to Chapter 12). Only really mature eggs (known as metaphase II or Met II eggs) can be frozen, so it's important that the follicles are good sizes (18–22 millimetres) before the final hCG injection (Chapter 11 tells you more) is given. After the egg collection, the eggs are assessed for maturity, the cumulus cells (the fluffy cloud-like cells around the egg) are removed, and the eggs are dipped in the sugar and antifreeze solutions.

A computer-controlled 'freeze machine' slowly takes the eggs down from body temperature (37 degrees) to absolute zero (−196 degrees centigrade). At this temperature all cellular activity stops and the eggs are 'frozen in time'.

Reaping the Benefits of Egg Freezing

Many different groups of fertility patients may benefit from the relatively new technique of egg freezing. As with all fertility treatment, remember that egg freezing does not offer a guarantee of a baby, but it does offer a chance.

Cancer patients

One in 1,000 young adults are survivors of childhood or adolescent cancer, and for many adolescent girls and young women in this group, egg freezing offers a chance of future genetic motherhood that can be of enormous psychological support to themselves (and their parents) during a difficult time of stress and potentially shattered ambitions.

Under UK law, the Human Fertilisation and Embryology Authority (HFEA) takes the view that 'the option most likely to result in pregnancy for adult cancer patients with impaired fertility who are unable to cryopreserve embryos is that of mature oocyte (egg) freezing'.

Egg freezing for young, single women who need cancer treatment offers them a chance of a future genetic pregnancy. At first, the types of cancers considered suitable for egg freezing were restricted to the blood cancers (leukaemia, Hodgkin's, and non-Hodgkin's lymphoma), or non-hormone dependent cancers (bowel, osteoma, or sarcoma). But now so many women are being diagnosed with breast cancer (25 per cent of diagnoses are in pre-menopausal women) before they have completed or even started their families, resulting in a relaxation of the previous rule that women with breast cancer must never be treated with gonadotrophins. Increasingly, many cancer doctors take the view that as long as chemotherapy begins immediately after ovarian stimulation and egg retrieval has been performed, high levels of oestradiol for a few days doesn't damage a patient's prospect of remission or cure.

Ovarian tissue freezing has significant theoretical advantages over egg freezing because ovarian cortical slices (the most active 'rim' around the ovary) may be obtained (at laparoscopy) and cryopreserved without any delay beginning chemotherapy. The cortical slices may be returned as an *in situ* graft to allow ovulation, fertilisation, and conception in the body, as 'normal'.

Two births in Belgium and Israel have been reported following this technique. Alternatively, the tissue may be implanted in an accessible place, such as the forearm (yes, that's the forearm!), where development of the follicles can be monitored by ultrasound and conventional egg retrieval for IVF performed. Although ovarian cortical tissue provides a good source of potential eggs, there's a theoretical risk of reintroducing malignant cells, and a general anaesthetic and laparoscopy may be considered too much to bear for a young woman struck down by cancer.

People with religious objections to embryo freezing

Egg freezing may also be a choice for couples who need IVF, but who may have religious or ethical objections to freezing excess embryos. If you believe that life begins at the moment of fertilisation then embryos have the moral status of people and just can't be put in the deep freeze. Freezing eggs (rather than embryos) may be seen as a way by which the costs and risks of ovarian stimulation and egg retrieval can be minimised and yet allow the couple a cumulative chance of pregnancy equivalent to that achieved with repeated transfer of frozen embryos.

We (co-author Gill) started egg freezing at our clinic in 2000 for young cancer patients, but the first time we needed to 'test the recipe' was in 2001 for a couple who had ethical objections to embryo freezing. We couldn't do a fresh transfer for this couple, so we froze the unfertilised eggs instead. Their second thaw cycle in 2002 produced the UK's first 'frozen egg' baby, a beautiful little girl called Emily.

Women with poor ovarian reserve

If you're worried that the ticking noise you keep hearing is your biological clock running down then 'poor ovarian reserve' may be the problem. Poor reserve, associated with a low response to ovarian stimulation and the production of only a few eggs, often of poor quality, is an increasingly common diagnosis in fertility clinics.

Early menopause runs (or sprints!) in families down the female line, so if you're thinking of delaying starting to try for a baby, remember to ask your mum and granny when their periods stopped. Don't forget that they were probably starting their families at a much younger age than today's would-be mums. Some, but not all, women with poor ovarian reserve will be trying to conceive in their late 30s or early 40s and many will be well aware that their eggs are 'past their sell-by date'. For these women, their best, if not their only, chance of having a baby, lies with the use of donor eggs.

Benefits of egg freezing techniques for donor egg programmes

In the UK, eggs for donation are usually used fresh, whereas donor sperm is always frozen.

The use of egg freezing techniques would:

✔ Allow 'egg banks' to be established just like sperm banks, and then the eggs could be quarantined for six months before use

✔ Enable better 'matching' of donor and recipient's characteristics

✔ Avoid the need for extended HRT to 'schedule' recipients' cycles. With frozen thawed eggs, recipients who were still ovulating could have the embryos created from frozen thawed eggs transferred in a 'natural' cycle and not need to take drugs during the first few months of pregnancy.

✔ Ensure anonymity. Egg donors participating in altruistic or 'egg share' programmes should not meet the women receiving their eggs but in small clinics it's often very difficult to schedule appointments at different times or on different days for donors and recipients.

The Bridget Joneses of the world

'Bridget Jones' is the stereotype of the goodtime girl who is too busy partying, drinking Chardonnay, and worrying about her weight to settle down and make babies the old-fashioned way (with a nice man who loves visiting IKEA and spends the weekends putting up shelves!). Today's poor Bridget faces a big problem. She knows she wants to have kids one day but she first has to pay off her student loan, save up for a deposit on a flat, work her way up the career ladder, *and* find Mr Right. And all that time her biological clock is running down. By the time she is ready to make babies she may well only have a few years left . . .

Getting pregnant over the age of 35 takes twice as long as under 35 and by the time Bridget (and Mr Darcy) have tried for two years, even high-tech fertility treatments may not be able to help.

Of course, most women who opt for 'social' egg freezing aren't business tycoons who 'forgot' to have children: Often they have been caring for elderly relatives, trying to get on the first rung of the housing ladder (or even to find out where the ladder is propped up), finding Mr Right or even, sadly discovering that Mr Right doesn't share her dreams of marriage and babies. If Mr Darcy decides at 36 that he isn't quite ready for parenthood, he has another 10 or even 20 years to think about it. Poor Bridget has only 3 or 4 years at best.

Completing the Job: Thawing, Fertilisation, and Transfer

Eggs (like embryos) can be frozen for up to ten years in the UK (and in special circumstances they may be stored for even longer). At the temperature of 'absolute zero' (–196 degrees Celsius) all biological processes come to a halt and when the eggs are thawed they're just as fresh as when they were frozen.

Thawing eggs is the reverse of freezing, but much faster. The antifreeze mixture is washed off and the shrivelled little egg is placed in a dilute solution to rehydrate it so it gets nice and plump again. When it has recovered it can be ICSI injected (refer to Chapter 13). The fertilisation rate is just as good as for fresh eggs. Embryo transfer is just the same as in conventional IVF or ICSI, as explained in Chapters 12 and 13. The chance of a pregnancy occurring from embryos created from frozen eggs is the same as from frozen embryos and, as ever in fertility treatment, varies with the age of the woman at the time the eggs were harvested.

Creating a Storm in a Test Tube – The Controversy over Freezing Eggs

When our (co-author Gill) clinic announced the birth of the UK's first 'frozen egg' baby in 2003, we were attacked on all sides by people who realised that egg freezing could allow women to 'beat' their biological destiny and possibly extend their reproductive life span until it was as long as a man's. My response was, 'And your problem is what exactly?'

The prospect of women who aren't in a position to start a pregnancy now, but who wish to become mothers in the future, choosing to have their eggs frozen as an 'insurance policy' against future subfertility, seems to have stirred up the greatest disquiet about of egg freezing.

Women need to be aware of the difficulties and dangers of late pregnancy: the delay in conceiving and the risk of miscarriage, and genetic abnormality. In the UK, 15 per cent of all babies are born to women aged 35 and over, and 9 per cent of all first live births are to women over 35. These women are the lucky ones that actually have babies. Many more conceive and miscarry, or never even conceive. Clearly, a woman is far more likely to achieve a successful pregnancy aged 40 and over with her own eggs that were cryopreserved in her 30s than with her own 'time expired' eggs in her 40s. You wouldn't try to make an omelette with a 40-year egg, let alone a baby!

Despite media warnings that egg freezing will encourage legions of career-centric alpha-females to freeze their eggs between botox appointments and test-driving their latest two-seater convertible, only a hundred UK women have opted for the procedure. And almost all of these still hope to conceive naturally, rather than schedule an appointment for the thaw and fertilisation of the eggs once they're 45 and have a seat on the Board.

It's early days for egg freezing and only a few hundred 'ice-babies' have been born worldwide compared to over a million babies born following IVF and ICSI. However, all the babies born to date have been healthy and there are no more reasons, scientifically speaking, to worry about freezing eggs rather than freezing embryos. Egg freezing is certainly not going to persuade all young women to delay settling down until they are over 40 because they have a few frozen eggs in the freezer, but the situation may allow a few more women to experience the joy of giving birth to their 'own' baby.

Chapter 15

Giving, Receiving, and Sharing: Egg Donor Treatments

*E*gg donation is a growing national trend, because one of the commoner causes of infertility now is women trying to conceive at older ages with eggs that are past their 'sell by' date.

Unlike sperm donation, which has been around for decades, the use of donor eggs is a fairly new phenomenon. The process required the invention and perfection of IVF (in vitro fertilization) in order to become practical.

The decision to move on to donor eggs can be a tough one. Your specialist says: 'You have a 5 per cent chance of a baby with your own eggs and a 40 per cent chance with donor eggs!' Easy decision? No! You and your partner need to have a long, hard think about why you want to be parents and quite how significant a complete genetic link to your child is to you.

Using Donor Eggs: The Whys and Wherefores

The reasons for using donor eggs are similar to those for using donor sperm. The recipient doesn't make any eggs, doesn't make enough eggs, or doesn't make good eggs. This lack of good eggs may be due to premature ovarian failure or age, or the woman may carry a lethal gene or chromosome disorder that she doesn't want to risk passing on to her baby.

Using donor eggs is fairly complicated; IVF centres usually try to coordinate the menstrual cycles of the egg donor and recipient so that the donor produces eggs that can become embryos at exactly the right time for the recipient's uterus to receive them. That way, the recipient can have transferred into her uterus *fresh* embryos that were created a few days before in the IVF lab. This transfer requires monitoring the recipient at an IVF centre to make sure that her uterus is ready to receive the embryos.

Finding an Egg Donor

Perhaps you're wondering how you can obtain donor eggs. You have three options: a woman who's going through fertility treatment at the same clinic as you, a friend or relative who's keen to help, or an altruistic egg donor – a woman without fertility problems who wants to share her good fortune (and egg-making capabilities) with others.

Of course, asking someone to be an egg donor for you is much more complicated than asking someone to be a sperm donor. Egg donation involves several weeks of injections, blood tests, and ultrasounds. You and your donor and partners can benefit from counselling. Plus, you'll need to explore the emotional and legal consequences, just as you would if you were using donor sperm.

This section runs through the major issues you need to know if you're considering egg donation.

Knowing your options: Who ya gonna call?

Finding someone to agree to give you some of her eggs is an unusual and huge request to make of anyone. Some women find this wonderful lady in her family or one of her dearest friends and welcome the 'family ties' of the known donor route. Others ask their clinic to source an anonymous donor because they prefer not to know anything about the woman who is giving this amazing gift. You have the following options:

✔ **Be matched with a fellow infertility patient at your clinic.** A woman who needs IVF (perhaps for male factor infertility) agrees to share half her eggs with you in exchange for your paying her IVF costs. Few women under 35 are infertile because they have 'bad eggs.' More often, the difficulty is due to sperm problems or blocked tubes, fibroids, or other uterine abnormalities. This type of 'egg sharing' can be a good solution for two women's fertility problems, and promotes a nice 'sisterly solidarity' about being able to help one another with a problem that you each understand so well. All the evidence is that sharing half her eggs doesn't reduce the chance of the donor becoming pregnant and the recipient has the same good chance of a healthy pregnancy. A real case of 'buy one, get one free!'

✔ **Find a willing friend or relative.** Some women are fortunate enough to have a friend or relative who offers to donate eggs. Having your younger sister donate for you brings blessings and problems. The woman who is your child's 'aunt' is actually her genetic mother. This scenario has advantages. Don't forget that your kid sister has half your genes, so if she is the donor, the baby is going to have three-quarters of the genetic make-up that your 'own' baby would have had. But her children won't be cousins to your child, they will be half brothers and sisters! This reason is why honesty and openness from the very beginning are so important in 'known' or 'inter-family' donation and why counselling is so vital. (See Chapter 20 for more on the emotional considerations of using egg donation.)

Although your friend or relative may be keen to help, she may not feel comfortable with knowing the outcome of the pregnancy or meeting her 'genetic' child. In these cases, your friend can donate to another woman on your behalf and you automatically go to the top of the waiting list.

✔ **Use an altruistic egg donor.** If you're interested in this option, your chosen clinic may be able to match you with one. Altruistic donors are usually young mums who have so enjoyed being a parent that they are keen to help other women share the joy. Sometimes they're women who have no desire to become mothers themselves but feel that they ought not to 'waste' their eggs when they could help someone else.

Considering legalities, duties, and other fun stuff

As well as considering your options about where to find eggs, you also have to consider the legal side of things.

Rights and responsibilities

You don't need a lawyer to draw up a detailed legal contract when you use donated eggs because, under UK law, the 'genetic' mother has no rights at all after the eggs have been 'used' (that is, embryos created from them have been transferred to the recipient's uterus). That doesn't mean, however, that the donor has no rights: The egg donor may withdraw her consent to you 'using' her eggs right up to the point of embryo transfer. Also, some egg donors may be unwilling to let 'spare' embryos be frozen or used later. Check that the donor has not placed any restrictions on the use of her eggs.

Donors are entitled to know whether a pregnancy resulted from their dona-tion. But not any other information, such as whether there was live birth or what sex or how many?

The donor does have some duties, however, the most important of which is to declare any significant family medical history that could indicate the risk of a genetic or inherited disease or disability.

Risks involved

One disadvantage of donor eggs is that, unlike donor sperm, you don't know what you're getting in advance. Because the egg donor is doing a stimulated IVF cycle while you're taking medication to be ready for embryo transfer, you won't know how many eggs you'll get, or their quality, until the day of their egg collection a few days before your transfer. And although you may assume that a young donor makes a good number of eggs in an IVF cycle, that doesn't always happen. Clinics usually have rules about what happens if your donor doesn't stimulate well; be sure to check with your clinic to see what its policies are.

In addition to dealing with the risk of your donor not producing enough eggs, you also have to deal with the possibility that her preferences and expectations don't align with yours. For example, egg donors can also refuse to have embryos created from their eggs frozen, or they may consent to only a short period of storage.

Preparing for a wait

The shortage of donor eggs means that most clinics in the UK have a waiting list and you may have little 'choice' about the donor. The more specific your request, the longer you have to wait. Clinics try to match for hair colour, ethnicity, and possibly build and eye colour, but most physical characteristics that babies inherit are the result of a complex genetic mix. If you really are looking for something very specific – say, a redhead because everyone in your family has red hair, or a mixed-race donor if you're both bi-racial – you may have difficulty finding a donor. Some centres have very few black donors; others have very few Asian donors.

Buying and selling eggs in the UK is illegal so don't be tempted to post or buy on eBay! Many couples unfortunately resort to 'fertility tourism' and go to clinics abroad that are allowed to pay egg donors; and therefore, may be able to offer you treatment. Ask your UK clinic if they have any links with overseas clinics. That way you can get most of your treatment cycle done in the UK (scans and blood tests and so on) and you can be confident about the level of care you are going to receive from your chosen clinic abroad.

Taking Steps to Egg Donation

Where to go now? Well, your donor is checked for her general health and genetic diseases, you all sign the paperwork, and then the embryo transfer occurs. This section explains these steps in more detail.

Checking out your donor: Necessary screenings

Not all women are suitable egg donors or sharers, which is a shame, because finding volunteers is so hard to start with. But to ensure the very best possible care and chance of conceiving for recipients (that is, women who use donor eggs to conceive through IVF or ICSI), all potential donors and sharers are tested for infectious diseases, chromosomal abnormalities, and possible hereditary genetic conditions. In addition, all donors and sharers are offered counselling before treatment to ensure that they've considered and have come to terms with all the implications of giving away their genetic material, which one day could be a real-live baby in someone else's family.

Consider the following for different donors:

✔ **Fellow patient at your fertility clinic:** Women who need fertility treatment can agree to share up to half their eggs in return for subsidised treatment (and the knowledge that they've helped another woman in an even more difficult fertility situation than she is!). The response to any previous fertility treatment or hormone tests will indicate if she's able to produce enough good quality eggs and whether egg sharing is in the woman's best interests. If so, such 'egg sharers' have to meet tough criteria, including being:

- Under 36 years old

- A non-smoker (for at least six months before egg sharing)

- Of normal weight (a body mass index of about 20–30)

- Free from a personal or family history of inherited illnesses or abnormalities, such as carrying the cystic fibrosis gene

- Screened for and free from syphilis, chlamydia, gonorrhoea, hepatitis B, hepatitis C, and HIV

- Clear of chromosomal abnormalities

✔ **An altruistic donor:** Most centres accept altruistic egg donors only if they're under 35 years old and have no major health issues or inherited family disease. Most centres also have the donor and her partner checked for all infectious diseases, such as HIV, hepatitis B and C, syphilis, and gonorrhoea. The clinic also contacts the donor's GP for family health information and some do psychological screening to make sure that the donor fully understands the implications of egg donation and is mentally stable enough to handle donating.

✔ **Friend or relative:** If you're bringing a donor that you've found yourself to the clinic, she'll most likely be required to undergo all the same testing. The 'only-under-36 ' rule isn't so rigidly enforced for 'known' donors and you may be prepared to accept some genetic traits (like being a carrier of cystic fibrosis) in order to be able to use a known donor.

Although the risks of IVF are quite low (about 1 per cent of treatment cycles results in hospital admission) every medical procedure carries some risk. Many clinics in the UK are reluctant to accept very young donors who have not started or completed their families as known or altruistic egg donors. These women, however, can be *egg sharers*, women who require IVF or ICSI treatment (possibly for male factor infertility) and who agree to donate up to half their eggs to another woman in return for subsidised treatment costs.

Signing the documents

The Human Fertilisation and Embryology Act (1991), and the Codes of Practice that derive from it, give very clear guidance about the duties, rights, and responsibilities of gamete (eggs or sperm) donors and recipients.

You and your donor must sign legal consents. The donor signs that she's voluntarily donating her eggs. This consent is required even if the donor is someone you know.

You sign that you're voluntarily using donor eggs to create a child. You also sign that you and your partner (if you're not a single parent) agree to be the sole legal parents of the child and assume all costs for bearing and raising the child.

At present, a child born from donor sperm, eggs, or embryos is automatically the child of the recipients and doesn't need to be legally adopted by either parent at birth. Under UK law, the 'birth mother' is the legal parent, wherever the eggs, sperm, or embryos have come from. If you're part of a married couple then the father has full parental rights, too.

If, however, you're a cohabiting couple then exactly the same rules apply as if the baby had been made by the conventional route. Putting your (unmarried) partner's name on the birth certificate does *not* give him full paternal responsibilities, unless he makes a formal agreement with the mother, obtains a court order, becomes the child's guardian (which only takes effect on the mother's death), or marries the mother. No such thing as 'common law' marriage exists in the UK, so if you both want full security then it must be wedding bells. However, after marriage to the child's mother, the father named on the birth certificate assumes all parental rights and responsibilities, just as if the child was conceived naturally from both their eggs and sperm. The 'non-mother' partner in a civil partnership may adopt their partner's child as long as the applicant has lived with the child for at least six months.

Synchronising your timing

Women who live together in a community (college, convent, or prison!) soon synchronise their menstrual cycles through some mysterious process that seems to involve pheromones (subtle chemical messages released in sweat glands). To make an egg donation cycle work also requires synchronising donor and recipient's cycles. Fortunately, you don't have to live with your donor for three months to achieve synchronicity; we can use routine IVF drugs to achieve the same thing. It works like this:

Step 1: You and your donor start your GnRH agonist drug (for example, buserelin or nafarelin) on cycle day 21. The recipient (you) starts first if your period dates are very different.

Step 2: You and your donor are both checked for 'down regulation' after 2–3 weeks on the agonist and when the donor starts her gonadotrophins (the stimulating injections like Merional, Menopur, Fostimon, Gonal F, or Puregon) while you start your HRT (oestradiol valerate tablets).

Step 3: By the time the donor has grown some nice follicles and is ready for the hCG 'late night' injection (usually after 9–12 days), you should have grown a nice thick endometrium (at least 8 millimetres in depth) and be ready to start your progesterone pessaries.

Step 4: Egg collection proceeds as usual (check out Chapter 14). If the donor is also an 'egg sharer' then the eggs are allocated 'in turn' by the lab, so don't worry whether you or the donor is going to get all the 'good' eggs.

Your partner has to produce his sperm sample on the day of the egg collection (as does the donor if she's an egg sharer), or the lab prepares any frozen partner or donor sperm sample.

Step 5: Embryo transfer takes place on the second, third, or fifth day after egg collection. If you're using an 'unknown' donor then the clinic takes great care to ensure that you and your donor are given appointments for ultrasound scans and embryo transfers at different times, so you're not sitting in the waiting room wondering whether the donor is the glamorous blonde with the handsome husband!

Step 6: After the embryo transfer, the donor has routine luteal support (usually Cyclogest pessaries), and you continue with your oestrogen tablets and pessaries. After a positive pregnancy test, you need to continue with the oestrogen and progesterone until the baby's placenta takes over (8–12 weeks). The donor (if she is an egg sharer) can stop her progesterone sooner. Altruistic donors need to be aware that they must use barrier contraception until their next period and that the next period could be a little delayed and/or a little heavier than usual.

Being an egg donor or egg sharer is one of the most fantastic things that any woman can do for any other woman. The process is time consuming, uncomfortable, and not entirely risk free. But the gift of life is the most precious gift we can give.

Getting Support

The National Gamete Donation Trust Web site has loads of information and reassurance for people who need donor eggs or sperm and is a useful starting point. Take a look at www.ngdt.co.uk. Alternatively, you can find numerous support groups on the Internet, not only for egg recipients but also for donors. Go to your favourite search engine, enter 'donor eggs,' and see what you get! If you have any questions or doubts about donating eggs or receiving donor eggs, you should be able to find plenty of people on the bulletin boards – try www.infertilitynetworkuk.com or www.fertilityfriends.co.uk – who can help you with your decision.

If you want a more one-to-one approach, a family counsellor who specialises in adoptions or other family situations may be very helpful; the phone book is a good place to look for family counsellors. You can also ask your fertility clinic for referral to a counsellor or contact one of the patient support groups, such as Infertility Network UK.

Chapter 16

Creating an Embryo: Amazing Teamwork in the Lab

So far, your fertility treatment has been in the hands of nurses, doctors, ultra-sonographers, administrators, and biomedical scientists. The embryologists and *andrologists* (sperm experts) who join the team at this point are skilled in working with the most precious of all human material: the eggs, sperm, and embryos that have the potential to become your child.

The latest point at which you meet your embryologist is just before your egg collection (that is, egg retrieval), after which the progress of your treatment is in the hands of the embryology team. They check your eggs, prepare the sperm for fertilisation, and help nurture those embryos in perfect condition until the day of transfer.

In this chapter, we tell you what goes on in the lab, what the embryologists want to see, and what they *don't* want to see in eggs and embryos. We also consider how many embryos you may want – and are allowed – to transfer, and how you get through the two-week wait afterwards.

Recognising a Good Egg

Before you go home after egg retrieval, the embryologist assesses your eggs and lets you know how many are mature, post-mature, or immature. Eggs need to be mature for fertilisation to occur, but immature eggs sometimes mature after retrieval. An egg retrieval may yield eggs that are both mature and immature, especially if you made a lot of follicles. If your eggs are post-mature, they may not fertilise, or may let in too many sperm; they also may be dark and grainy looking.

A mature egg has:

- A fluffy cumulus layer.

- A dense outer layer called the corona, which a single sperm needs to break through for fertilisation to occur.

- A polar body: *Polar bodies* (the egg originally has two) are the 'leftovers' after an egg has completed its final cell division, which leaves it with just 23 chromosomes. The first polar body is eliminated at the time of ovulation, and the second at the time of fertilisation. A mature egg is ready to be fertilised because it has already completed one of the last stages of cell division, called *meiosis*; it now contains 23 chromosomes. (Refer to Chapter 14 for a picture of a mature egg.)

- No *germinal vesicles* (immature cells): An immature egg usually doesn't have a polar body (described in the preceding paragraph), and it has germinal vesicles, meaning that it hasn't yet completed the division to 23 single-stranded chromosomes.

Sorting Suitable Sperm

While the eggs are counted and checked (see the preceding section), an *andrologist* (sperm expert) prepares the sperm for insemination. If you're using fresh sperm, your partner is asked to provide the sample when you arrive at the clinic for your egg collection. The sample is then washed, counted, and the *motility* (movement) and *morphology* (shape) of the sperm are checked. The sperm sample is then graded through a fine 'filtering' process to isolate the very best sperm – the 'gold-medal swimmers' – for use in the treatment. The best quality sperm are then washed and counted again and stored in an incubator ready for insemination.

If you're using a frozen sample, the washed and sorted sperm are removed from liquid nitrogen at −196 degrees centigrade, then thawed, and washed again to remove the cryoprotectant, making them ready to use.

IVF: Making an Embryo 'in Glass'

Almost 30 years after the birth of the world's first test-tube baby, the wonder of fertilisation using the IVF technique is now often referred to as 'normal' or 'standard' insemination to distinguish it from ICSI.

Normal insemination

The embryologist removes your eggs from the incubator and places about 150,000 (just a droplet) washed, good-quality sperm in each of the wells containing one or two eggs. Under the microscope, the sperm are checked to see that they're still swimming and then they're put back into the incubator for one sperm to find its way into each egg for fertilisation to happen overnight. Imagine the eggs and sperm, together at last in a warm, quiet, dark place . . . It's almost romantic! The next morning the embryologist checks the eggs for fertilisation success rates; the first step to getting embryos.

ICSI: Injecting for male factor

If you need to do ICSI for male factor (very low sperm count), using a microscope, the embryologist removes the cumulus and the coronal layers from the egg, while the sperm is washed, graded, and sorted by the sperm expert.

The embryologist then sits at an ICSI rig – a high-powered microscope equipped with 'micromanipulators' – which is used to 'catch' the best sperm and break their tails. The embryologist then uses needles ⅒th the width of a human hair to pick up the sperm and inject them right into the jelly-like centre of each mature egg, which is held steady at the correct orientation so that the delicate structure isn't damaged. This procedure gives the very best chance of fertilisation for sperm that may otherwise not be able to penetrate the egg. ICSI requires very steady hands and a good eye for picking the best-looking sperm. The injected eggs are then placed back in the labelled section of the incubator for fertilisation to happen overnight. If the eggs don't fertilise, ICSI can't be redone using those eggs.

Some studies have shown that ICSI embryos have a higher than normal rate of *aneuploidy*, or abnormal chromosomes. This higher rate may occur because men with severe male factor have more chromosomal abnormalities, such as Klinefelter's syndrome.

Going pronuclear: Getting good embryos

The day after the retrieval, the embryologist takes the dish out of the incubator to check the eggs and look for embryos at the 'two pronuclear' (2PN) stage, that is, embryos that have two visible circles lined up next to each other (see Figure 16-1). If they're visible at this stage, congratulations! You've got embryos! These embryos contain the genetic material from each parent.

If you're planning to freeze some or all of your embryos for use at another time, your clinic may freeze them at the 2PN stage. Some centres may prefer to freeze embryos at the cleavage stage (4–6 cells) or at blastocyst stage.

Good fertilisation depends on the quality of the sperm and egg. At most centres, the fertilisation rate is about 65–70 per cent. When embryologists look at the other 30–35 per cent of the eggs, they may see things they'd rather not. For example, your embryos may be *polyploid*, meaning that they contain more than two pronuclei. This can occur when more than one sperm has entered the egg, or when the egg doesn't throw off the second polar body (which should occur at the time of fertilisation). These embryos are never normal, because the egg or the sperm that created them isn't normal.

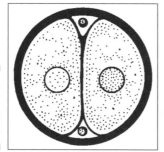

Figure 16-1:
A 2PN
(pronuclear)
embryo.

Taking the Call from Embryology

An embryologist usually calls the morning after your egg retrieval to let you know how many embryos you have and how they're developing. The embryologist also lets you know if any are suitable to freeze and confirms whether you'd like to go ahead with freezing. If you have a high number of embryos, the embryologist may suggest freezing some of them at the 2PN stage.

Embryologists may sometimes call with bad news – very few or no embryos are suitable for transfer. Although this occurrence is unusual, the embryologist is going to suggest that you return to the clinic for a follow-up appointment, where your treatment can be reviewed and options can be considered for any future treatment.

Deciding which embryos to freeze and at what stage is a real challenge for the embryo experts. The embryos that are frozen after a few days usually have four to eight cells and their thaw rate may not be as good as 2PN embryos (embryos frozen the day after egg retrieval). But (and this is a big but!) delaying the freezing decision may help to select the best embryos. But (another big but!), 'late' frozen embryos also have the potential to turn into beautiful babies . . . Sometimes you simply have to leave the decisions to the experts and go with the flow!

Two days after retrieval, embryology may call again, this time to tell you how your embryos are growing. Hopefully, they've now reached the four- to eight-cell stage. Figure 16-2 shows a four-cell embryo. Each cell – or *blastomere* – contains the entire genetic blueprint to make a baby.

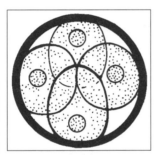

Figure 16-2: A four-cell embryo.

You may get another call from embryology the third day after retrieval, if you're doing a day-three transfer. Some centres do most transfers two days after retrieval, and some, five days after retrieval – when the embryo should have reached the blastocyst stage. (We discuss blastocyst transfer in the section 'Blast Off! Considering a Blastocyst Transfer,' later in this chapter.) If your embryos are now four to eight cells, they're ready for transfer.

Occasionally, if you're doing a day-three transfer, your embryos may already be *morulas*, or embryos that have 10 to 30 cells. Morulas usually have a very high rate of implantation, similar to blastocysts; in fact, they're the embryo stage right before blastocyst.

Many centres give you pictures of your embryos to take home with you. And no, it's not crazy to treasure these images in the same way as you're going to treasure your first baby scan! When your baby is born, what an amazing image to show them when they're older!

Grading an Embryo

Does a great-looking embryo improve your chance of getting pregnant? Most embryologists would say a cautious 'yes', depending on your age, uterine cavity, general health, and many other factors. For IVF centres, a great-looking embryo has a few standard characteristics:

- ✔ It has cleaved (divided) at the right rate.
- ✔ Its cells (blastomeres) are regular and equally sized.
- ✔ It has little or no fragmentation (cell break up pieces).
- ✔ The 'gloop' (cytoplasm) is nice and clear.

Latest research suggests that analysing the chemical structure of the fluid the embryos are in, to see what they are 'eating' and 'excreting' can help select those embryos with the best chance of survival. Identifying the most 'metabolically fit' is more accurate than the visual ID still used in most clinics. This idea is new, but it may become common procedure to 'drop' the embryo beauty pageant in favour of the new physical assessment. (Although I (co-author Jill) felt both proud and reassured to be told that our two embryos, about to be transferred into my uterus, were both 'beautiful'!)

Fragmentation

Embryos are also graded by the equality and roundness of the cells and by the amount of fragmentation, or broken pieces, that are in the embryo. Figure 16-3 shows an embryo with a high degree of fragmentation.

Although a funny looking embryo doesn't create a funny looking baby, most embryologists do feel that an embryo with less fragmentation and more even-looking cells has a better chance of implanting. If you do get pregnant from fragmented embryos, the fragmentation does *not* mean that your baby is going to be abnormal in any way. Some centres remove the fragmented pieces before the embryo is transferred. As long as the embryo has less than 50 per cent fragmentation, it has a chance of implanting and developing into a baby. Highly fragmented embryos can't be frozen.

Is it wise to transfer that embryo?

Not all embryos are perfect. In fact, most aren't. But most embryos that are at least four cells and not too fragmented have a decent chance of implanting, and every embryologist has seen terrible-looking embryos that went on to become beautiful babies. Embryologists suggest discarding the following types of embryos, however, because they're generally chromosomally abnormal:

✔ Multinucleated embryos, which contain three or more 'bundles' of genetic material: At least 75 per cent are abnormal.

✔ Embryos with uneven pronuclei: About 85 per cent are abnormal.

✔ Embryos that develop too rapidly: Many of these have an abnormal number of chromosomes.

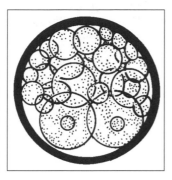

Figure 16-3:
An embryo with a lot of fragmentation.

Looking at Your Uterine Lining

Embryos implant only if the uterus is ready for implantation. Fertility centres use ultrasound to look at the uterine thickness and also the appearance of the lining, called the *pattern,* to decide whether your embryos have a good chance of growing:

✔ **Triple lined (tri-laminar):** This pattern description is shortened to TL in most centres and describes the lining most clinics like to see before embryo transfer. Fertility centres differ on what's considered a good thickness, but most prefer to see a thickness of at least 7 millimetres before transfer. The endometrioum will seem light and bright.

✔ **Isoechogenic (IE) pattern:** This type of pattern is the next best lining. The contrast with the myometrium or muscle layer of the uterus may not be so great.

✔ **Homogenous hyperechoic (HH) pattern:** The HH pattern has the lowest implantation rate. The endometrium looks a little 'immature' or dark. This is the time to trust to the experience of your clinic.

Different clinics place varying amounts of importance on lining patterns, so don't be concerned if they don't comment on your endometrium. Your centre's emphasis on the importance of the lining thickness or pattern will vary (refer to Chapter 10).

Hatching Embryos – Come on Out, Guys

Around 1994, embryologists came out with a new technique called *assisted hatching* to help human embryos implant in the uterus. The majority of good IVF centres do hatching on at least some of their embryos.

Assisted hatching (AH) is carried out just before the embryos are replaced in your uterus. The principle of assisted hatching is to help your embryo break through the zona pellucida and attach to the nourishing layer of the uterus. The embryologist takes a tiny needle with an acid solution on the end of it and barely touches the shell of the embryo, creating a small hole. This helps the embryo 'break through' the zona pellucida, or hard shell, and attach to the uterus, an action that must happen a day or so after the embryo reaches the uterus in nature. Embryos created in the lab often have harder shells than those in natural conception, so the little hole can help them break out and bed down where they belong. Some clinics use a fine laser beam to make this little hole in the zona.

Although some clinics don't offer assisted hatching at all, others may use it regularly. Usually though it's offered to:

- ✔ Patients over age 37 whose embryos may have a harder time breaking out of the *zona pellucida* shell
- ✔ Women with more than three failed embryo transfers
- ✔ Women with high FSH levels
- ✔ Women having frozen embryo transfers

Blast Off! Considering a Blastocyst Transfer

A few years ago, IVF centres became alarmed at the large number of higher-order multiples (triplets or more) their patients were delivering, and they looked for ways to transfer fewer embryos and still maintain the all-important high pregnancy rates.

Across the UK the average percentage of live-birth twins is about 25 per cent of total births, and triplets is less than 1 per cent, but pressure has been applied for clinics to bring the total number of multiple births to less than 10 per cent of all live births.

Subsequently, because of this concern, the *blastocyst transfer* – the transfer of a five-day-old embryo – was instigated. During natural conception the embryo doesn't normally reach the uterus until day four or five after fertilisation and, by delaying transfer, the blastocyst can be placed into the uterus at the same stage that it would arrive naturally. Because only 30 to 50 per cent of embryos grow to blastocyst stage (see Figure 16-4), centres felt that only the best embryos were going to be transferred. As it turned out, blastocyst transfer of two embryos results in pregnancy rate about 40 per cent of the time in those under age 35, compared to 30 per cent in a day-three transfer of two embryos.

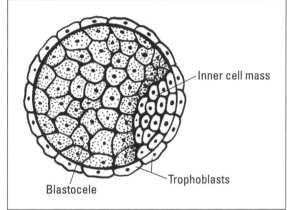

Figure 16-4:
A
blastocyst.

Inner cell mass

Blastocele

Trophoblasts

Blastocyst transfer isn't the solution to IVF failure. Blastocyst transfer isn't for everyone and can't turn weak embryos into strong ones. Because blastocysts are more complicated to create than day-three embryos, requiring multiple media changes to keep up with their increased nutritional needs, many embryos fail to get to blastocyst stage. So if your centre transfers only blastocysts, you may end up with nothing to transfer.

The second problem comes from the blastocysts themselves. Because they may be already 'hatching' out of their shells at the time of transfer, blastocysts seem unusually likely to split into identical twins. Although on the surface, having identical twins doesn't seem much different than having fraternal twins, the fact is that identical twin pregnancies are much more problematic than fraternals. Because identical twins may share the same placenta and sac, *twin-twin transfusion syndrome*, in which one twin gets too many nutrients and the other not enough, is more common. The incidence of identical twins is about four to five times higher in blastocyst transfer than in normal conception. Of course, if you transfer two blastocysts and one splits, you're right back to the problem of high-order multiples again. For these reasons, some centres have stopped doing blastocyst transfer on all patients and instead use it selectively, for patients who have had several IVF failures with standard two- to four-cell embryo transfers.

'One Embryo or Two?'

Current practice in the UK, as directed by the Human Fertilisation and Embryology Authority (HFEA), is to transfer one or two embryos in women under 40 and up to three embryos for women who are older. If you're using donor eggs, these have been given by a woman who is no more than 35 years old, so you can only have up to two embryos transferred (remember that it's the age of the egg, not the recipient's uterus that determines the quality and viability of the egg).

In 2006, one in four IVF pregnancies resulted in twins – more than 10 times higher than the rate of twins born from natural conception. And because a multiple birth is the single biggest risk to the health and welfare of both a child conceived by IVF and its mother, fertility experts are calling for the number of transferred embryos to be reduced to just one.

So maybe you won't have a choice, but until that legislation is brought in, make sure that the issue of the number of embryos is discussed at your first treatment planning appointment (that is, after you've had all your baseline tests and they know that you will need IVF or ICSI). Every UK clinic has an obligation to explain the benefits and risks of a single, two-, or three-embryo transfer to every patient to allow you to make an *informed* decision about the number of embryos you would like to be transferred. If you're part of a couple, both of you need to give written consent agreeing to this number in advance of the transfer. A phone call or e-mail isn't sufficient and the absence of your partner's signature before embryo transfer may cause it to be abandoned and rescheduled as a frozen embryo transfer, postponed indefinitely, or cancelled altogether.

Transferring Your Embryo

When you arrive for your embryo transfer, you'll be taken back to the egg collection suite. Most clinics prefer your partner to be with you – as he would be if you were able to conceive naturally! Some centres ask you both to change into sterile gowns and coveralls, but in others your normal clothes are just fine – it makes no difference to the clinical safety of the procedure. You don't require drugs before your treatment, unless the procedure may be deemed unusually difficult, that is, you've had surgery to your cervix. If this is the case, most clinics carry out a trial embryo transfer earlier in the treatment cycle. The following sections explain the implantation procedure.

Getting comfy

You'll be instructed to lie on a couch that can be tilted. The worst part of the transfer in most clinics is that you're lying there with a full bladder. A full bladder, although uncomfortable, makes seeing your uterus under ultrasound guidance that much easier, and most centres now do embryo transfers under ultrasound guidance in line with NICE (National Institute for Clinical Excellence) guidelines. A full bladder also straightens the cervical canal in the 80 per cent of women with an anteverted or forward-tilting uterus.

Your bladder, lying right under the uterus, pushes your uterus up when it's full; it also straightens the path into the uterus, making the transfer easier. A full bladder isn't needed if you have a retroverted uterus.

Talking to the embryologist

An embryologist may come in to speak with you before the transfer and tell you how your embryos look today. They confirm your identity and the number of embryos that you want to transfer. They may even show or give you pictures of these cell clusters – baby's first portrait. You are asked to sign to confirm your identity, that you agree to transfer one or two embryos (or three, if you're over 40), that you understand the risks of multiple birth, and that you realise that you may not become pregnant after an embryo transfer.

Time to transfer

If your clinic uses ultrasound guidance for embryo transfers, a nurse or ultra-sonographer places the probe on your abdomen so that the uterus can be seen on the monitor. The doctor or nurse doing the transfer inserts a speculum into your vagina to see the cervix. They gently wipe your cervix to remove any mucus from the opening, then, leaving the speculum in place, they let the embryologist know that everything's ready. Here come your embryos!

The transfer doctor or nurse then slides the catheter through your cervix, which may cause a little cramping. If your clinic uses ultrasound guidance for the transfer, the transfer doctor or nurse sees how far away from the top of the uterus the catheter is before slowly injecting your embryo(s) into your uterus. The catheter is slowly removed and handed back to the embryologist, who examines it under a microscope to make sure that no embryos are still in the catheter.

For most women, an embryo transfer isn't physically very different from having a smear test – no sedation, lie down, knees apart, the use of a speculum, and 20 minutes later it's all over. A transfer that's traumatic in any way, causing bleeding or severe cramping, may decrease your chance of pregnancy. If you've done a mock transfer (in a mock transfer, a soft catheter is inserted into the uterus, and the depth of the uterus and the angle required to get into it are recorded) before starting IVF, the doctor has a 'map' of your cervical canal and uterine opening, so trauma is less likely. Ultrasound guidance also makes the process easier by showing the curves in your anatomy, so your centre may not do a mock transfer if it's using ultrasound guidance for your embryo transfer.

Putting your feet up

After your embryos are in the uterus, you may need to stay on the couch with your feet tilted up a little while. Clinics vary widely in their bed rest requirements, and they may keep you anywhere from no time at all, to up to four hours. Your clinic will give you written information and possibly a list of 'do's and don'ts' after embryo transfer.

Embryos are placed directly into your uterus and emptying your bladder or bowels isn't going to dislodge them! In fact, not going to the toilet when you need to can increase uterine cramping, which *can* have a negative effect on your getting pregnant.

Keeping Your Feet and Your Spirits Up after the Transfer

After you're safely home, you may be on restricted activity for a period of time, depending on your clinic's policies. Try not to compare what you're doing to what anyone else is doing, because different centres have different policies. If you don't follow your centre's advice, you're bound to feel guilty if you don't get pregnant, so follow your instruction sheet. Also ensure that you continue with the hormone medication you're given after your transfer to help your embryos implant in your uterus. (Head to Chapter 17 for more on post-transfer luteal support.)

Restricting your activity

Clinics may advise you to rest for a few hours to a whole day and night, depending on their policy. But all clinics advise you not to do any heavy lifting (over 1 stone or 2 kilogrammes, typically) or strenuous exercise for the two-week wait before your pregnancy test and, if that's positive, for the next two weeks before your six-week scan. Shopping for clothes and jewellery is fine, but not groceries! You may also have sex – but nothing strenuous!

The heavy lifting advice can be a problem if your job requires you to do so, or if you have a small child. Most clinics gladly write you a note restricting your work activity, but your 1-year-old probably won't understand a note saying that you can't lift him into his high chair. If you have to lift a child, bend with your knees, trying to keep your back straight when you lift, rather than bending at the waist and straining your abdominal muscles.

For the two-week wait after your embryo transfer, mild exercise, such as a leisurely walk, is fine, but forget about aerobics for a while. Use common sense about yoga, pilates, or whatever else you do to decrease stress and increase endorphins. If you feel guilty doing it, you probably ought not to be doing it!

Swimming pools, hot tubs, Jacuzzis, and saunas are forbidden after embryo transfer, until you either have a negative pregnancy test or have your baby – although swimming in a chlorinated pool can be resumed after 12 weeks into your pregnancy and is very beneficial exercise while pregnant.

Dealing with your partner

Most women recuperate from their transfer at home, while some who are travelling for the procedure may find themselves in a strange hotel room. Either way, the same rules apply. Generally speaking, making plans at this time to entertain your relatives is not a good idea. The truth is you'll probably spend much of the transfer day itself relaxing, which helps calm you and your uterus. Right now, it's okay to feel excited, nervous, restless, nervous, optimistic, pessimistic, or apprehensive – or all the above. Take time to relax now because over the next two weeks leading up to your pregnancy test, you're going to get increasingly anxious.

If your partner isn't great at the old bedside manner, now's not the right time to try engaging in long, meaningful conversations. Your partner has also experienced a range of emotions as a result of all the activity leading up to this point. He may need a bit of his own time and space to relax as well, in a way best suited for him. I (co-author Jill) registered the delight on Gwyn's face when I 'let' him go skydiving as usual, the day after my second transfer.

Do's and Don'ts for the Two-Week Wait

The two-week wait (2WW) is one of the most stressful times of your treatment – more so, because there's very little you or anyone can do to affect whether you get a positive pregnancy test at the end of the 2WW. But here are a few suggestions:

- Do try to carry on as normal – see friends, socialise, work!

- Take the progesterone pessaries for 14 days, even if you spot or bleed.

- Don't keep dashing to the toilet to check for spotting or bleeding.

- Do take gentle exercise – but avoid swimming, hot tubs, or saunas.

- Do take plenty of fluids – lots and lots of water.

- Do contact your clinic if you are:

    - Drinking lots, but not passing urine

    - Feeling bloated or breathless after 24 hours

    - Have a headache or abdominal discomfort that won't go with painkillers more than 24 hours after transfer

- Don't do your pregnancy test until day 14 – anytime sooner can give a misleading result.

- Do your pregnancy test on day 14 even if you've started to spot or bleed before that, to confirm the outcome of your treatment.

- Do contact your clinic to let them know the outcome of the treatment.

Part V
Post-First Cycle: How You May Feel and What You Can Do

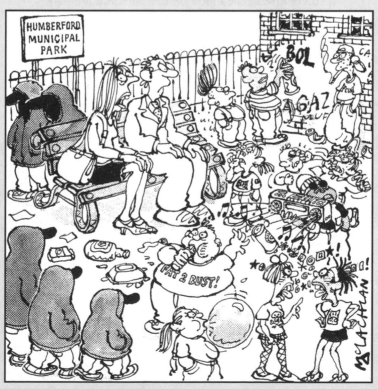

'I don't think I really want to try
for a baby any more.'

In this part . . .

After all the effort of 'big-time' assisted conception, you're now in the limbo time of the dreaded two-week wait where you're unable to do anything to affect a positive pregnancy test. This is a testing time and in this part we offer advice on how to deal with either getting through to the test, or coping with the arrival of your period or a negative pregnancy test. If you're not pregnant, we look at your options, including having no more treatment, opting for a frozen embryo transfer, or another full cycle of IUI, IVF, or ICSI.

Chapter 17

Waiting and Hoping: Surviving the Two-Week Wait after Embryo Transfer

*L*eaving the clinic after the embryo transfer at the end of your (IVF) cycle brings a whole host of emotions. You have one or two embryos on board, so you're pregnant, right? Wrong! Right or wrong, you're about to embark on the longest fortnight of your life.

Now it's time to wait for your pregnancy test. Because the test results won't be accurate for almost two weeks after your embryo transfer, this time period is often referred to by patients as the *two-week wait* (2WW). In this chapter, we review some of the do's and don'ts of the two-week wait, and peek a little into the future when you'll have an answer to the big question – am I pregnant or not? – and what you'll be doing in either case.

Technically, You're Pregnant – Waiting for the Proof

From a purely technical viewpoint, after the embryos are placed into your uterus, you're pregnant – in the loosest sense of the word, at least. You have embryos floating around where they belong, and all they have to do is attach and grow.

This is probably the first time in your fertility history where you can say without a doubt that you've formed an embryo and that it's where it needs to be in order to grow. You may have known that you made a follicle, and been fairly sure that you got sperm where it needed to go at the right time, but you never knew for sure that the egg and sperm got together. Now you do. Now comes the waiting period. The two-week wait is a time of 'what ifs' and 'if onlys' like no other time you've probably experienced.

What happens at the end of the 2WW is literally in the hands of a 'Higher Power'. By the time you get to this waiting game, you've done everything you can do to get pregnant. Some clinics do blood tests in the midluteal phase (meaning, after week one of the two-week wait), and high oestrogen and progesterone levels may be more suggestive of a pregnancy but aren't reliable indicators. In the words of a famous fertility doc, 'If midluteal numbers were so accurate, we'd call it a pregnancy test.' So, whether you're visiting the clinic for midluteal tests or not, you're pretty much left with your thoughts and just your progesterone to keep you company.

Dwelling on the possibility of success or failure and worrying do you no good, and have no impact whatsoever on the final outcome. Enjoying yourself and keeping busy with your day-to-day responsibilities is going to keep your life manageable and puts you in a better place for whatever news you receive.

Try to plan as many activities as you can manage (after your post-transfer rest period). If you work, consider the opportunity a blessing and immerse yourself in your responsibilities. Maybe a good book, film, or television show can distract or relax you but try to keep the subject matter as far away from the topic of fertility as possible. Exercise is also a good way to keep busy, but this isn't the time to take up hang-gliding. Most doctors recommend keeping your heart rate less than 140 while trying to conceive. Many couples find that the two-week wait is a great time to take a holiday. What better way to distract yourself than with a little rest and relaxation? Make sure that your holiday destination includes reliable drinking water supplies and doesn't require you to take antimalarials, or other potentially toxic medications. Remember that alcohol is a definite no-no for the 2WW and extremes of temperature and pressure (skiing, camel safaris, deep-sea diving, and so on) are not good ideas for the almost pregnant.

Some women say that the optimism of the two-week wait can make this a great time to check in with pregnant friends or friends with children who may have been difficult to talk to during the trials of fertility treatment. During the two-week wait, fertility patients go through essentially the same thing that any other woman trying to conceive goes through. Fertility patients' stakes may be a bit higher, but their impatience is similar.

Don't think that waiting as a couple is any easier. And don't be cross with your partner because he's apparently taking the situation all in his stride. There may well be nothing you can do to influence the outcome, there is even less that he can do! Just be grateful he's not down the pub every night boring his mates with his injection technique or what the andrologist said about his sperm count! Many choose to pass the two-week wait talking with fertility friends online, through support groups, or visiting one of the many Web sites that list all the standard pregnancy symptoms, such as www.pregnancyandbirthmagazine. co.uk, which gives you at least a symptom a day to obsess over.

If the tension does begin to run too high, assemble your backup plan. What are you going to do next, pregnant or not? This type of planning often alleviates the fear and uncertainty that accompany the two-week wait.

Seeking support during an uncertain time

Going through the two-week wait is something best done with lots of support. Your doctor takes care of the medical end of this equation, but you're undoubtedly going to need a little help from your friends to keep your mind on track. If you've shared your story with friends and family, you can hopefully lean on them during this period of waiting. If you've kept those around you in the dark, consider sharing your anxiety with a professional, such as a counsellor or a religious figure (your minister, priest, or rabbi, for example), or a support group.

If anonymity is your bag, consider the online resources discussed in Chapter 9. Many online bulletin boards have specific sections devoted to the two-week wait, which reassure you that you're not alone. You can find one such example of this at www.iVillage.co.uk, or your clinic may have a message board where you can e-talk to other folk going through the same thing! At sites such as this, you can share your hopes, fears, and daily symptoms with legions of women going through the same thing. This type of camaraderie can actually make waiting fun.

Making your to-do or not-to-do list

Taking care of yourself during the roller-coaster ride of trying to create a baby is crucial. For some women, this may mean a trip to the hairdresser, manicurist, gym, or all the above. But you need to consider a few limitations as you wait out these last few weeks before your pregnancy test.

Colouring your hair

For those whose follicle challenges begin at the top of their heads, hair colouring is more than just a luxury; it's a way of life. To colour or not to colour has been a long-time topic of discussion among the newly pregnant. According to fertility experts, hair colouring *is* safe during pregnancy. Based on this opinion, colouring your hair during the two-week wait is also presumed to be safe (unless of course your colourist turns your hair orange!). However, keep in mind that the two-week wait is only two weeks. If you're at all concerned, staying off the bottle (of hair colour, that is) for the time being may be the best advice for you.

Manicures and pedicures

The greatest danger that we know of in manicures and pedicures is for those who give them. You may have noticed that many manicurists now wear masks to protect themselves from the fumes and toxins generated by the products. A simple polish-and-go won't hurt you during the two-week wait. Those with acrylic nails are advised to refrain from having this service during the two-week wait, and those who don't have acrylic nails but want them are best waiting until after the two-week wait, and after the first trimester of pregnancy for that matter. If you already have acrylic nails, don't panic, but you may consider having them removed before your cycle.

Get your exercise

Exercise can be a great way to take your mind off your waiting and your worries during the two-week wait. Three basic rules to remember with exercise during this time are

- ✔ **Don't start up a brand-new routine during the two-week wait.** In other words, if you're not a runner, don't become one now. Keep your exercise routine consistent with what you engaged in before.

- ✔ **Keep your heart rate equal to or lower than 140 beats per minute.** This rate is also recommended during pregnancy, so this is a good time to get used to keeping track of it. Most fitness stores sell inexpensive heart rate monitors, and certain exercise machines (such as particular brands of treadmills) have a built-in monitor that can read your heart rate when you grasp the metal sensors on the handle bar.

- ✔ **Saunas, jacuzzis, and steam rooms are absolutely forbidden during the 2WW.** Take showers rather than baths during the first few days after embryo transfer (ET).

Keep in mind that moderation must become your middle name, in judgement and in exercise. You may feel fab and that you can 'climb any mountain' but it would be best to leave that to the Von Trapp family and concentrate on being sensible! The emotional toll of having fertility treatment is quite great and it's *normal* to feel tired, crotchety, emotional, and even slightly mad during the 2WW. The two-week wait calls for maintaining the status quo. Leave the new stuff for later.

Having sex during the two week wait

For those going through the two-week wait after in vitro fertilisation, sex is a big issue. A theoretical concern is that the female orgasm could cause uterine contractions, which aren't ideal in creating a hospitable environment for baby embryo until he/she/they have safely implanted (2 to 5 days after ET). IVF is stressful and good sex is a great stress buster and the risk is only a theoretical concern. I (co-author Gill) was asked by a husband, after I had just done the embryo transfer for his wife, when they could have sex again. I said, 'Wait till you get home!' Seriously, you'll probably feel a little sore after your egg retrieval and maybe a little bloated if you had a good response to the stimulating drugs. Now may be the time to re-discover the delights of the old-fashioned cuddle.

Sensing Every Little Twinge: The Truth about Pregnancy Symptoms

Of course you're anxious. Of course you're minutely examining every twinge, cramp, and tingle you have for some indication of whether you're pregnant. The hormone swings of the cycle, the stress, tiredness, and sheer frustration of not being able to do anything that could improve the outcome for two whole weeks after you've had so much to do for so many weeks can drive quite sane women to distraction. But remember that any symptoms or no symptoms can mean good news, so just keep busy.

Signs, omens, and other portents

If you're taking progesterone, as you most likely are after an IVF cycle, the symptoms of pregnancy can easily be confused with symptoms of progesterone supplementation, because an increase in progesterone is associated with many common pregnancy symptoms. Some symptoms you may experience and what they mean are as follows:

- **Sore breasts:** Tender breasts are almost a universal sign of pregnancy, with or without feelings of heaviness or tingling in the nipples. Unfortunately, sore breasts are caused by increased progesterone and oestrogen, so sore breasts may be caused by your pessaries and your hormone levels rather than by a growing embryo.

- **Spotting (light vaginal bleeding):** This symptom is very common in very early pregnancy, whether or not you've undergone fertility treatment. Spotting may be caused by an embryo burrowing into the uterus and causing leakage of blood from small blood vessels. If you're taking progesterone suppositories, irritation from the suppositories can also cause some spotting.

- ✔ **Cramping:** This discomfort is typical in the two-week wait and may be caused by the enlarged ovaries if you've done a stimulated cycle (taken ovarian-stimulating medications, as discussed in Chapter 11).

- ✔ **Fatigue:** This symptom is often related to higher than normal levels of hCG (human chorionic gonadotrophin, the injection given 36 or so hours before an egg retrieval) and progesterone, both of which can be from the growing embryo, or from your hCG trigger injection. Progesterone pills are particularly noted for causing extreme fatigue. Progesterone also raises your temperature, which may make you more sluggish than usual.

- ✔ **Nausea:** This symptom is fairly common with progesterone, especially in pill form, and also with high levels of hCG. Higher than normal levels of oestrogen can also cause nausea.

So how can you tell whether you're pregnant in the two-week wait? You can't! Continue taking your medications even if you're *sure* that you're not pregnant, because there's a good chance you're wrong!

Don't be so sure that you're not pregnant!

Patients who stop taking their medications, such as progesterone, because they assume that they're not pregnant make me (co-author Gill) want to pull my hair out. I usually only find this out when a patient who inexplicably never came in for her pregnancy test a week or so ago, or rang us with the result, phones to book a follow-up consultation. When I ask her why she never contacted us at the end of the 2WW, she says, 'Oh, I got my period, so I assumed it hadn't worked.' At this point my hair starts to stand on end, and I ask if she got a 'proper' period. She may say yes, but more often she says no – it was lighter than normal and she feels a bit weird. Some women have a very light period even though they're pregnant, so I keep calm and suggest that she does a pregnancy test.

Don't stop taking your medications until you've done your pregnancy test! When you've had two embryos transferred, what happens quite often is that initially both can implant and then one comes away, and you bleed a bit like a period, but you're still pregnant. Even if the period is just as heavy as normal, if you have odd symptoms, do the test! That extra progesterone is so important. Progesterone is the hormone that keeps the lining of the womb (the endometrium) stable until the placenta takes over. In a stimulated cycle plenty of natural progesterone should be around, but all the clinical trials show that extra progesterone (pessaries, tablets, gel, injections) is vital in the first few weeks after ET.

Preparing for 'But What If?' – Having a Plan B

So you're as positive as the day is long. You've kept yourself active and busy. You've benefited from the support of everyone, both in real life and in cyberspace. Still, the question keeps coming back: But what if you're not pregnant after the two-week wait? As you turn over this question for the 40,000,000th time, we suggest that you develop an answer. Having a Plan B can provide you with a sense of direction and confidence.

Will you try again? Will you continue down the high-tech highway or go back to more intermediate measures? (Many women have failed at IVF only to find themselves pregnant naturally or by lesser means in the months to follow.) Will you consider other alternatives, such as donor egg, donor sperm, or adoption? Do you want to just get away from it all for a while? Any and all of these thoughts are acceptable courses of action. You may decide on one path and find yourself veering off in another direction. That's okay. Sometimes, the mere process of just choosing something – anything – can be a relief as well as an acceptable backup plan.

For the more immediate future, we've found that having a Plan B is a good idea in preparing for the day when you receive your news. If the news is positive, you'll no doubt celebrate. But what if it's not? Consider planning a comforting alternative for the day. A great movie, a soothing meal, or a night on the town may help you and your partner deal with the news. Just having a direction can help you cope with the uncertainty of a situation that doesn't go as planned. This day is neither the beginning nor the end of your life. It's simply a day to use as you choose. Choose wisely.

Saying 'No' to Home Pregnancy Tests

Most women find the temptation of a home pregnancy test (HPT) impossible to resist. Those little packaged sticks promise immediate results and an answer to the question 'Am I pregnant or not?' Many clinics supply their patients with a test kit because they're so keen that they do the test even though they have had some bleeding. But before you go out and buy up an industrial supply of home pregnancy tests, consider the following:

✔ Many home pregnancy tests require a minimum amount of hCG in your system in order to register a positive (usually 25–50 mIU per millilitre). Early pregnancy may not result in this level, leaving you with a negative result, even in a positive situation.

✔ You were most likely given an hCG shot to trigger ovulation before your IVF retrieval. That shot of 10,000 units of hCG doesn't leave your system overnight. Furthermore, it's the same hormone (the pregnancy hormone) measured in home pregnancy tests. For some women, the traces of the hCG shot can take 10 to 15 days to disappear. Your HPT doesn't know that though! This can result in a false positive and a big let-down when the moment of truth arrives. Some clinics use injections of hCG for luteal support, which is even more likely to lead to 'false positives'.

✔ Home pregnancy tests generally require the morning's first urine, which contains the highest concentration of hCG, for greatest accuracy. Many women, pregnant or not, awake in the middle of the night to urinate, making the first morning's urine not the first after all. If you're 'really' pregnant this won't make a difference.

✔ Home pregnancy tests are, first and foremost, over-the-counter devices. Modern urinary tests are very accurate but they don't replace a blood test that measures the level of hCG in the blood stream. If your urinary test is ambiguous you must get a confirmatory check at the clinic.

Many women get on the HPT roller coaster, allowing their emotions to rise and fall with every test. It isn't worth it. Wait for the real thing at least 14 days after your embryo transfer, as hard as the waiting may be. You've no reason to subject yourself to a test that may very well yield incorrect results.

Waiting for the phone to ring

Some clinics may want to do a blood pregnancy test and then phone you with the result. Waiting for the phone to ring is almost always an unpleasant experience, whether waiting for a date to call or a nurse to deliver news of whether or not you're pregnant. Confidentiality is such an important part of UK IVF treatment that no clinic will leave such a vital message on an answerphone or voicemail. The clinic needs to know that they're talking to you and this requires a name check at least – they may also want your date of birth and clinic number!

You can't control the news you'll hear, but you can control the way you hear it. If you don't want to wait by the phone, arrange a time slot to call your nurse.

Responding to Positive News

After you get the call from your clinic that your test was positive, your initial elation may quickly change to worry: Will everything go well? Should you tell anyone yet? Having longed for one baby, what if it's two? After almost constant contact with your clinic for weeks or months, you may feel scared that you'll soon be leaving the people you've come to know and trust.

Don't panic. Most clinics continue to see you for a few weeks after your first positive test to make sure that your pregnancy is going well, and many undertake the first magic pregnancy scans.

Continuing the tests

Some clinics continue to check your hCG and your progesterone levels for several weeks to make sure that your pregnancy is progressing normally. The six week scan (two weeks after your positive pregnancy test) will hopefully show that all is well. Close monitoring ensures that if you have an ectopic pregnancy, you'll be diagnosed promptly, to avoid life-threatening complications.

hCG levels

Your clinic usually wants to see your hCG level double every two to three days for the first few weeks. The following numbers are typical milestones based on a day-three embryo transfer (three days after the egg retrieval). If you transferred blastocysts on day five, subtract two days. Obviously, many exceptions to the 'rules' can apply here. This list gives only the averages.

- **9 days post-transfer:** Average hCG 48; range 17–119

- **10 days post-transfer:** Average hCG 59; range 17–147

- **11 days post-transfer:** Average hCG 95; range 17–223

- **12 days post-transfer:** Average hCG 132; range 17–429

- **13 days post-transfer:** Average hCG 292; range 70–758

- **16 days post-transfer:** Average hCG 1061; range 324–4130; yolk sac may be visible

- **By the sixth week of pregnancy:** Average hCG 17,000; heartbeat seen by end of sixth week

- **End of sixth week:** Average hCG 30,000; embryo seen

Understanding chemical pregnancy and false positives

False positives are rare in pregnancy tests. You're most likely to get a false positive result on a home pregnancy test or a blood test if it's been less than two weeks since you took hCG to 'trigger' ovulation. Some doctors give hCG 'boosters' as luteal support during the two-week wait instead of prescribing progesterone because it stimulates the corpus luteum, the remnant of your follicle that produced an egg, to put out more progesterone.

Sometimes the blood test comes back positive, but it's a very low positive, less than 50 IU (international units). Some doctors don't consider a result 'positive' if it isn't at least 20 or so, while others consider anything over 5 to be positive and may keep you on progesterone supplements in hopes of keeping a tentative pregnancy going.

Although anything over 5 IU is a positive test, the chances of a pregnancy with such a low starting level succeeding are less than if the test result was higher. However, sometimes a pregnancy may implant a few days later than normal, giving an initial low positive. These pregnancies may pick up steam quickly, and the level starts rising appropriately.

A blood test hCG level that's positive for only a few days may be called a bio-chemical pregnancy by your doctor; a *bio-chemical pregnancy* is one in which the embryo starts to implant but fails to grow normally, so that a low level of hCG may be picked up for a short time. The level in these cases may be negative a few days later if you repeat the test.

Most clinics urge cautious optimism if the first level is lower than they would like to see it. Don't broadcast the news to anyone except those closest to you if your initial result isn't very high.

If your hCG level isn't rising appropriately, no one can do much but wait to see what happens. Some clinics monitor your progesterone levels and add more progesterone if your numbers are a little low, but adding progesterone won't save a bad pregnancy if the issue isn't a lack of progesterone.

A blood hCG level that's rising much faster than normal may indicate a *molar pregnancy*, one in which no embryo is present, only very fast-growing placental tissue. (Chapter 5 has more info on molar pregnancies.)

An hCG level that rises very quickly may mean a twin or triplet pregnancy.

Measuring crown-to-rump

One of the most accurate ways of making sure that your baby is growing the way it should is to measure the crown-to-rump length. The embryo can first be measured around five and a half weeks, when it's 2 millimetres long. Fetal growth in the first 12 weeks is very exact, and your baby's exact age can be determined from the crown-to-rump length (obviously, if you've had IVF, you know exactly when you conceived!). The measurements at the different stages are shown here. These time frames are based on your last menstrual period for spontaneous conceptions. With IVF you're already four weeks pregnant when you have a positive pregnancy test:

- ✔ **Six weeks:** 4 millimetres
- ✔ **Seven weeks:** 10 millimetres
- ✔ **Eight weeks:** 16 millimetres
- ✔ **Nine weeks:** 23 millimetres
- ✔ **Ten weeks:** 31 millimetres
- ✔ **Eleven weeks:** 41 millimetres
- ✔ **Twelve weeks:** 54 millimetres

Ultrasounds

When do you get to see your baby on ultrasound? Some clinics schedule an ultrasound around six weeks, or two weeks after the 2WW. Don't expect to see much at this point. The enthusiastic ultrasonographer or fertility nurse may be able to point out the fetal pole (the embryo) and the yolk sac to you, and you can usually see a rapid little 'blip', which is the baby's heart beating, but these features resemble a blob much more than a baby.

At this point, you know whether you have more than one baby, but keep in mind that very often one twin or triplet disappears by the next ultrasound. Very early losses of one or more embryos are very common (the 'disappearing twin' syndrome), so wait until 12 weeks or so before you tell all the neighbours you're having twins. By six to seven weeks you should be able to see a heartbeat, which you may actually recognise on ultrasound as a little flicker, and the embryo is visible. At this point, your baby resembles a fish more than a human being. No one will be willing to guess if you're having a boy or girl for another seven to eight weeks. Remember that ultrasound guesses aren't always accurate, so don't decorate the nursery in pink or blue just yet!

Celebrating your success, within limits

Congratulations, darling, we're pregnant! How will you celebrate? If you can't have sex or alcohol, is there anything left to celebrate with? How about a nice dinner out? Of course, now that you're pregnant, you're going to be eating a healthy diet and watching those empty calories!

The first few weeks of pregnancy can be dangerous for your embryo's health, because the rapid cell divisions mean that normal development can be disrupted by a number of outside influences. During this time, you need to be vigilant about what you ingest, breathe, or otherwise come in contact with.

Fetal heartbeat and health

In the IVF world we date pregnancies form the date of embryo transfer plus two weeks. When you miss your period and have a positive test you're four weeks pregnant (yes I know that you only had the ET two weeks ago, but we have to fit in with the all the folk who got pregnant the boring old-fashioned way and only have a date of their last period to go on). The first fetal heartbeat is sometimes detected around five weeks (positive pregnancy test plus one week), and averages 97 beats per minute. By six weeks, the heart rate is about 120, and by eight weeks, the baby's heart beats about 160 times per minute. The heart rate should increase 3.3 beats per minute on average during the first week a heartbeat can be detected. Several recent studies have indicated that a heart rate of less than 90 beats per minute in the first 12 weeks is associated with a high (80 per cent) miscarriage rate. By the end of your pregnancy, the baby's heart rate ranges between 120 and 160 beats per minute.

Don't forget that most women who are pregnant and didn't have IVF don't even know that they are pregnant yet, so *try not to worry!* However, be sensible when considering:

- **Medications:** Prescription medications are usually classified as to whether they're definitely, probably, or possibly safe in pregnancy. Some drugs known to cause birth defects are Ro-Accutane, an acne medication, and Thalidomide, used in the 1960s to treat morning sickness. Generally speaking, a drug should be safe to take as long as your doctor is aware that you're pregnant when taking it. All prescription medications are listed in the *BNF (British National Formulary)* and can be checked for safety before being prescribed for you. Don't take anything that wasn't prescribed for you by a doctor who knows you're pregnant.

- **Illegal drugs:** There are *no* safe illegal drugs! Some drugs are linked with prematurity or an increased chance of miscarriage; others may cause your baby to be born addicted and to go through painful withdrawal. Cocaine can cause the placenta to separate from the uterus, so that the baby loses its blood supply and must be delivered immediately.

- **Alcohol:** You're better eliminating drinking alcohol in pregnancy altogether. A very occasional glass of wine in the last trimester is unlikely to cause harm, but daily heavy drinking, especially in the first few months of pregnancy, can cause fetal alcohol syndrome, which causes lifelong physical and behavioural problems.

- **Sex:** Many clinics worry that orgasm may cause uterine contractions, which can 'push' a tentative pregnancy over the edge. The likeliest times to bleed in early pregnancy are when you would normally be having a period, so avoid sex in weeks 4, 8, and 12. If you have any bleeding in pregnancy, take that as a warning and resist the temptation until you've had at least three days without any bleeding.

✔ **Cigarettes:** Smoking is linked with increased miscarriage rates; babies whose parents smoke have more respiratory problems and are more likely to suffer from asthma.

Saying goodbye to your fertility doctor

Some fertility clinics monitor you through the first few weeks after you become pregnant; others wave goodbye with your first positive test. Most clinics don't want to keep you too long as a pregnant patient because your GP wants to get involved. Your clinic is probably happy to do your first two scans (at 6 weeks and 8 weeks) and sees you again if you've had bleeding or other problems. But you may have a hard time getting an appointment with an obstetrician until you're 18–20 weeks pregnant or so, leaving you in sort of a no man's land of medical care.

Tell your GP you're pregnant as soon as possible. This way, if you have any problems in the first few weeks, such as spotting, cramping, or severe pain (as in a possible ectopic pregnancy), your GP can arrange to take care of you, if your clinic doesn't deal with these issues.

Defining high-risk pregnancy

Don't think of yourself as a high-risk pregnancy just because you had IVF to get pregnant. Most of the time, IVF doesn't increase the risk of complications in pregnancy unless you have a multiple pregnancy. The complications come from whatever caused your infertility, such as your age, uterine shape, or other health issues.

Most doctors consider you high risk for the following reasons:

✔ You're over age 35.

✔ You have a uterine malformation (fibroids or a unicornuate or septate uterus) that may make conditions hard for you to carry the pregnancy.

✔ You're expecting multiples (twins or higher).

✔ You have a health history of cancer or a disease such as diabetes, lupus, high blood pressure, or heart disease.

✔ You have a history of incompetent cervix (see Chapter 5).

✔ You've had previous caesarean sections.

✔ You're significantly overweight.

✔ You've had bleeding in early pregnancy.

CVS or amniocentesis?

For many years, the only way to evaluate chromosomes in an unborn child was to wait until the uterus grew large enough for the fluid surrounding the baby to be withdrawn through a needle under ultrasound guidance. This procedure, called *amniocentesis,* generally wasn't possible until after 16 weeks of pregnancy; if a problem was found, the fetus was too large to be aborted with a dilatation and curettage, and a mini-labour was needed for the baby to be delivered. A newer technique, done between 10 and 12 weeks of pregnancy, is called *chorionic villus sampling* (CVS). Your doctor aspirates a small amount of the tissue that attaches the sac to the uterine wall. This procedure can be done through the abdomen or through the vagina. If you have a tipped or retroverted uterus, the procedure may be safer to do abdominally. The risk of miscarriage is small, less than 1 per cent. CVS was done earlier, before ten weeks, when the technique first came into use, but a small percentage of babies born had limb defects. Now CVS is done after ten weeks, and the risk to the fetus has been negligible. The risk of miscarriage after amniocentesis is less than 0.05 per cent, or about 1 in 200.

If you're a high-risk patient, you'll probably see the obstetric consultant more often than once a month in the first trimester. You may do additional testing, such as chorionic villus sampling (CVS), to check for chromosomal abnormalities in the first three months.

Considering the Next Step If IVF Doesn't Work

Every day, a patient asks me (co-author Gill) how it can be possible that she's *not* pregnant. 'But my embryos looked perfect. My lining looked great, and I did everything I was supposed to. How could it not work?' women say.

Unfortunately, most of the time the answer is, 'We just don't know.' Statistically speaking, even if everyone does everything perfectly, you've at best a 30–40 per cent chance of getting pregnant, which means you've an equal 60–70 per cent chance of not getting pregnant, but this isn't the answer a disappointed patient wants to hear. You want an answer, something that you can fix in the future. But the truth is that medicine doesn't have all the answers.

Figuring out what happened

What happened? What went wrong? One of several things happened if your pregnancy test was negative.

✔ **The embryos may not have implanted at all.** Sometimes this happens because the lining of the uterus and the embryo were *asynchronous,* meaning that the lining and the embryo weren't developed in synch with each other. Like a flower planted in January, an embryo planted at the wrong time won't grow. Because IVF is an artificial process, you can't be sure that your lining is at the exact right stage for implantation when the embryos are transferred. The doctors can look at the lining with ultrasound, but the only way to truly tell what stage the lining is at is to do an endometrial biopsy, a procedure in which a little piece of lining is scraped off and sent to pathology to see if it was growing properly. Obviously, a biopsy can't be done if you're trying to get pregnant at the time, because the bleeding caused by the biopsy disturbs the lining.

✔ **Another possibility is that the embryos started to implant and then stopped.** Usually this happens because the embryos are abnormal chromosomally. The older the woman, the more likely she is to have embryos that have abnormal chromosomes. The only way to tell whether embryos have the right chromosomes is to do preimplantation genetic diagnosis (PGD), a procedure in which one cell is removed from the embryo before implantation and its DNA is analysed for abnormalities. This procedure is expensive, and not all centres do PGD.

✔ **Sometimes embryos stop growing because of the level of progesterone, a hormone that helps the uterus nourish the embryo.** Progesterone supplements are usually given after an IVF cycle, and the leftover corpus luteum also produces progesterone, but some people need much higher doses than others to keep the lining optimal.

✔ **Because IVF is a mechanical procedure, the embryos can be damaged during the process of growth in the lab and in the actual transfer itself.** Man-made processes are never going to be as effective as nature intended, and occasionally, a bad batch of medium, which is used to nurture the embryos before transfer, can prevent the embryo from growing the way it's expected. Before you're tempted to blame the lab, remember that half of all 'naturally' made embryos also fail to implant successfully.

Questions for God and your doctor (who are not one and the same)

An unsuccessful attempt at IVF can be devastating financially, physically, and emotionally. The situation opens up the floodgate for a host of worries and fears that can be overwhelming. For this reason, your best thinking probably doesn't come on the day of, or the day after, an unsuccessful attempt. You need to put some time and space between the cycle and your next steps. Remember that your hormone levels are probably off kilter as well. They'll eventually return to normal and probably your mood will, too, as the days pass.

Your doctor may refrain from any immediate action. Don't panic if your doctor doesn't schedule your follow-up visit for a few weeks after receiving your results. Your doctor has experienced this scenario time and again and is probably giving you time to heal, as well as a chance to collect your thoughts and your questions. Give yourself and your partner a break, and take advantage of this time, before rushing to ask, 'What went wrong?' You may find that the more immediate questions you have become less important in a week's time, while other, more pertinent questions come to the surface.

Your doctor is preparing as well during this time. The lab reports have to be completed and compiled before your doctor can review them. Give your doctor the necessary time to do a thorough examination of your cycle so that you can have the best possible explanation.

As you prepare your list of questions for your doctor, try to be as specific as possible. 'What went wrong?' may be a good question to start with, but you're better off breaking this broad question down into more specific questions, such as the following:

- Did I respond as expected?
- How was my egg quality?
- What particular stage in the process did you feel posed the most problems?
- What did you learn about me and my situation through this process?
- What would you recommend as a next step? Why?

As you prepare your questions, think of your cycle in stages as well. Ask your doctor about your particular preparation for your IVF cycle (Did you respond well to 'down-regulation?), your follicular phase (as the eggs mature during stimulation), ovulatory phase, and luteal phase (the stage in which your body either accepts or rejects the embryo). What area would your doctor focus on or change for your next cycle? Why? Would your drug protocol be different? How and why?

You may find that your doctor has collected a great deal of information about your body and its reproductive abilities through this IVF cycle. Those findings may suggest a different course of action, perhaps less technological (if your doctor feels that IVF isn't warranted in your case) or more technological (through the use of third-party reproduction, a topic we discuss in Chapter 20). Your follow-up consultation is a good time to inquire about this and find out what your doctor believes is the best plan for you.

Remember that your doctor isn't God and doesn't have all the answers. Fertility is a numbers game, under the best of circumstances. If doctors knew exactly why or why not it all worked, they would save you and themselves a lot of time, and make a lot more money. Unfortunately, medicine doesn't have all the answers, for anything, especially fertility.

Your doctor may also be a great source of comfort, but consider taking the 'Why me?' question to a therapist, a religious person, or God. Your doctor is undoubtedly well aware of your pain and would do anything in her power to relieve it. Like all of us, however, your doctor has limitations. Use your doctor for the knowledge that she does have and seek other avenues for the answers that your doctor doesn't have.

Going through the grieving process

Perhaps the best way to deal with the morass of emotions brought on by an unsuccessful cycle is by looking at the grieving process. You can treat this disappointment as a loss, and some women even liken it to miscarriage. Consider the following stages and how they may apply:

- **Denial:** 'Maybe the test results are wrong, and I really am pregnant,' you may say. Denial is perhaps one of the most time-honoured human traditions in dealing with painful situations. Although denial provides you with a brief respite from your pain, this emotional tool isn't something that can successfully carry you out of your grief. Accepting that you're not pregnant (after your doctor has confirmed it), no matter how much you want to be, is the first step.

- **Anger:** 'My doctor doesn't care,' or 'Somebody messed up,' may be a typical response. Anger is also a perfectly natural and understandable response to grief. Perhaps your anger is justified, and you do need to take some action. Now is probably not the best time to do so. Instead, work on taking the sting out of the anger. If you do need to take some action, you can wait for a few weeks. You may find that, as your emotions (and hormones) subside with time, your anger may not seem as urgent. Remember that physical force or verbal intimidation is never appropriate, no matter how angry you are. If you feel this way, you need some time to cool off and perhaps some professional help to do so.

- **Bargaining:** 'If only I can be pregnant, I'll never again (pick one) yell at my partner, slack at work, speed, or engage in any other bad habits.' Bargaining is a normal reaction to grief, albeit not a very useful one. Allow yourself time to move through this stage (as with all the stages that you experience). This too shall pass.

- **Depression:** 'I'm not pregnant. I'll never have a baby. My life is worthless.' Also known as 'stinking thinking,' depression can cast a cloud over your thoughts and feelings. This emotion is another (normal) stage of grief that often doesn't let you take into account the positive realities in your life. Try to remember that, when depressed, you're likely to paint your circumstances in a particularly dull shade of grey. If your depression lasts longer than two weeks, consider seeking professional help, whether from your doctor or a counsellor. They may prescribe antidepressants to get you through this difficult time. Your feelings are real, but they're also temporary.

✔ **Acceptance:** Remember that acceptance doesn't equate to agreement. You may accept your circumstances as they are today and yet continue to feel that the situation is unfair – and it is. Remember that you can change your circumstances now that you've passed through your period of mourning.

You may go through these stages of grief more than once. You may skip a stage or repeat it twice before you come to accept what has happened. Regardless, don't rush yourself. You'll get there when you get there, and not a moment sooner.

Taking time out for you and your partner

While you're grieving, your partner may be grieving as well. Or he may be stuck in a particular stage of the process, such as denial or anger. Keep an eye on him. Look for signs that he may need some additional help to work through his feelings.

After you're both past the initial shock and grief, consider taking some time out to relax and regroup, in that order. Although you may be tempted to resume your normal routine, your body, mind, and spirit will benefit from a little rest and relaxation. Your relationship will, too. Grief can be a very personal thing and one that isolates you from the most important people in your life, including your partner. Take the time to reconnect with one another and appreciate those things that you love in each other. This time is a great opportunity for taking a fertility free holiday, whether that is an exotic destination, or your own back garden. Either way, give yourselves the time off to relax. A one-month hiatus doesn't make a difference to the big picture. However, not taking the time to recoup, and renew yourself and your partnership, can have lasting effects.

Use your follow-up doctor's visit as a springboard to discuss your future plans with your partner. Remember that you're both playing in the same team. If your goals appear to be different at this point, give one another the space and time to consider both sides. If you need help to arrive at a mutually agreeable decision, you may want to consider visiting a counsellor, or a religious adviser. If your partner appears to be reluctant to try again, listen to his point of view and give him some time. More than likely, time will help to bridge differences in opinion, and heal hurt feelings.

Chapter 18

What's in Your Freezer? Frozen Embryo Transfers

*E*very busy housewife and working woman knows what a godsend her freezer is! The ability to rustle up a tasty meal in minutes when she gets in from work, or to have one big cooking session and freeze the dishes in portions to eat later, or enjoy 'out of season' produce from her garden in the depths of winter all demonstrate how useful freezing is in speeding things up, avoiding waste, and preserving things when they're at their best. The same is true with IVF embryos. Embryo freezing or 'cryopreservation' has transformed the prospects for success with IVF for many couples. But don't worry that the embryology team ever forgets that they are working with the most precious of all biological material: The embryos that have the potential to become your child.

In this chapter, we tell you what your chances are of having surplus embryos to freeze, what goes on in the lab, and what the embryologists want to see, and what they *don't* want to see in embryos. We consider different strategies for performing frozen embryo transfers (FETs) and tell you about success rates. We also review the tricky ethical issues that arise when considering freezing, storing, and transferring surplus embryos.

Before you have IVF you may consider an embryo to be just a little 'cluster of microscopic cells' that are invisible to the naked eye. When your first IVF baby is born following successful transfer of that little 'cluster' you may think of the other clusters in the freezer in quite a different light. They could be your baby's potential brother or sister.

Facing a Few Facts about Frozen Embryos

We all know that fish fingers and chicken nuggets won't keep indefinitely even in the freezer because they start to deteriorate after a few months. IVF freezers contain liquid nitrogen at −196 degrees, the temperature at which all cellular activity stops. This means that embryos aren't damaged by the freezing process and when they're thawed (whether two months or 20 years later) the cells that make up the embryo and the genetic blue-print they carry are just as good as when they were frozen. The embryos are literally frozen in time.

Healthy babies have been born from embryos that have been stored for over 20 years, but in the UK the normal period of storage is five years maximum but that can be extended to ten years if your doctor believes that your fertility is permanently impaired and the frozen embryos represent your best, or only, chance of having a child.

Who uses them

Embryo freezing is a very important part of an IVF programme and 30–70 per cent of IVF and ICSI cycles yield surplus embryos suitable for freezing. This surplus not only reduces wastage of valuable embryos but also maximises the number of conception attempts in each stimulation cycle. Embryo freezing also increases the cumulative pregnancy rates and reduces the health risks, costs, and inconvenience of repeated fresh cycles.

Success rates with 'frosties'

Worldwide pregnancy rates with frozen embryos are just a little lower than with fresh embryos but the simplicity and much reduced cost of a frozen embryo transfer makes it a very good idea for couples who are lucky enough to have embryos to freeze. Some couples believe that if their fresh embryos didn't make a baby then they have no chance of success with a frozen one. This simply is not the case, because many women only get pregnant with frozen embryos and never with their fresh ones. This may be due to the lower and more stable hormone levels that operate in a natural cycle or HRT controlled cycle (see the later section 'Natural cycle or hormone control for embryo transfer?').

Although a funny-looking embryo doesn't create a funny-looking kid, most embryologists do feel that an embryo with less fragmentation and more even-looking cells has a better chance of implanting. If you do get pregnant from fragmented embryos, the fragmentation does *not* mean that your baby is going to be abnormal in any way. Some centres remove the fragmented pieces before the embryo is transferred.

Discovering Why Embryos Are Frozen

Freezing embryos is done for many reasons and in this section we describe some of the usual ones. The basic principle is that we want to safeguard the health of the woman having fertility treatment and to maximise the chance of a healthy pregnancy and healthy baby.

Freezing excess embryos created during IVF

IVF is much more successful if the ovaries are stimulated with gonadotrophins. These drugs promote the growth of multiple follicles within the ovaries resulting in the production of many eggs, and hopefully many embryos. Currently, we can only transfer a maximum of two embryos to women under 40 (it's three for the over 40s) and some young women having a first cycle of IVF may be advised to reduce the risk of twins and just have one embryo transferred. With modern freezing (cryopreservation) techniques you're almost as likely to get pregnant from frozen embryos as from fresh ones and freezing any good quality embryos for possible future use makes good sense because they can give you a second chance of a pregnancy if the fresh cycle doesn't work (or the chance of a second baby if it does!) without needing to go through the whole stimulation and egg retrieval process again.

Creating a complete family from just one stimulation cycle is possible. I (co-author Gill) like to tell the story of one of the luckiest couples that had treatment at our clinic. From their first NHS-funded IVF cycle they got twins from the fresh transfer and had eight spare embryos frozen. From these 'frosties' they got two separate singleton pregnancies: one two years later, and one four years later!

Saving younger eggs for ageing women

Older women may also benefit from embryo freezing because their embryo quality (which is largely determined by the age of the egg) is literally 'frozen in time' at the age the woman was when the eggs were collected. So a woman who has a first IVF baby at 38 and has embryos frozen can delay trying for baby number two, secure in the knowledge that, even though she may be ageing, her embryos aren't.

Preserving the possibility of parenthood for those facing medical issues

Sometimes we need to freeze embryos created during an IVF or ICSI treatment cycle for compelling medical reasons:

- **Ovarian hyperstimulation syndrome (OHSS):** Sometimes a fresh embryo transfer can't be undertaken because the risk of ovarian hyperstimulation syndrome (OHSS) is too high. (Refer to Chapters 11 and 12.) This occurs if you over-respond to the drugs that stimulate the ovaries and produce too many follicles. Because pregnancy almost always makes OHSS worse, the best course of action is to postpone the fresh transfer and freeze all the embryos at zygote (two pronucleate, or 2PN), cleavage (four to six cells), or blastocyst stage.

- **Problems with the uterine lining:** Embryo freezing may also be advised if you develop an abnormality in the endometrium (uterine lining), such as a polyp or fibroid, that could interfere with successful implantation or if the endometrium fails to develop properly.

- **Other health concerns:** If you're about to have surgery, chemotherapy, or radiotherapy that may affect your future fertility, the possibility arises to create and freeze embryos for you to have transferred in the future.

Understanding the Process of Cryopreservation

Freezing embryos is a technical process that wouldn't look out of place in a science-fiction film! This section describes the stages involved.

Freezing the embryos

Freezing embryos requires that the embryos be dehydrated (partially dried out) to stop ice crystals forming inside and shattering the delicate structures within the embryo. (Do you remember those experiments you did in science class with potatoes and sugar solution when you were learning about osmosis? Now don't you wish you had paid attention!)

The embryos are placed in solutions containing increasing concentrations of sugar and an 'anti-freeze' mixture called a *cryoprotectant* for a period of 30 minutes. They're then placed in fine plastic straws each labelled with your name, date of birth, clinic identity number, and a unique freeze-cycle number. The embryos are then loaded into a computer-controlled freeze machine that cools the embryos slowly over a period of two hours. The straws are removed from the machine and stored in tanks of liquid nitrogen.

Embryos can be frozen at one of several stages:

- ✔ **2PN:** The earliest stage after normal fertilisation has been identified the morning after the egg collection. Embryos at this stage are quite robust and freeze well.

- ✔ **Cleavage:** Four–six cells. This is the stage at which embryos are normally transferred at ET (embryo transfer).

- ✔ **Blastocyst stage:** Blastocyst freezing occurs five–six days after egg retrieval.

If you're planning to freeze some or all of your embryos for use at another time, your clinic may freeze them at the 2PN stage. Some clinics freeze the embryos the morning after your fresh transfer and some centres try to grow all your embryos on to the blastocyst stage and freeze only those that make it to blastocyst.

Not all embryos are good enough quality to withstand the freeze-thaw process. Freezing embryos that are very slow to develop, or full of fragments or little blisters called *vacuoles*, is pointless. You may be very disappointed to start off with a good number of eggs and embryos only to find that nothing is suitable for freezing. However, freezing poor quality embryos just gives false hope and couples should focus on their fresh transfer, and regard having 'frosties' as a bonus.

Thawing the embryos

When the time comes to use the embryos, care must be taken because if re-warming is carried out too slowly, ice crystals could form as the temperature rises. Normally 2–3 minutes at room temperature is enough: Then the straws are opened and the embryos are placed into four different solutions in turn to remove the anti-freeze whilst gradually warming them to 37 degrees Celsius (98.6 degrees Fahrenheit).

On average, three-quarters (75 per cent) of early embryos (2PN) survive the process of freezing and thawing. Of those embryos frozen later (cleavage stage) about two-thirds (65 per cent) survive. Sometimes one or two of the cells or *blastomeres* become damaged or die and appear as little dark fragments within the embryo. Since each blastomere contains the entire genetic 'blueprint' to make a baby, as long as some healthy cells survive, the embryo has the chance to continue to develop and can be transferred.

Using natural cycle or hormone control for embryo transfer?

The two options for transferring 'frosties' is during your natural cycle, or during a hormone-controlled cycle.

Natural cycle

If the woman has a good, regular, ovular cycle then her frozen embryos can be replaced in a 'natural cycle'. This option is suitable if there's no anxiety about the development of the womb lining; and it has the advantage that you don't need to take high doses of hormones during the first few months of pregnancy. An ultrasound scan on cycle day 8–9 confirms whether a good follicle is developing and the lining (endometrium) looks normal. Urine testing sticks (LH sticks or OPKs) can then be used to identify the day of ovulation. On the appropriate day, the embryos are thawed and cultured for a little while to make sure that they're viable and dividing; after that, they can be transferred in the same way as fresh embryos. Most clinics suggest that you take additional progesterone in the form of vaginal pessaries, tablets, or injections until the pregnancy test.

Hormone-controlled cycle

If you have irregular, unpredictable cycles (such as occur with PCOS or in the years leading up to the menopause) then a hormone-controlled or HRT cycle may be recommended. This can be done in a 'down-regulated' cycle where you take GnRH analogue drugs such as buserelin, or nafarelin (just like in a 'long protocol' IVF cycle). When you're 'down-regulated' then you start taking the oestrogen (oestradiol valerate) tablets in a 'step-up' system until you're taking 6 milligrammes a day. When the endometrium is thick enough (ideally more than 8 millimetres) after about 12 days, you start the progesterone and the embryos can be transferred. If the pregnancy test is positive, the oestrogen and progesterone must be continued until the 12th week of pregnancy, as no natural *corpus luteum* is present to support the pregnancy until the placenta takes over.

On a personal note, I (co-author Gill) introduced a simpler system of HRT-controlled cycles that we call 'the Swedish recipe' in honour of a friend who runs an IVF clinic in Stockholm in Sweden. On cycle day 2, you start taking 6 milligrammes a day of oestradiol valerate tablets and when the endometrium has a well-defined pattern and is 8–10 millimetres deep then the progesterone can start. The embryos (depending on their stage of development) can be transferred 2–5 days later.

The 2WW (refer to Chapter 17) after a frozen embryo transfer is just as long (and difficult!) as the 2WW after a fresh transfer. If these 'frosties' came from a batch of embryos that gave you your darling son or daughter then the wait can seem even harder. The build up to a frozen embryo transfer (FET) cycle is not so physically demanding but emotionally you can feel far worse.

Dealing with the Ethical Issues of Embryo Freezing

Although embryo freezing does make a big contribution to the cumulative pregnancy rate, embryo freezing isn't for everyone. Give the following considerations some serious thought before you decide to freeze your embryos:

- ✔ When do you believe that life starts? If you believe that life begins at the point of fertilisation, the possibility of creating supernumery embryos and freezing the spares is not an ethical option for you.

- ✔ What happens to frozen embryos that you don't use? Signing the forms that say you agree to have your spare embryos frozen isn't a mere formality. You and your partner need to think what to do with frozen embryos if you do not choose to use them in your own treatment within the time frame allowed. Will you choose to donate them to another couple, or to help medical research? Or will you both be prepared to accept that they should be allowed to perish if either one of you (or both of you) no longer want to use them but would be unhappy with either of the other options? For some couples, the delight of knowing they had 'frosties' at the time of their fresh embryo transfer turns into a very difficult dilemma.

- ✔ What do you want to do with the embryos in the event of personal crises? The HFEA consent forms ask difficult questions about what you would want to happen to your embryos if one of you died or became mentally incapacitated.

✔ What happens if your relationship with your partner ends? All couples believe that their marriage or partnership is together forever, but what if you do split up? Under UK law, the continuing consent of both partners that contributed to the creation of an embryo is required for that embryo to continue in storage, or be used. If either of you withdraws consent, the law says that the embryos can't be transferred and must be taken out of storage and allowed to perish. The heart-rending legal cases that are really 'custody' battles over frozen embryos are a constant reminder of the moral, ethical, and personal dilemmas that the science of cryobiology has created.

That tiny dot of frozen gloop is potentially a son or daughter, a brother or sister. Frozen embryos are potential people and everyone who works in an IVF clinic is very well aware of your anxieties on this issue. If you have ethical concerns or just need a little support, have some sessions with the counsellor or consult your own religious leaders.

Chapter 19

If at First You Don't Succeed: Trying IVF More than Once

*M*aybe your first attempt at in vitro fertilisation (IVF) failed, and you're wondering whether it's worth trying a second time. Or maybe you got pregnant first time, have a brand-new baby, and wonder whether you should get started right away on number two, just in case getting pregnant again takes a while.

In this chapter, we look at the decision to try IVF two, three, four, or more times. We also look at some really high-tech additions to the IVF mix that may increase your chances – or just leave you still childless, and a lot poorer. The jury's still out on some of the controversial therapies so we help you decide which ones to consider and which to avoid.

Calculating the Odds: Success Rates per IVF Cycle

If your IVF cycle ended in a negative pregnancy test, your first question, after 'Why didn't it work?' may be 'What are my chances next time?' Most doctors feel that your chances of success don't drop in your first three cycles; in other words, if you're in an age group in which 30 per cent get pregnant doing an IVF cycle, your chance of getting pregnant is 30 per cent in each of your first three tries. After three failed attempts, something more may be preventing you from getting pregnant, and your doctor may want to change your protocol, or do more testing. Nearly 50 per cent of all IVF babies get made in the first cycle, but this fact doesn't mean that if it doesn't work first time you're doomed to be unlucky. Success rates stay pretty constant for the first three cycles because the clinic learns things about you from an unsuccessful cycle that helps the next time.

Statistics are averages. A 28 per cent per cycle pregnancy rate means that of 100 couples having a cycle of IVF or ICSI, 72 won't even get a positive pregnancy test. Don't get hung up on numbers, but recognise that low means low.

Having IVF isn't like rolling the dice and hoping for a six. Don't settle for 'better luck next time!' Although many people do get pregnant on their fourth or fifth attempt without changing anything, the 'one-size-fits-all' approach to IVF (where everyone follows the same protocol) is old-fashioned and ineffective. Tailor-made always fits better than off-the peg. So review the entire cycle with your doctor to see what went well (you got a good number of eggs?) and what went badly (the fertilisation rate was low?) so that you and your doctor can consider alternatives that may work better (shall we try ICSI next time?).

If you're over 40, the three-tries rule may not apply because your chance of getting pregnant in each cycle decreases due to you getting older. If you're over 40, the secret of success may be getting a chromosomally normal embryo, and that's more difficult to achieve because so many eggs are chromosomally abnormal at that age. For this reason, you're allowed to transfer three embryos at a time, hoping to get at least one good one in the bunch.

Going Back for Seconds? Considering Your Options

If you've had one failed cycle, you may be anxious to try again right away. This step is pretty simple if you have frozen embryos; without frozen embryos, the task is a bit more complicated:

- ✔ **With frozen embryos:** If you have frozen embryos, you're monitored during a natural cycle, or you take medication to thicken your endometrial lining for a few weeks and then transfer the embryos back. The monitoring is much less frequent than a stimulated retrieval cycle (refer to Chapter 18), the drugs cost relatively little and the cost of the transfer is usually much less than the cost of an egg retrieval cycle. If you have frozen embryos, many clinics let you start a frozen embryo transfer cycle soon after your first failed cycle because the protocols for frozen transfer are fairly standard.

 ✔ **Without frozen embryos:** If you don't have frozen embryos, you need to go through the entire IVF process again, with frequent monitoring, daily injections, and an egg retrieval. If you need another egg retrieval, most clinics ask you to make another appointment with your doctor or fertility nurse to talk over what may have gone wrong and what can be changed. Remember that even if everybody (doctors, nurses, scientists, and even you!) did everything right, IVF still only works 25–40 per cent of the time.

If you get pregnant and have a baby (or two!), you may want to go back for seconds in another sense: baby number two. Most clinics want you to have an appointment with your doctor and re-do some of the blood tests; if you still have frozen embryos, you'll probably use them up instead of doing another fresh cycle. A frozen embryo cycle involves far less medication and less monitoring.

Deciding when to start another cycle

How soon you want to try IVF again depends on your clinic, your emotional state, and your finances.

Your clinic's standards

Whether your clinic encourages another cycle straight after a negative pregnancy test depends on your clinic's thinking. Although little evidence supports this position, some doctors believe that taking stimulating gonadotrophins back to back (two or more months in a row), doesn't allow your body to recover, and this may decrease your response to the medications in the next cycle. IVF can be very demanding (physically, psychologically, and financially), so taking a few months off from constantly having to think about injections, scans, and hormone levels is a good idea. Far more couples than you'd expect conceive spontaneously after a failed IVF cycle, so don't think of the next month or two as wasted time in your quest for a baby.

If you're going back for your second child and have no frozen embryos left, most doctors won't want you to do an IVF cycle until your first child is no longer breast-feeding because the prolactin hormone that breast-feeding women produce can interfere with ovarian response. Some doctors want you to have resumed regular periods, but other doctors don't consider this important as long as you have one period, which can be brought on artificially, before starting again.

Many couples embark on pregnancy number two with the attitude that they may take a long time to get pregnant again, and then they're shocked when the very next attempt ends with a positive pregnancy test. Be sure that you're really ready for baby number two before you get started again!

Your emotional health

You also need to consider your psychological health. A life that's a continuous sequence of injections, blood tests, scans, and consultations can rapidly become lacking in pleasure. Remember to make time for some fun and for your partner. Many couples plan a holiday to coincide with the end of their IVF cycle to compensate for the negative pregnancy test that they're dreading. This is okay as long as the test *is* negative. That camel safari or hanggliding course that seemed so exciting before looks very different if you have morning sickness and twin fetuses on board! For more detailed information on how to judge how you're doing emotionally (and how your relationship with your partner is faring), head to the section 'I'm Okay, You're Okay – Checking on the State of Your Union'.

Your finances

What price a baby? In an ideal world the answer is 'unquantifiable', but we're living in the real world. If you've spent £4,000 on your first IVF cycle and are still not pregnant, money matters become important for most people. If you have frozen embryos, a frozen embryo transfer costs much less than a full treatment cycle (around £750 to £1,000 instead of £3,000 to £6,000, depending on the clinic), plus the cost of any drugs (which is much less than the 'full' down-regulation and follicle-stimulating drugs required for a new treatment cycle). But if you have no frozen embryos, you have to pay the whole cost for a second, or further, full treatment cycle. Consider your options:

- ✔ Can you get NHS-funded treatment? If not, can your GP agree to pay the cost of your drugs (which can save you around £350 to £1,000)?
- ✔ Do you still have savings?
- ✔ Are the doors of the Bank of Mum and Dad still open for business?
- ✔ Are you willing to egg share (refer to Chapter 15) to reduce the cost of your next treatment?
- ✔ Are you prepared to get a bank loan or flex your credit card further? (But bear in mind the repayment issues with the additional costs and possible reduced income you'll face in future months if you do have a baby!)
- ✔ How many cycles are you prepared to try and how many can you really afford?

Other health issues discovered along the way

Most women start infertility treatment in reasonably good health. During an IVF cycle, you'll probably be under more medical scrutiny – at least certain parts of you are going to be – than at any other time during your life. Diseases such as diabetes or lupus sometimes are diagnosed while women are undergoing ultrasounds and blood testing. Women have also discovered ovarian cancer, breast cancer, or cervical or uterine cancer after those areas were scrutinised for infertility.

Frozen embryos and their expiry dates

Embryos are frozen in liquid nitrogen in −196 degrees Celsius, the temperature at which all cellular activity stops. This technique means that embryos frozen up to fifteen years have produced healthy babies. In the UK, embryos can be frozen for five years in the first instance and the storage period can be extended to ten years, or beyond, if two doctors agree that the circumstances are right to do so.

If you have frozen embryos, you'll probably pay a storage fee each year. Most centres send out a letter (or invoice) reminding you that your embryos are still there. If several years have passed since your last transfer, in addition to seeing your doctor to make sure that everything's okay to proceed with an embryo transfer, you can also contact the embryology department to confirm how many frozen embryos you still have.

Even if you have twins or triplets and don't think that you'll ever want more children, don't be too quick to decide to discard or donate your remaining embryos. The 'quality' of frozen embryos is higher than 'fresh embryos' created five years later (because you'll have aged), and more likely to produce a pregnancy.

If you find out that you have another disease in addition to infertility, will it put your conception plans on hold? That depends on the disease and treatment required to cure or control it. Some examples include:

- ✔ If a cancer is found, you may need to put your fertility plans on hold while you receive radiation or chemotherapy. On the other hand, your doctor may allow you to do a cycle of stimulating medications before treatment so that you can have some eggs or embryos frozen, especially if your cancer treatment may make you permanently infertile.

- ✔ If you're found to have diabetes, your blood sugars need to be controlled before you start treatment. After your diabetes is under control, you may then be able to proceed. Your pregnancy is at greater risk if you're a diabetic.

- ✔ If you're diagnosed with thyroid disease, you'll need treatment to regulate your thyroid. Without treatment, you probably won't be able to get pregnant. Regulating your thyroid can take several months and may require readjustment of your medication if you do get pregnant.

- ✔ If you find out that you have an autoimmune disease, such as lupus, you'll need to be evaluated for problems with your kidneys, lungs, or other organs before trying to get pregnant. Your pregnancy will most likely also be treated as high risk.

Switching clinics and protocols – or not

When something doesn't work, many people go from one extreme to the other: They either do nothing and just keep trying the same protocols at the same clinic, or do something entirely different and rush round to other clinics expecting that second, third, and even fourth opinions will transform their chances. Remember that you chose your clinic for good reasons in the first place (personal recommendation, good published success rates, flexible hours, geography). Those things are still true even if you got a negative pregnancy test result.

Changing protocols

If you're curious about a new method or protocol, raise the subject with your doctor at your follow-up consultation. If you've found information online, or in a magazine or journal describing this new technique, bring it with you. Many doctors are willing to look at something new and even try it, *if* they believe that it's going to benefit you. Recognise that your doctor may determine that this new protocol is a valid one, but not likely to be effective with you. Whether you like or agree with your doctor, he or she has significantly more experience in the field than you do, if based only on the number of patients they've seen!

Cutting-edge protocols may turn out to be the greatest thing since sliced bread. They also have an equal probability of being totally useless, or even detrimental. New isn't always better. Other people's protocols may not be the answer for you, either. Every woman's body is different, as is her response to medicines and techniques.

You may, however, feel that you've given your current doctor enough time and opportunity. You may have found that your doctor is unwilling to think outside the box and try anything different. Perhaps it's time for a change of clinic.

Trading clinics

Even if everything goes really well, the odds are still stacked against you. Because the difference between success and failure when a fertility treatment doesn't work can be indefinable, keep in mind the positives as well as the negatives before you decide to leave your old doctor in favour of someone new. Nevertheless, if you believe that you've taken advantage of all that your current clinic has to offer, and decide to move on, consider these points:

- ✔ **NHS-funded patients:** If you're an NHS-funded patient you may feel that you have little choice about where you go for fertility treatment. In fact, if you're eligible for NHS-funded treatment, you're entitled to a choice of clinics. You may need to write several letters and get quite cross, but hang on in there and eventually the suits are going to see things your way!

> ✔ **Private patients:** If you're a private patient, be a savvy shopper. Don't just fall for any doctor who tells you that they can bring you a baby. On the contrary, these claims ought to strike you as suspicious. Instead, ask your doctor for data, published articles, studies, and sample protocols to support their proposal.

Arrange a consultation with a new clinic before kicking the old one into touch, but always be suspicious of doctors that attack other doctors' practices. Hindsight is wonderful, but was not available to your previous doctor at the time they were doing your cycle. It may be very clear now that you over-responded or under-responded, or had an unexpectedly difficult embryo transfer and that may be why the cycle didn't work, but a first cycle of IVF is always an experiment!

An unsuccessful cycle merely reflects the low odds that you're dealing with, not necessarily the ability of your doctor. Each time you switch doctors and practices, your new team must relearn everything about you. Sure, they can review your records, but doing so doesn't take the place of hands-on experience and the knowledge that your former doctor had been accumulating. Remember, the 'best' doctors generally take their information and knowledge from the same pool available to all doctors. They also may be a great deal busier than the doctor next door, resulting in less personal time and attention to your individual case.

Reaching out for more help

Whether you're trying to decide if you want to stay with your current doctor, or contemplating how, when, and why you're going to try again, remember that you don't have to go it alone.

This moment is an ideal time to reach out to relatives, friends, online resources, your medical network (including your family doctor), or a professional association to help you determine the next right thing to do. Some sites (www.highfsh.org, www.hfea.gov.uk, and www.healthcarecommission.org.uk for example) publish reviews where you can check out your current and potentially future caregiver. Online resources such as PubMed (www.pubmed.com) offer a search engine where you can check out medical publications about a variety of protocols, conditions, or clinic studies, and www.britishfertilitysociety.org.uk contains useful information about key issues in fertility and patient fact sheets. Online forums can be a big help at this stage. Many of the regular contributors to www.infertilitynetworkuk.com, www.fertilityfriends.co.uk, or www.midlandfertility.com have experienced failed treatment and the dilemmas about going again, so make use of these willing confidantes.

Some people say that 'it takes a village' to raise a child. I (co-author Gill) believe that it also takes a village to *make* a baby. Patients have told me that when they were trying to conceive, one of the most helpful people was not a formal part of our medical team. Rather, it was their homecare pharmacy, who helped them decipher much of the medical lingo, provided them with their medications at the proper time, came through with last-minute requests, and encouraged them along the way. Consider infertility as an opportunity to widen your network and recognise just how important the people in your life are, whether they play a big role or not.

I'm Okay, You're Okay – Checking On the State of Your Union

Where's your partner in all of this treatment process? The state of your union must remain an important component throughout the process of baby makes two, three, or more. The idea is to *add* to your life, not have a baby at all costs, including your sanity, your health, or your relationship. A baby doesn't transform a miserable existence or relationship into a blissful one. It merely provides a temporary diversion from whatever relationship issues you face today, and adds a significant amount of responsibility into your life and/or partnership.

Before rushing out to interview the next world-renowned specialist in fertility or researching the latest, greatest advances in the field, consider a quick (or not so quick) check on your own feelings and state of mind, as well as that of your partner's. Ask yourself these questions:

- How are you really doing? Have you been taking care of yourself throughout this stressful process, getting enough exercise, eating well, and having some fun? Depriving yourself of daily self-care only results in more problems. Perhaps this is the time to take a breather and pamper yourself with a long walk, a good book, or a dinner out with friends.

- How are your partner and partnership doing? Are you spending time doing things other than trying to conceive (whether that be doctor's appointments, required reading, or timed sex)? Consider spending some fertility-free time with each other.

- Did your partner or your relationship get a year older with neither of you having noticed? Maybe it's time to shift the focus a little bit.

- How does your partner feel about continuing treatments? How do you feel about continuing treatments? Take time to consider your feelings on this topic. Make sure that you're on the same page or at least reading the same book. You're more powerful as a cohesive team. Make sure that all the positions on that team are intact.

- How does your bank manager feel? Now is a good time to also take stock of your finances.

Exploring Some Controversial Fertility Treatments

If standard fertility treatments have failed you, you may be interested in moving on to some of the more controversial methods. These methods all involve manipulation of the immune system. Human beings have a fantastic ability to recognise the difference between our own cells and other cells, such as bacteria and viruses. If a transplanted kidney isn't perfectly genetically matched then it's rejected. If the body makes a mistake and starts failing to recognise its own cells and attacks them, *auto-immune diseases*, such as lupus and rheumatoid arthritis, can occur. So how come a woman's body can tolerate and even nurture an embryo that is 50 per cent not her genetic material and, in the case of a donor egg, 100 per cent 'not self'?

This question lies at the heart of all the controversial therapies we outline in this section. These methods are considered controversial because only a few doctors support them or because they're considered to be risky in some way. Immune issues are generally believed to be responsible for less than 5 per cent of infertility, but some doctors feel that this condition is under diagnosed, because the testing for immune factors is expensive and done only in a few labs.

Leukocyte immune therapy (LIT)

The idea that some women's bodies reject an embryo isn't a new one, but the methods for overcoming rejection are fairly new. One method, leukocyte immune therapy (LIT), looked very promising initially but proper clinical trials failed to demonstrate its effectiveness. The process was simple: White blood cells from the woman's partner or a donor were washed and injected under the woman's skin. The theory behind LIT is that some women don't have the right number of blocking antibodies that keep them from rejecting a growing fetus as a foreign piece of tissue. By giving proteins from your partner or another person, some of the proper blocking antibodies are introduced into your body, and the embryo hopefully is not then rejected.

Intravenous immunoglobulin (IVIG)

Because LIT has been questioned, some doctors recommend intravenous immunoglobulin (IVIG) therapy as a substitute. Unfortunately, IVIG must be administered as an intravenous infusion, which takes two to four hours, and must be done by a doctor or nurse.

IVIG has two major drawbacks:

- ✔ A single infusion may cost between £2,000 and £3,000, and if you get pregnant, your doctor is most likely to recommend at least two or three more infusions.

- ✔ Unlike the proteins injected from your partner in LIT, IVIG is a commercially produced blood product from strangers, so you have a small chance of transmission of HIV or hepatitis through the infusion.

Use of IVIG therapy in infertility is extremely controversial. Many doctors don't see any benefit at all to IVIG; other doctors believe that good prospective, randomised, studies on IVIG treatment in infertility are few and inconclusive.

Side effects of IVIG can range from fairly common side effects, such as rash, fever, headache, dizziness, and nausea, to small risk but severe conditions, such as anaphylactic shock.

Steroids

Steroids (prednisolone tablets, for example) have been used for many years to damp down the body's immune response in autoimmune diseases, such as lupus, asthma, and rheumatoid arthritis. Some fertility doctors believe that steroids taken around the time of conception can increase the chance of an embryo implanting or possibly reduce the risk of early miscarriage.

Very little evidence shows that steroids improve the chance of implantation following embryo transfer (ET), but they are used in conjunction with antibiotics in assisted-hatching protocols in IVF. Steroids are powerful drugs with significant side effects, so never take them without medical supervision.

Gearing Up for More Cycles

Another thought process to consider is how you view your less-than-positive results. Not getting pregnant isn't a failure, like failing an exam or messing up an important project at work. It's not your fault, nor is it in your control to will your body to conceive. Reframing your vocabulary may indeed help your spirit. Phrases such as 'less than perfect' or 'not successful yet' are much better for your psyche than 'failed'. Remember that your thoughts help dictate your feelings. What are you thinking today?

The hardest decision

Gwyn and I (co-author Jill) had a year's break between the last frozen embryo transfer of our first cycle and the start of our second cycle. This was determined by when the NHS funding we were lucky enough to receive became available, and also allowed us some time for normality. However, I just remember waking up every Monday morning during that year thinking there must be more to life than this. I couldn't imagine that I wouldn't have the chance to have a child – or children – and that the comfortable lifestyle we had achieved so far would continue week-in, week-out, for the rest of our lives. It also allowed us to consider how many more times we could go through it again. Following our first self-funded cycle, we had generous NHS funding for up to two full cycles. We decided that we would see how we got through the next before starting possibly our third: If it was successful, we wouldn't need to go again, and if it failed and was all too emotionally traumatic, maybe we couldn't face going again. Thankfully, the birth of Connie from that second treatment cycle meant we didn't have to make that ultimate decision about 'no more treatment' after no success. To this day, I don't think I could have handled it.

How many times do most people try before stopping treatment? In the clinic where I (co-author Gill) work, patients frequently ask this question. Of course, no single right answer exists. Some patients have tried ten cycles and have finally become pregnant, and other patients have changed their game plan and decided to look into adoption or other options after just one failed cycle. Some patients adopted and then got pregnant naturally, and some patients were just getting ready to do an IVF cycle when they had a positive pregnancy test.

When should you keep going? Consider these possibilities:

- ✔ When you can afford it.
- ✔ When you still have a chance of success.
- ✔ When you can't bear *not* to try again.
- ✔ When you and your partner are in agreement that continuing is the right thing to do.

On the other hand, when should you take a break, temporarily or permanently?

- ✔ When you just can't afford another cycle.
- ✔ When you've been told by a realistic doctor that you've next-to-no chance of getting pregnant.
- ✔ When one of you wants to stop.
- ✔ When trying has become unbearable.

The most difficult consultations I have (co-author Gill) are the 'low hope' but not 'no hope'. I always say that the right time to stop IVF is when the stress of IVF (emotional, financial, and personal) is worse than the stress of not being a parent.

Giving Up on Fertility Treatments? Considering When to Let Go

'When to say when' may come sooner for some infertility patients because of basic reasons: a lack of money, time, or opportunity. But even for those who've figured out ways to juggle limited resources a little bit longer, knowing when to say 'when' still isn't easy. Sometimes deciding that you've given IVF your best shot can be almost liberating. Making a positive decision to stop trying, puts you back in control of your life. If you're fortunate, you have alternative options (education, career, travel . . .) and a relationship that will have been strengthened by your shared endeavours.

Part VI
Different Strokes for Different Folks: Options for Non-Traditional Families

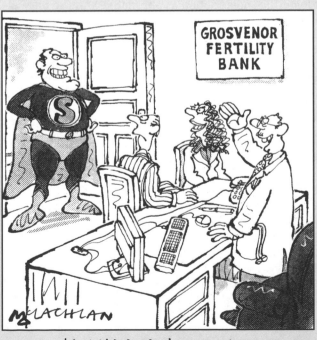

'And this is Nigel, our number one sperm donor.'

In this part . . .

Families today do not all conform to the 'average' mum, dad, and 1.7 bio-kids. In this part, we address fertility issues for single men and women, gays and lesbians, and also consider the surrogacy and donor eggs, sperm, and embryo routes to having a baby. We also look at fostering and adoption as alternative ways to have a family, and also at living child-free. Finally we look at some amazing – although sometimes controversial – developments in the future of treating infertility.

Chapter 20

Third-Party Reproduction: You and You and Me and Baby Make . . . Four!

*T*he traditional happy family picture of mum, dad, and two children (preferably a boy and a girl) and a dog named Spot has changed somewhat over the past few decades. Happy families today may contain biological children, adopted children, children born with the help of third parties from donor eggs, sperm, or embryos, as well as children carried through pregnancy by their grandmother, their aunt, or a total stranger.

Although most of the families created through third-party reproduction are perfectly happy ones, the legal and emotional issues involved in using eggs, sperm – or both – from someone else can be tricky. In this chapter, we explain how you can decide whether third-party – or even fourth-, or fifth-party! – reproduction is right for you, and how to proceed after you make your decision.

Preparing Yourselves for Using a Donor

Deciding to use donor eggs, embryos, or sperm is rarely an elective decision and always a difficult one. The issue raises not only a host of emotional issues but also a host of legal issues.

Getting ready to ride the emotional roller coaster

Usually, you make the decision to work with a donor because you have to – because one or both of you has a fertility issue that can't be fixed. Or you make the decision because you're a same-sex couple or want to be a single parent; obviously, you need some type of donor in these cases.

If you're moving to donor eggs or sperm because you have an unfixable problem, you need to come to terms with your loss before moving on. You may have difficulty coming to terms with the fact that you have a fertility problem and need fertility treatment. But dealing with the double whammy of knowing that you don't even have the raw materials (eggs and sperm) and need to use someone else's is going to be hard. As a fertility doctor, I (co-author Gill) have seen couples move on too quickly to donor eggs and sperm and then struggle with their feelings about being pregnant with a child that's not biologically their own. Using donor eggs, sperm, or embryos is a big decision; don't jump in before you're sure that you're emotionally ready. Counselling isn't compulsory, but it really can help you explore these difficult issues, and under UK law, all clinics must offer counselling services.

If you decide to use donor eggs or sperm, the child created will be biologically related to *one* of you. The non-biological parent is the legal parent, but is this fact going to be a problem if you and your partner separate down the road? Is this issue something that one of you might fling in the other's face if the child has a serious health problem, or ends up in trouble with the law? Will the fact that one of you can see family features in your child's face while the other can't, become a source of friction? You need to consider these questions, as well as any others that cross your mind, before you make the leap.

Understanding the legal issues

Finding donor eggs, sperm, and embryos isn't so simple a task as it was before April 2005 – and even then, these were in short supply.

In 2005, the law regarding donor anonymity changed so that any child conceived after 1 April 2006 from donor sperm, eggs, or embryos from donors registered after 1 April 2005 can, on reaching the age of 18, or sooner if they are to marry – access information revealing the identity of the donor. The information won't be given to the recipient or the patient couple, and being identified to any child resulting from the donor treatment depends on them:

✔ Knowing that they were conceived from donor sperm, eggs, or embryos.

✔ Having the inclination to seek their biological parent.

There's no legal requirement for parents to tell their offspring about the circumstances of their conception and no risk that they could find out unless the family all underwent DNA 'finger-printing'. But secrets in families can be difficult to keep and secrets that emerge at the wrong time in the wrong place can be very destructive. Don't feel ashamed about needing to use donor eggs, sperm, or embryos to become a parent. Most children would like to think that they were wanted that much!

Although the donor has no financial or legal responsibility for any child conceived with the use of their *gametes* (eggs or sperm) or embryos, the ending of anonymity legislation has considerably reduced the number of available donors. Young students no longer see donating sperm as 'easy' beer money, when a knock at the door in their early 40s and the words 'Hello biological daddy', may be a very unlikely, but very real consequence. Equally, some potential egg sharers have been put off because of the risk of their treatment cycle failing, but the chance that their eggs produced a baby in another woman's successful treatment and them having to deal with the emotional consequence of this outcome if ever they were identified to the child.

Protecting yourselves – the least you can do

Before entering into any type of donor situation that we describe in this chapter, whether it involves eggs, embryos, or sperm, you need to do several things:

✔ **Do some soul searching.** Only you know how you really feel about using another person's eggs, embryos, or sperm. Think the situation *all* the way through – past the cute baby stage into the teenage years and beyond. Make sure that you're really ready to take the donor step. You may be temped, when you long for a baby so much, to believe that the much higher success rates using young donor eggs (40 per cent + per cycle) compared to 15 per cent per cycle using your own 40-year-old eggs make the decision a 'no-brainer', but only you know whether you're ready to give up on the chance of biological parenthood. For men with severe sperm problems a difficult decision, too; ICSI means your partner going through time-consuming, stressful, and uncomfortable medical procedures because *you* have poor sperm. A simple treatment like donor sperm insemination can seem very tempting. Make sure that you're making the right decision for the right reasons.

✔ **Decide who, when, and how to tell.** Counsellors and social workers are certain that honesty is the best policy and that trying to keep secrets in families is always a bad idea. Legislative changes in 2005 in the UK mean that children born as a result of donor gametes (eggs or sperm) or embryos may apply for identifying information about their donor at the age of 18 (or 16 if they plan to marry). This assumes that these children know about the circumstances of their conception. Research suggests that the majority are never told and never suspect. Only you as a couple can decide about telling. You may change your mind later about divulging (or not) to your child, and others, that you used donor eggs or sperm. If you didn't tell anyone, you don't have to explain anything. If you must reveal your decision to someone, make sure that the person or people are supportive and can keep a secret until you're ready for the news to go public.

If you're using a gestational carrier or surrogate (see 'Surrogacy: Borrowing a Uterus for the Next Nine Months,' later in this chapter), make sure that everything is in writing. *Everything.* Legally controlling another person's actions is very difficult, so bring up just about any possibility you can think of. Having something in writing may save you from heartbreak down the road.

Borrowing from the Sperm Bank

Donor sperm has been used for artificial insemination (AI) for more than 100 years. The method can be an extremely effective treatment for couples where the man produces no sperm, or carries a genetic disease that he doesn't wish to pass on to his offspring. Donor sperm can also allow single women and women in a lesbian relationship to become mothers. The ending of donor anonymity in the UK has reduced the willingness of men to become sperm donors but new recruitment campaigns may ease the shortage.

Why fewer couples are using donor sperm

Use of donor sperm has decreased since 1992, when it became possible to inseminate an egg with a single, carefully selected 'ideal' sperm (as ideal as existed in the male's sample, anyway) in a process known as *intracytoplasmic sperm injection*, or ICSI (browse Chapters 10 and 13 for more information on ICSI). Men whose sperm counts are very low, or those with poor sperm motility, or movement, can now become biological parents – as long as they can afford to do in vitro insemination.

Many couples, however, can't afford the cost of the treatment, which is about £3,000–6,000, so they still use donor sperm. Also, those men who have no sperm at all, such as those with Sertoli cell-only syndrome, or who have received chemotherapy or radiotherapy, still depend on donor sperm to become parents.

Picking a 'dad' from a catalogue

All sperm that's used for donation in the UK must have been quarantined and frozen for six months, so a donor must have better-than-average sperm because some are lost in the freeze-and-thaw process.

The donor is tested for all significant infectious diseases (such as hepatitis B and C and HIV) as well as certain genetic diseases such as cystic fibrosis (CF). He's also required to fill out a very detailed questionnaire about his background, his family background, his interests, and his likes and dislikes. He is asked to write a 'pen portrait' about himself and also a letter to any child that may be born.

Because the risk of disease transmission is too high, sperm banks no longer use fresh sperm. Instead, sperm are now frozen and the donor retested for infectious diseases before the sperm are released for use – after a quarantine period of six months.

Donor sperm can be frozen nearly indefinitely. They're kept in liquid nitrogen containers and shipped out when requested. UK legislation permits a donor to 'father' a maximum of ten 'birth events' (twins count as one) but the same donor can be used to create full siblings for an existing donor child. Sperm banks routinely follow up with questionnaires to centres using donor sperm to ask whether the donation resulted in a live birth.

When ordering sperm, you can choose between sperm that's ready for intracervical insemination (ICI-ready) or sperm that's ready for intrauterine insemination (IUI-ready). The technique for IUI, which injects the sperm directly into the uterus, is more complicated, but most clinics report a higher pregnancy rate with IUI than ICI. Pregnancy rates for women under 35 are about 10 to 15 per cent per insemination; rates decrease for women over 40 to 5 to 10 per cent per insemination.

Estimates show that only one child in ten is ever informed that he or she is the result of donor insemination, but times may be changing. The rights of children to know their genetic 'identity' are considered to be more important than the rights of the donor to keep their anonymity.

Asking someone you know to donate

Some parents-to-be choose a donor they know, perhaps a brother or close friend of the intended dad.

You must be aware of the dangers of 'DIY insemination'. Fresh sperm have a higher pregnancy rate than frozen, and this fact may be a consideration if you have a relative or friend who's willing to donate. But keep in mind that the donor needs to be tested for sperm quality and infectious diseases, and that a waiting period of six months is required before the sperm can be used. This gives the clinic time to retest for infectious diseases – many infectious diseases take six months to show up in the blood. Unless a clinic is involved and the strict rules of the HFEA Act are followed then no protection is available for donor or parents. If all the rules are followed then the 'social' father of the child born is the 'legal' father and the donor has no rights or responsibilities. If the arrangement is 'unofficial' then the mother can come after the donor for child support!

With known-donor insemination of course, the chance of the child finding out the truth about his conception is much higher, because more people are involved in the process. For some couples, the psychological issues may be too complicated for them to handle. However, couples who want a genetic match that's as close as possible, and who can handle the psychological problems, may find this method to be a good solution.

Although such a topic may be difficult to bring up, you really ought not to go with a known donor until some type of legal document is drawn up. This document must address such issues as how much say the donor is to have in the child's upbringing, how much contact he'll have with the child, and whether he'll have legal rights to the child if anything happens to you.

Of course, you may never experience any emotional or legal problems as a result of this donation. The donor may see your child as just another niece or nephew and never give their genetic relationship a second thought. You know your own family best, but covering the possibility of interference down the road is always a good idea.

What if your partner's *father* is interested in being your donor? This happens more often than you think. He *is* a genetic link, but remember that grandparents in general can be too outspoken about your child's upbringing. Also 'old' sperm is not as good at making healthy babies (for this reason 'altruistic' donors in the UK must be under 45 years of age). Ask yourself whether his being the silent 'parent' as well as the grandparent may cause problems in your relationship.

Using Donor Eggs

Donor eggs from an altruistic egg donor (possibly some of the most generous people on this planet!) or from an egg sharer (women who require IVF anyway and who run a close second in the generosity poll) mean that women with too few or poor quality eggs have the chance to conceive and give birth.

Using donor eggs includes all the usual emotional, clinical, and financial hardships of IVF or ICSI, and then multiplied! But couples who do have babies from donor eggs are not only eternally thankful to the unidentified donor but also often relish in the comments of 'doesn't he/she look like his/her mummy', from friends and families who are not aware of the details of the baby's conception – or maybe even who are!

(Chapter 15 has more information on sharing, giving, and receiving donor eggs.)

Receiving Donor Embryos – Embryo Adoption

Some clinics maintain lists of couples who want to donate their frozen embryos to another couple, usually because the donating couple has one or more children through IVF and doesn't want any more. Screening is just as thorough as for sperm or egg donors and you also receive information about the donating parents, and usually some type of family genetic history. If you tell your child, at the age of 18 they can find out identifying information about his or her 'genetic' parents, and whether he or she has any siblings.

When you use donor embryos, you're essentially adopting a child, hence the other name *preimplantation adoption*; the difference between this and traditional adoption is that you get to experience the pregnancy and delivery just as if this were your genetic child. Your name is on the birth certificate, and unless you share the information, no one will know that you used donor embryos. Some couples find that having a child who's not related to either one of them, rather than using donor eggs or sperm, is a much easier situation to deal with emotionally.

Of course, this method again brings up the possibility of legal questions, moral issues, and possible complications a few years down the road. Many of these issues are similar to those raised by adoption but some are more complicated. Although very many thousands of frozen embryos exist, relatively few are donated. Couples donating embryos often have difficulty imagining 'their' child' being brought up by another couple and never knowing that their IVF child or children have full brothers and sisters somewhere else in the country. Using donor embryos is technically fairly simple. The procedure requires doing a frozen embryo transfer at an IVF clinic. In a 'natural' cycle transfer this requires minimal medication, usually just oestrogen pills before the transfer and progesterone after the transfer to maintain the pregnancy for the first few weeks until the placenta takes over and sustains the pregnancy.

Surrogacy: Borrowing a Uterus for Nine Months

Asking a woman for some of her eggs is one thing; she only has to commit to a few weeks of time and discomfort. Asking someone to commit to your cause for nine whole months by being a *gestational carrier* is quite another.

The use of gestational carriers has grown with the advent of IVF. Women with serious health issues, women who lack a uterus, and women with a history of recurrent miscarriage are among those who use friends, family, or total strangers to carry and deliver their biological children.

Finding a willing woman

Some women love to be pregnant, and other women love to be pregnant as long as they're getting paid for it. Either type may be suitable as a gestational carrier (also known as a 'full' surrogate). Many women ask immediate family members first, but remember that a 'no' doesn't mean that person doesn't love you or want to help. Some women see pregnancy as a nine-month misery and wouldn't go through it if you begged them; others truly enjoy being pregnant and welcome the chance to help you out as well.

If your sister and best friend turn you down, you need to look a little farther. What if your mum wants to do this act for you? Would you feel funny about her giving birth to her grandchildren? How would you handle the local press? If all possible friends or relatives are out, you may want to look on the Internet and contact 'self-help agencies such as COTS (visit www.surrogacy.org.uk). Under UK law, the clinic isn't allowed to find a surrogate for you and the surrogate can't be paid to carry your baby. You're allowed to pay them reasonable expenses for travelling, loss of earnings, maternity clothes, and so on.

Don't sign up with the first wonderful-sounding candidate who offers to be your surrogate without doing *a lot* of research. Get to know her and understand her motivation for wanting to help you. Make sure that she has a good obstetric 'track record' and agrees with good health advice about smoking, alcohol, and medication in pregnancy. If she has children, make sure that they're aware and happy about their mum's plans to have a baby for someone else. Remember that under UK law, the birth mother *is* the legal mother and the genetic parents (also known as the commissioning couple) don't have any right to be the child's parents if the surrogate decides that she doesn't want to hand the baby over.

The commissioning couple must be married and at least one of them must be genetically related to the child for the fast-track adoption or Parental Order rules to apply. The baby must leave the hospital with its genetic parents and after six weeks they can apply through a Guardian ad litem for the child to be issued with a new birth certificate and be formally adopted by them. The Guardian ad litem checks with the clinic that all the rules have been followed.

Another slippery slope that you need to address *before* a pregnancy occurs is the view that you and your surrogate have about multiple pregnancy. You may want to maximise your chance of pregnancy by having two embryos transferred. She may be quite happy to carry one baby for you, but not two! Another difficult area is genetic testing during the pregnancy, and pregnancy termination if a serious problem is found. Even though the baby is genetically yours, the decision to undergo testing and/or end a pregnancy is that of the carrier, *regardless of legal contract*. Make sure that you and your carrier are on the same page on this difficult and touchy issue. If you're not, consider it a deal breaker.

Going through the surrogacy process

You'll have to do IVF to use a gestational carrier, because you'll be transferring embryos to her uterus. The law regards you as her egg donor and your partner as her sperm donor; therefore, his sperm has to be quarantined for six months before you can do IVF and create embryos. The surrogate usually takes an oestrogen pill, to thicken her uterine lining, for several weeks. The embryos are then transferred to her uterus. You and your carrier can do synchronised cycles, so that the embryos can be transferred to her a few days after your egg retrieval without first being frozen. Or you can do an egg retrieval first, and freeze the embryos to transfer to the carrier six months, or even later, down the road.

Legal nightmares: They can and do happen

Everybody remembers the nightmare surrogacy cases but they're very rare. Cases debated in the courts in the last few years have involved donor embryos, donor eggs, and gestational carriers, which shows how complicated these cases can be. In one case, a couple used donor embryos and a gestational carrier. The prospective father asked for a divorce several months before the baby was born, and he didn't want to pay child support because he wasn't the biological or adopted father. The courts ruled that he 'showed intent' to be a parent when he signed consent forms for the embryo transfer to the surrogate.

UK clinics insist on proper legal contracts being drawn up to cover things such as:

✔ Who pays for child care if the surrogate is admitted to hospital?

✔ What happens if the obstetrician recommends a Caesarian but the surrogate doesn't want one?

After the surrogate gets pregnant, her pregnancy and delivery proceed just like any other; she is not subject to any additional physical pregnancy risks. Most couples are in fairly close contact with their surrogate during the pregnancy, so that any problems that arise can be dealt with jointly. If you've chosen a previously unknown surrogate, rather than using a friend or relative, have a clear schedule about how much contact you have agreed on before doing the embryo transfer. Because surrogate pregnancies are still quite rare, the antenatal visits to the hospital may be a little awkward! Trying to explain why four people (the surrogate, her partner, and the commissioning couple) all need to see the first scan can be difficult.

In most cases, the surrogate agrees to let you be present for the delivery, so you can see and hold the baby right away. Your surrogate's name is shown on the first birth certificate and the baby is only 'genetically' yours. After a short hospital stay, you take the baby home with you.

Traditional Surrogacy – The Road Less Travelled

Unlike gestational carriers where the surrogate has no genetic link to the baby she is carrying, 'traditional' or 'straight' surrogates are both the egg donors and the pregnancy carriers. The good thing about traditional surrogacy is that it often doesn't require doing IVF. The bad news is that you're asking for more than nine months out of a woman's life – you're also asking for her biological child. Because the child born is the natural child of the surrogate, most clinics do not cooperate with this type of surrogacy. Legal agreements, no matter how complete, don't hold up in court if the birth mother changes her mind.

If the surrogate is a relative, you may have a greater trust in her to keep her promise to give the baby to you after she delivers. But keep in mind that if she does change her mind, you're looking at a family nightmare that you may never recover from.

Because of the risks of traditional surrogacy, many couples use donor eggs from one person and find another to be the gestational carrier, in order to avoid the risks of using a traditional surrogate. This route is more expensive, but it may buy you some peace of mind about the likelihood of your surrogate changing her mind and keeping the baby.

Telling the Family or Keeping It to Yourself

Will you tell your family? That depends on you, your family, and a host of other factors that only you know. Some people don't even let their families know that they're doing IVF, much less explain that they're using donor eggs.

Donor sperm has been utilised for more than 50 years, and evidence shows that most parents *do not* tell the child that their father isn't their biological parent. It seems likely that some families won't talk about using donor eggs, either, although in a recent study, just over half the parents surveyed indicated that they planned to let the child know, eventually.

It's possible that somewhere down the line, your child may find out that they're the product of donor eggs or sperm, even if you don't want them to. It may happen in a school biology lesson, where students often test their blood types. Or it may happen when your child develops a rare inherited disease, and you need to go back to the biological family for information.

Keeping a secret like this one is difficult, but dealing with negative family reactions, if there are any, is difficult, too. If you tell your child, you'll cry inside every time they say, 'You're not my *real* mother!' and if you don't tell, you'll cringe every times they say, 'I wish I had a different mother!' All children say things like this, whether they're adopted, biological, or whatever;

take it on the chin. Grandparents may treat their 'real' grandchildren differently and this can cause great distress. Children who know that they are the product of donor sperm but are unable to find out anything about their biological father also can be very unhappy. At least 5 per cent of children are not the offspring of the men they believe to be their biological fathers anyway, so a lot of unofficial 'donor' insemination is going on out there. Wherever you stand on the 'Nature' versus 'Nurture' debate, you and your partner need to explore all these issues before you start treatment.

Chapter 21

Safe Options for Same-Sex Couples and Single Mums

. . . .

In This Chapter

▶ Having a baby as a gay or lesbian couple

▶ Adopting a baby as a gay or lesbian

▶ Having a child or adopting as a single parent

. . . .

*G*ay, lesbian, bisexual, and transsexual couples are often as eager to build families as their heterosexual counterparts. Others looking to be parents aren't part of a couple at all; they're singles who forgo or just put aside the search for Mr or Ms Right in lieu of the quest for a child.

Both gays and singles need a little help to achieve their dream of a family. Welcome to the brave new world where options exist whatever your lifestyle. If you want to be a parent, if you long for a child, hang onto the dream because it can happen. In this chapter, we discuss how to achieve parenthood when you're not a member of a traditional family unit.

Examining the Issues That You May Face as a Same-Sex Couple

As a gay or lesbian couple looking to have children of your own, you need to find an outside source of eggs or sperm. After you overcome that obstacle, and a child is on the way, you'll most likely want the child legally to belong to *both* of you.

The biggest problem for same-sex couples who both want to be listed as parents of the child is that the law does not recognise *both* partners as parents. The birth mother is considered the legal parent, and her partner may not be allowed to adopt. If they have a civil partnership, things are more straightforward or the lawyers can arrange shared parenting and custody rights.

Male couples who father children using egg donors and/or surrogates face an uphill struggle to establish their parental roles. Best advice is see a good specialist family lawyer before you put 'make me a daddy' into your favourite search engine.

If you're a lesbian or gay couple with children, you *both* must have Wills that are up to date. If something happens to one or both of you, unless you're both listed as legal parents of your child, you could easily end up in a court battle if someone else in your partner's family sues for custody. Same-sex couples have gone to court and lost custody purely on the basis of their sexual orientation.

Gay couples

Gay men can be considered 'egg-and-uterus-challenged'. That is, they lack two of the major necessities of childbearing and, one way or another, must 'hire out' the pregnancy – in other words, get a surrogate or gestational carrier.

Because of the possibility that a traditional surrogate, a woman who both conceives and carries the child can decide to keep a child that's biologically hers, many gay men have opted to use both an egg donor and a *gestational carrier* (a woman who has no genetic link to the child).

The egg donor may be a friend, relative, or someone who has been located by a fertility clinic or private agency.

If a couple wants to maintain a genetic connection to both partners, they may chose an egg donor related to one partner – a sister, for example – and use the other partner as the sperm donor.

In this new age of technology and the Internet, you may even find egg donors abroad online. Gay men from Britain who wish to become fathers often have to resort to foreign shores to fulfil their dreams of fatherhood. The US is expensive, but egg donors and surrogates can be found via the Internet and legal contracts about handing over the resulting child are more likely to be enforced in some states in the US than in the UK where the birth mother *is* the mother until she voluntarily gives up that status.

Creating the embryo

After the donor has been tested for infectious diseases or other obstacles to pregnancy, she goes through a typical IVF cycle; she's treated with gonadotrophins to produce eggs and monitored through the maturation process of the egg follicles until the time of the egg retrieval (refer to Chapter 12 for greater detail on what the IVF cycle entails). However, instead of the eggs being fertilised by the woman's partner or husband, or by donor sperm, they're fertilised by sperm obtained from the gay couple, and the embryos are ready to be implanted.

Implanting the embryo

After the eggs are harvested and fertilised, the embryos are then implanted in a gestational carrier who has no biological connection to the child she's carrying, or into the egg donor herself if that's what the couple decides.

The person who'll be carrying the baby needs to be tested to determine whether her uterus can carry a pregnancy. Most centres want the surrogate to have a hysterosalpingogram (HSG) (find out more about this test in Chapter 7) to rule out the presence of any fibroids or polyps that may prevent pregnancy.

Lesbian couples

Lesbian couples have eggs and uteri to spare – they're merely 'sperm-challenged'! They need another part to complete the baby equation, although obtaining sperm isn't nearly as complicated as obtaining an egg and borrowing a uterus.

Finding sperm

Regardless of the method of conception, a third party's sperm is vital to the equation. Here are your options:

- ✔ You can purchase this necessary component through a sperm bank. Some clinics also provide access to donor sperm.

- ✔ You can work with known sperm donors, men you know who are willing to donate their sperm. Known sperm donors may or may not retain a role in the life of the baby.

All HFEA-licensed clinics in the UK – HFEA stands for the Human Fertilisation and Embryology Authority – use sperm that has been frozen for six months to ensure that the woman (and her baby) is not at risk of any transmittable infectious diseases. If you're using sperm from a friend, it's vital to have him tested too for infectious diseases, such as

HIV and hepatitis, before using his sperm. The semen specimen is frozen for six months, and then his blood is tested again. If he's still negative for infectious diseases (some take a while to show up in the blood), then you can safely use the frozen specimen.

Currently a quick Internet search reveals various sources through which lesbian women can obtain sperm. This option is very dangerous and risky compared to approaching a licensed fertility clinic. The European Tissue Directive is soon to outlaw the importation of 'Internet sperm', and the selling of 'fresh' sperm within the UK. Lesbian couples and single women will then need to access sperm from the better-regulated and safer resource of licensed fertility clinics.

Working together

Some lesbian couples have decided to take turns being pregnant, inseminating one partner the first time and the other partner the next time. Legally, this results in children who are considered the child of the partner who gave birth only, unless the couples have a civil partnership that allows same-sex parents to adopt the other partner's children.

Some couples have used IVF to get pregnant so that the eggs of one partner can be carried during pregnancy by the other. This way, both partners are involved in the conception and birth of the baby. If one of you is the egg donor and the other is the gestational carrier, you'll need to have your menstrual cycles coordinated by your clinic; this process usually involves taking birth control pills to synchronise your cycles.

Finding the right clinic

You may have to search a little to find the right clinic, one that's going to treat you with care and respect. Clinics aren't allowed to discriminate on the grounds of sexual orientation, but the current HFEA Act does allow the clinic to 'consider the welfare of the child that might be born' and the 'need of the child for a father'. Some clinics may use these concerns as a way of avoiding offering treatment to certain groups. NHS funding is also unlikely to be available to single women or lesbian partners seeking to conceive.

After you've got together your list of possible clinics to call, mention your specific circumstances during your first phone call. You want to make sure that your chosen clinic is supportive of your situation before you make an appointment.

Adoption in the Gay and Lesbian Community

So perhaps you and your partner have decided that a biological connection to either one of you isn't particularly important. Or perhaps through your passage of fertility rites, you've discovered that a biological connection requires more medical attention, time, or money than you're willing or able to spend. Adoption is often a great alternative and one that provides a home for a child in need of one.

Adoption, whether domestic or international, comes fraught with its own processes, procedures, and waiting periods. But for a gay or lesbian couple, the red tape may be a little stickier.

Generally, the process is easier for an individual to adopt a child than for a gay couple to adopt a child together. For many gay couples, one partner adopts the child, and the other partner asks a court if he or she can also adopt the child through a second legal procedure. Although *second-parent* adoption (also known as *co-parent adoption*) does, eventually, accomplish the goal of official parenthood by both partners, the route involves more steps and more money than joint adoption. *Joint adoption* allows both parents to have a legally recognised relationship to their child in just one step.

If you're a single gay or lesbian individual, you'll probably run across the same hurdles that a single heterosexual would face, and more. Another thing to consider is that even though you may be allowed to try to adopt a child as a homosexual single or couple, the authorities may still give *preference* to married couples, or even to single heterosexuals. Young children, let alone healthy babies available for adoption, are very few and far between. Our children's homes are full of older children, children with special needs and handicaps, children who have been abused, and children in complex sibling groups, that are all desperately in need of good, kind, supportive parents to adopt them and love them. You may need to face the fact that you're not going to be given a cute, newborn, but you could become the parent of an older child that needs the type of parenting that only you can give.

Whatever part of the country you're in, you'll most likely find judges and social workers at either extreme when considering gay and lesbian adoption, although those in favour may be a great deal harder to find.

If you're interested in adopting from a foreign country, you need to be aware that your sexual orientation may render you ineligible to adopt in particular countries. Many foreign countries with children available for adoption, including China, are adamantly opposed to lesbian and gay adoptions, although they do allow single-parent adoptions. Often, the agency you work with is aware of your sexual orientation and can advise you how to find countries that will consider your application fairly. However, after your child is admitted into the UK, the adoption proceeds according to our laws, not those of the foreign country.

Going It Alone: Fertility Issues for the Single Parent

If you're a single parent, you're far from alone; 25 per cent of new-born babies in the UK leave hospital to go to a home that doesn't have a functioning father figure. If you want to be a single parent, the road may be a little more complicated, but the difficulties are far from insurmountable.

Today, the process of adopting as a single parent is much easier than ever before. And if you want to give birth to your child, you've the option of using donor sperm.

If you're a woman alone

If you're a single woman, having a baby is much easier for you than a single man – you've got the right equipment! All you need is the sperm, and sperm is something that is available, whether you want to use an anonymous donor or a close friend.

Using a friend as a sperm donor

If you're considering using a friend as your donor, here are some of the benefits:

- You're most likely aware of the person's personality traits.
- You know what he looks like.
- You probably like the person, or you wouldn't be asking him to do this for you.

Alas, where you find pros, you also find cons. Here are some of the potential complications that come from using a donor you know over one who remains anonymous:

- ✔ How involved does he want to be in your child's life? No involvement, holiday visits, or heavy involvement?

- ✔ If your parenting techniques differ, how much input is he going to have on how you raise your child?

- ✔ If something happens to you, is he to be the legal guardian?

- ✔ You must both be aware that unless he is a registered sperm donor, then he has no escape from his 'parental' financial responsibility if your 'friendly' relationship breaks down and you decide to pursue him for child maintenance.

If you're using fresh sperm from a known donor, you need to be aware of the risk of contracting an infectious disease such as HIV or hepatitis. You're much wiser using a frozen specimen that's come from your donor who's tested at the time the specimen is frozen, and then tested again six months later. If he's still negative, you can use the frozen specimen.

Using an anonymous sperm donor

If you're thinking of using an anonymous donor, consider the following pros:

- ✔ You won't have to worry about the father wanting to be involved with the child.

- ✔ You can match basic physical characteristics such as build, ethnicity and hair and eye colour.

On the con side, consider these issues:

- ✔ You'll have to rely on what the clinic says about the donor, with no way of knowing how accurate the information really is.

- ✔ You won't be able to tell your child much about his paternal heritage.

- ✔ Your child may have difficulty contacting the birth father, should they decide to do so, although at the age of 18, they will have the right to access identifying information. (Refer to Chapter 20 for more information on donor gametes and anonymity.)

Inseminating at home

If you plan to do an insemination at home, you can find home insemination kits that are sold over the Internet that can probably help you get the job done. The kits may contain little more than a small cup, something like a cervical cap, which holds the ejaculate.

If you're using a known donor who's making a contribution outside of a fertility clinic, do not 'catch' the ejaculate in a condom because they contain spermicides. Ask your donor to masturbate into a small clean container where the ejaculate will liquefy after a short while (keep the pot at body temperature during this time). The semen can then be drawn up into a medical syringe (without a needle!) and inserted into the vagina near to the cervix.

You absolutely positively must *not* try to insert the sperm into the cervix itself or, even worse, into the uterus. Sperm need to be washed before going into the uterus, and this procedure is *not* a DIY project! You can do yourself some real harm if you try to insert fresh sperm into the uterus. For that reason, never try and do an intracervical or intrauterine insemination at home! You can place the sperm near the cervix but not inside it!

If you're a man alone

Things are certainly more complicated if you're a man trying to have a baby by yourself. You just can't do it alone! Your first problem in the UK is to find a clinic that's willing to help. If you want to be a father, you need to find a mother – or at least a woman (or women) willing to donate an egg and a uterus.

You may want to ask a friend, or you may want to find a surrogate who'll carry the baby for you and then relinquish all parental rights to you. A *traditional surrogate* is both the biological mother of the baby and the person who carries the baby throughout the pregnancy; a *gestational carrier* isn't the biological mother of the child, but is the carrier for the nine months of pregnancy. (You can read more about these options in Chapter 20.)

If you want to use a gestational carrier, you'll have to use IVF (in vitro fertilisation); the eggs of one woman can be fertilised, and the resulting embryo can be transferred to the gestational carrier. This method, of course, is much more expensive than traditional surrogacy, because you have to pay the expenses of the gestational carrier and the egg donor, not to mention the IVF centre. You're looking at spending £15,000 or more.

If your surrogate is married, the child, when born, may be presumed to be legally her husband's. You may have to adopt your own child.

The Surrogacy Arrangements Act applies only to married couples, so no automatic right exists to adopt the child just because DNA fingerprinting can show that he or she is your flesh and blood. (For a copy of the Act, see www.surrogacyuk.org/surrogacyact1985.pdf)

Adopting a child as a single parent

Over the last 20 years, the fastest growing trend in adoption has been the increase in the number of single-parent adoptions. About 5 per cent of all adoptions are by single parents, and an even higher percentage – about 25 per cent – of all 'special needs' children are adopted by singles.

However, as gay and lesbians trying to adopt very often find, just because the law doesn't prevent it doesn't mean that bias doesn't preclude it. Singles trying to adopt may find themselves viewed as second-class citizens to their married counterparts.

Find an agency that specialises in single-parent adoption, or consider international adoption as another option. Foster parenting may also be an easier route that's also less discriminatory, but in many cases, the State tries to find a two-parent family first before letting you adopt your foster child. (Head to Chapter 22 for more information on fostering and adoption.)

To make yourself as appealing as possible to an adoption agency, prepare some information about yourself and your lifestyle before you start your home study. An agency, typically, wants to see the following information:

- **Financial security.** You don't have to be wealthy, but you do have to have the means to provide for a child.

- **A well-thought-out childcare plan.** If you work and intend to continue to work, this plan is essential.

- **Backup plan in the event of your death.** To whom would you leave the care and responsibility for your child? Is your designated person agreeable to this?

- **A plan for having a 'male figure' (or female figure, if you're male) in your child's life.**

Leaning on the network

If you've an existing network of friends with children, coupled or not, lean on them for advice relating to pregnancy and child care, and get their input on the struggles and joys of parenthood. If most of your friends are still footloose and fancy free, now might be a good time to acquaint or reacquaint yourself with people with children, whether you do so through work, social groups, or religious organisations. Your life as a parent will be drastically different to what it was as a single person. Make sure that you're familiar with the unique struggles that you'll face when you truly are the sole provider.

A formal home visit by a social worker is *not* the best place to trot out your latest beau or, worse yet, beaux. Stability, whether in or out of a relationship, is key, and you don't want to appear as though your home has a revolving door of Mr or Ms Rights. If you're introducing a romantic partner into the picture, make sure that he or she is someone who's been a constant in your life for some time. If this person is to be a significant other in your child's life, he or she is subject to the same judgement criteria as you. The investigation could include fingerprinting, background checks, and more – not exactly fodder for a brand-new relationship!

✔ **Evidence of emotional support for both you and your future child.** Letters from potential aunts, uncles, grandparents, or close friends indicate that you have a strong support system.

If you're interested in foreign adoption, be aware that many countries require you to spend two to three weeks in their country. Can you take an extended amount of time off work?

If you're considering adopting a special needs child because you think this option may be an easier route, really think this idea through. It takes special people to raise special children, and only you know whether you're really adopting a special needs child for the right reason. If you're interested in a child with a particular disability, visit other families with a similar child, preferably an older child. Parenthood doesn't end at the baby stage, and handling an infant with a handicap is very different than managing an older disabled child. Some people are born to take care of special needs children; make sure that you're one of them before jumping in.

If you're interested in a private adoption of a healthy Caucasian newborn, keep in mind that you've an incredible amount of competition.

Chapter 22

Ready-Made Families and Other Choices

. . . .

In This Chapter

▶ Adopting different attitudes

▶ Fostering the right spirit

▶ Deciding to be happily child free

▶ Finding ways to spend time with children

. . . .

*F*or some people, the road to biological childbearing closes early. Severe male factor infertility (such as a total absence of sperm), lack of a uterus or ovaries, or other structural problems may make biological parenthood impossible. Other couples invest months or years, along with huge sums of money, seeking biological parenthood, only to end up at the same roadblock. If surrogacy or donor sperm, eggs or embryos aren't suitable for you – by choice or availability – you've reached the point where you may want to consider other alternatives.

In this chapter, we help you evaluate your choices and find the path that's right for you – when you're ready. The information on adoption and fostering is intended as an overview and directs you to alternative definitive sources.

 Working through the grief process of never having a biological child takes time. You pass through denial, anger, guilt, bargaining and, finally, acceptance – just as you do with any of life's crises. After you work through your sorrow, you can be ready to move on.

Opting to Adopt

A life without biological children doesn't mean a life without any children. Many children in the UK and abroad need parents to love and care for them. The adoption process can be emotionally draining, overburdened with paperwork and red-tape, and can make the intrusion of fertility treatment into your lifestyle and relationship seem a walk in the park. But for many, it offers a wonderful and fulfilling alternative to biological parenthood.

First, consider the basics. Adoption is a way of providing a new family for children who can't be brought up by their birth parents. It's a legal procedure where all the parental rights and legal responsibilities are transferred to the adopters. After an adoption order has been granted, it can only be reversed in rare circumstances.

If you're part of a couple, are you both equally willing to consider adoption? If not, one partner's intent to adopt may damage the relationship. Consider what your priority is – a child at the cost of your relationship, or finding a life together where the baby you want is no longer the main focus?

Children available for adoption

Around 4,000 children in the UK are waiting for permanent new families – although homes are never found for about 40 per cent of any children available for adoption. They range from newborn babies to teenagers, are from a variety of ethnic backgrounds, and more than half of them are in family groups of brothers and sisters who need to be placed together. They include physically disabled children and children whose emotional and intellectual development is unclear. Some have experienced neglect or physical, sexual, or emotional abuse and some have challenging behaviour.

In England and Wales 4,038 children were adopted from care in the 12 months up to March 2005 (equivalent figures were not available for Scotland and Northern Ireland). Of these:

✔ 5 per cent were under 1 year old

✔ 60 per cent were aged 1 to 4

✔ 29 per cent were aged 5 to 9

✔ 5 per cent were aged 10 to 15

✔ 1 per cent were aged 16 +

The gender split was exactly 50/50. (Source BAAF)

The growing number of single parents, an increase in abortions, and a falling birth rate all mean that, compared to 30 years ago, fewer babies are currently available for adoption. This changing situation means that many more approved adopters are available than infants. Compounding the problem is the fact that many approved adopters want a single, white, healthy baby, further limiting their chances of adopting successfully. But considering adopting an older child, possibly with siblings or maybe with special needs, may speed the match-making process and create a family for the benefit of you and your new child – or children.

Adoption agencies and organisations

Adoption in the UK can be arranged through a local authority's social services, a voluntary adoption agency, a family placement consortium (in Scotland), or privately – but only with a member of your close family. In the UK, a parent arranging the adoption of their child themselves is illegal. All adoptions must be arranged by an approved adoption agency, which can assess and verify the new parents, and must be approved by the courts.

The key adoption organisations in the UK are as follows:

- ✔ **The British Association for Adoption & Fostering (BAAF)** is a UK-wide organisation for setting standards, raising awareness, influencing social policy, and managing adoption and fostering services. Visit www.baaf.org.uk or more information.

- ✔ **Adoption UK** provides advice and support services for prospective adopters, adoptive parents, and long-term foster carers. Check out www.adoptionuk.org to find out more.

- ✔ **NCH** is a leading children's charity and provider of children's services in the UK, including finding homes and families for some of the UK's most vulnerable children. Look on their Web site at www.nch.org.uk for a full description of their services.

- ✔ **The Adoption Register for England and Wales** is run by BAAF on behalf of the Government's DfES and the National Assembly for Wales to match children requiring adoption and families. Their Web site www.adoptionregister.org.uk tells you more about the Register.

- ✔ **The Adoption and Fostering Information Line (AFIL)** claims to be the most popular adoption Internet site in the UK. It offers advice on how to adopt, details of children who are looking for new parents and families, and has a search facility for regional adoption agencies. Go to their site at www.adoption.org.uk to register your interest.

Adoption can be arranged for any of the 4,000 children waiting for new families in the UK, or with an agency that specialises in arranging adoptions abroad (see the 'Adopting abroad' section later in this chapter for more information).

Who can adopt?

Agencies require a variety of possible adopters to match the (special) needs, and ethnic and cultural diversity of the babies and children waiting for new parents, and so they welcome adopters who are single, and those in all types of relationships, including married couples, or heterosexual, gay, or lesbian partners or unmarried couples. Since September 2005, unmarried couples in England and Wales can apply to adopt jointly. Adopters can be from any religion or ethnic background, already have children, and be disabled or have experience of disability.

One restriction is age. Adopters need to be at least 21 years old and ideally no more than about 45 years older than the child to be adopted – although there's no legal upper age limit. You also don't need to own your house or have a garden. As amenable as adoption agencies and laws are, however, a couple of scenarios do present a problem for potential adoptive parents: If you have some criminal offences – especially those involving children – or you smoke. In either case, you may not be considered 'suitable' to become an adopter.

Most agencies won't process your application for adoption while you're having fertility treatment, and you need to demonstrate your commitment to adopting, rather than pursuing this option as 'insurance' if treatment doesn't work.

The cost of adoption

If you live in the UK and are planning to adopt a child who is also a UK resident, through a local authority or voluntary agency, you will usually incur no fees for the preparation, home study, and assessment stages (check out the later section 'Assessment – more hurdles to clear' for more on what these stages entail). Part of the process may require you to undergo a medical assessment and this check can cost from £74 per adult, depending on the GP surgery.

However, if you're planning to adopt from abroad, you have to pay a fee for a home study. If this is carried out by an accredited voluntary adoption agency, the cost starts at £5,000. Fees may differ if the home study is conducted by your local authority social services.

Voluntary adoption agencies depend on financial contributions from individuals, businesses, and government to support their work. Although voluntary adoption agencies may not charge for their services, any contribution to help their work continue is most welcome.

Matchmaking you and your child

Adoption is all about finding families for children, not finding babies for childless couples.

Would you want to adopt an older child or one with physical disabilities, or learning difficulties? Are you willing to adopt siblings and take on the rewards and challenges of a true ready-made family? Are you interested in a child from a different ethnic background to you or your partner?

Your preferences concerning the age, gender, and number of children are the basics when finding the right family for a child, but increasingly agencies try to place children in families with a similar background. This includes considering matching ethnic groups, culture, and diversity and also accounting for the child's age and attachment to their birth mother and any wishes of the child and birth mother. Although agencies always strive for a 100 per cent match, often adopters and agencies – on behalf of the child – are prepared to compromise, providing evidence exists that the adopters have a commitment to developing the child's identity.

The adoption process can be a frustrating time for both the adopters and social workers and is often referred to as a marathon rather than a sprint, because continual sustained effort is required instead of a short sudden burst of activity.

Some agency Web sites include details of 'available' children. If you can bear to visit them (these sites can be heart-breaking), they are a good starting point to see if your commitment and perceptions match the reality of adoption.

Getting through the assessment – more hurdles to clear

If you've experienced the assessment to be treated at a fertility clinic, and the questions about your lifestyle and private life, you're well placed to tackle the hurdles of the adoption process. The assessment process involves regular visits by your appointed social worker – usually over about six months – to discover more about you and what you have to offer a child. Lots of cleaning and tidying are involved (although probably not necessary!) and you're asked to consider issues such as discipline, the availability of strong support systems, and protecting your child from harm. You're also required to attend preparation groups and must be able to demonstrate that you can provide a safe, secure home and meet the emotional and physical needs of the child.

In addition, confidential enquiries are made about you to the police and to your local social services, and you must be examined by your GP, and are asked to provide personal references.

The home-study process is completed within about six months of the agency receiving your completed application form. Review panels are available for applicants who are not approved to adopt, and can be contacted through your adoption agency.

Moving in and getting legal

Once the assessment process is complete and you have been matched to the particular needs of a child, the excitement can begin! You and your social worker plan a series of introductions and contact sessions with the child over a few weeks or months, depending on the child's needs. After a date has been agreed for moving in, social workers continue to support your family and the child until an adoption order is made – and often beyond that time.

The child lives with you for a minimum of 13 weeks before your adoption application can be heard in court. The exact timing depends on the child's age, the progress of your relationship, and the legal situation. If you adopt a newborn, this period can't start until the baby is 6 weeks old, so no order is ever made before an infant is 19 weeks old. A court official checks that the birth parents understand that their child is to be adopted, and witnesses their agreement to the process. If the birth parents don't agree to the adoption, the court can still make an adoption order, but the process takes longer, and legal guardians have to be appointed to advise on whether the order can be finalised.

Being aware of adoptive-family issues

Every family deals with individual and distinct situations, but issues about the original identity and early life of the adopted child are universal. Here are some tips about being honest about how, and when, your child came in to your life.

- ✔ **When and what to tell your child about the adoption:** Best advice is that children can never recall the actual time they were told they were adopted – instead it needs to be something they've always known. Agencies recommend that adopted children are also told why they can't live with their birth family.

✔ **To contact or not?** Some contact between the child and the birthparents is often advised – even it is an annual letter via a third party. Occasionally your child may retain contact with siblings or grandparents, and, rarely, you may have direct contact with the birth parents. Whatever the contact plan, the feelings of the adopter parents are always considered.

✔ **Obtaining original birth certificate:** Most adopted children are curious about their birth family and they have the right at the age of 18 (16 in Scotland) to see their original birth certificate. Following up these questions can be a tough time for the child, the adopter parents, and the birth mother, but the adoption agency or another third party, such a priest, can offer guidance and support through this process.

Adopting abroad

Adopting a child from abroad, at its extremes, can be perceived as a wonderful humanitarian act or as selfish über-consumerism that puts the wishes of the adopter before the child's needs for a family that can help nurture its cultural identity.

Following the 'Romanian Baby' scandal in the early 1990s, The Hague Convention implemented new international regulations that require the country of origin to prove that

✔ The child is available for adoption.

✔ No family is able to adopt them in their own country.

✔ Necessary consent is preceded by counselling, is in writing, has not been induced by payment, and in the case of a mother, is given only after birth.

The receiving country must establish that

✔ The adopter parents are eligible and suitable.

✔ The adopters have received counselling.

✔ The child is able to enter and live with them in their home country.

Adopting a child from another country can take years, and adopters are likely to have to comply with follow-up requirements; for example, reports on how the child is doing. It's not a soft alternative to UK adoption.

Do's and don'ts for adoptive parents

Here's a collection of ideas based on the experience of people who have already adopted. This list is not definitive or prescriptive. Some are common sense, others a little more imaginative. They may help you and your new child through your first days and weeks together.

Do:

- Set up some parts of your new child's room; doing so helps make everything seem more real, and passes the time!

- Get involved with a group of waiting parents. This support helps beforehand, when you're waiting together, and afterwards, when you're frustrated together!

- Start a journal of everything you're experiencing, recording your impressions of the waiting time and your child's first days with you.

- Read up on whatever age group your new child fits into, especially if you don't have any children yet. You'll get a better idea of what to expect.

- Buy some clothes ahead of time, if you know whether you're getting a boy or girl – but show some restraint (see below).

- Find out and practise a few words of their language if your child is coming from abroad. Your pronunciation may be terrible, but it may help settle the child in the crucial first days.

- Record your child speaking their first language if you're adopting a child from abroad. It will be a family treasure for them for the future.

Don't:

- Expect instant love on either side. Many children have known trauma or instability in their lives, and may have already been with a foster family. Your excitement and delight may overwhelm your child and you may be disappointed by their neutrality, or even hostility.

- Buy too many clothes ahead of time. Your child may be smaller than you're expecting or your taste may not suit the personality of any older children you welcome into your family.

- Buy too many toys ahead of time. Wait until you know your child a little better and have a better idea of what he or she likes.

- Be surprised by temper tantrums, backsliding in toilet training, and other challenging behaviour. Lots of older children test you out a little to make sure that you're going to keep them. Babies' schedules may be in complete turmoil, and they may take several weeks to adjust.

- Get discouraged. *All* parents, no matter how they became parents, have moments when they just plain don't like their kids and wonder for a few moments why they ever did this to themselves! This moment too shall pass!

- Deny having a real problem. Not all adoptions end successfully; if things aren't going well, talk to your social worker as soon as possible – they've probably seen all manner of problems before.

For definitive information on adopting from abroad, visit the Intercountry Adoption Centre (IAC) at www.icacentre.org.uk. The IAC is a UK-registered charity that aims to ensure that, if people do contemplate adoption from another country, they have the means of making informed decisions, with a clear understanding of the issues involved.

Trying Out Foster Parenting First

Some couples look at foster parenting as a way to test their ability to love another person's child before considering adoption. Although you may possibly be allowed to adopt a foster child, the majority of children in foster care aren't available for adoption. Other people foster many children over many years with no plans to adopt. Fostering is an equally important and possibly even more challenging way of having children in your life! There are many types of fostering, including:

- **Emergency:** Where children need somewhere safe to stay for a limited time.

- **Short-term:** Where carers look after children for a few weeks or months.

- **Short-breaks:** Usually for children with disabilities or special needs to enjoy a short-break while their usual carers get the chance to do the same.

- **Remand fostering:** Where children in England and Wales are placed by the courts with a specially trained foster family while waiting for a court hearing.

- **Long-term:** For children who don't need or want to be adopted and who retain regular contact with their family, but who need somewhere permanent to live until they're old enough to live independently.

Who can foster?

Married and cohabiting couples, single and divorced people, gay men, and lesbians can all provide foster families, although the requirements in Scotland are specific and need to be clarified with a local foster agency.

Foster parents usually need to train to be registered with agencies and social services. They're also subject to home inspections and supervision from social workers. Although no upper age limits apply, foster parents need to be both mature and physically fit enough to handle the demands of the role.

If you're interested in fostering, visit the Web site of the British Association for Adoption and Fostering at www.baaf.org.uk and check the agencies database for those in your area. Advisers outline the preparation, assessments, support groups, and training that's all part of becoming a foster parent.

Don't think of fostering as 'adoption lite' – it takes huge commitment and you may be caring for vulnerable children, and young adults.

Foster grants

Many foster parents are volunteers, but increasingly they're seen as professionals and receive a self-employed fee, based on their skills and expertise, the needs of the fostered child or children, and the length of their foster experience. You can receive tax relief on your foster income up to a maximum of £10,000 and pension benefits are also available.

Foster parenting can be very rewarding, but it can also be heartbreaking to see children that you've come to care about go back to environments that were harmful to them in the first place. However, a real need exists for good foster parents, and if you want to be truly instrumental in the life of a child – or more than one – foster parenting can be a good place to start.

Deciding to Live Child Free

So here you are. You've tried and tried to conceive your child, and you've run out of money, time, hope, or all the above. Third-party reproduction (donor eggs or sperm) isn't an option for you. Adoption is neither financially nor emotionally feasible at this time. So what are the initial do's and don'ts? Here are a few things to keep in mind:

✔ **Visit the More to Life section of www.infertilitynetworkuk.com for 24/7 mutual support from people with the same experience.** They aren't going to think that you're 'moaning' or 'oversensitive', but instead give constant reassurance while you're trying to re-frame what you want from life.

✔ **Don't blame yourself or your partner.** Your bodies have done the best they can to cooperate with your childbearing plans. You have no more control over your reproductive capabilities than you do over your ability to digest food. Inability to conceive isn't anyone's fault. You're dealing with biology, not punishment.

✔ **Don't harass your doctor or the clinic staff.** Even if they have appeared to be rushed, doubtful, or just plain insensitive, they, too, wanted to see you succeed with having a baby. The medical teams are on your side! They feel your disappointment, albeit with a bit more detachment. They have seen cases better, and worse, for years, and sometimes their experience may cause them to arrive at conclusions long before you do. Let this mix of care and practicality guide you in your decisions.

✔ **Don't commit yourself to a life of misery.** Whether you have a child or not, happiness is still within your power *and* your responsibility. It's up to you to make it happen, one way or the other.

My clinical role (co-author Gill) often includes consultations with couples who feel that they have reached the end of the road with fertility treatment and are still childless. I find that reviewing the treatment cycles with them, emphasising the positive, such as the strength and commitment they've shown as a couple during their treatment, reassuring them that they have tried everything that can be tried, and giving them 'permission' to stop trying, can help bring resolution – even though I also understand that the pain of being involuntarily childless may never really go away.

Okay, so now that you're in the right frame of mind, what do you do next? Take stock in your life as a child-free individual or couple. Think that living a life without children sounds depressing? Well, consider a few benefits of being child free:

✔ **Extra money.** Can you figure out a fun way to spend £166,000? We thought so! We discuss the costs of child rearing at the beginning of this book, but, in short, child-free couples have a 'spare' few hundred thousand to play with. Maybe you've always wanted a second home, or to travel far and wide. And maybe you just like the idea of being able to go out to dinner whenever you want and not worry about whether you can afford the extra starter or bottle of wine.

✔ **Extra time.** Most parents today find themselves 'time-deprived', forcing them to skip many former activities, such as hobbies and working out. Former pleasures, such as putting your feet up after a long day at work or enjoying a relaxing dinner with your partner, quickly become a thing of the past for most parents, new and old.

✔ **Spontaneity.** Are you the type who enjoys a last-minute holiday or even a last-minute movie? Spontaneity of this sort doesn't fit in well with raising children, particularly when they're young. Child-free living, however, leaves plenty of room for spur-of-the-moment plans and quick turnarounds. Whether you're talking about a romantic interlude in the living room, or a decision to chuck dinner and eat out instead, as a child-free adult, you can freely indulge in these activities.

No one can flip a switch where suddenly that longed-for baby is no longer your priority but, instead, you're planning a life spending your income on you alone. Coming to terms with living child-free takes time and – often – help. Nothing is all good or all bad, and child-free living does have its high points. Make it a point to figure out all the positives of the situation and go on from there. Also keep in mind that not having children of your own doesn't mean that you have no children in your life whatsoever. You probably have nieces or nephews or friends' children to spoil and care for. (No, we won't mention the old platitude about 'giving them back' at the end of the day because it doesn't help!)

Working with Children

Of course, you can work with children as a teacher or a social worker, but you have other, less known ways of becoming important to the life of a child. Here are some other options that you may want to consider:

- ✔ **You can volunteer at a hospital.** Hospitals may need committed adults to read or chat to children.

- ✔ **You can become a *Guardian ad litem*.** These volunteers represent the child's best interest in the legal system. A training period is required and volunteers are expected to spend a minimum number of hours each month in this position.

- ✔ **You can be a coach, a music teacher, part of a children's theatre group, or a school volunteer.**

- ✔ **You can work with any number of other organisations that work with special-needs children.**

- ✔ **You can volunteer at your church, mosque, or synagogue, work in the nursery, or teach a Sunday school class.**

- ✔ **You can be a Big Brother or Sister to a child in need.** You can be as involved as you want to be with 'your child' and his family. You may see 'your child' as many as several times a week or as little as once or twice a month.

- ✔ **You can become the best aunt or uncle in your family.** If your siblings have children, become involved with them. Often a special aunt or uncle can be a child's mentor or confidante for life.

Chapter 23

New Advances and Ethical Dilemmas

· ·

In This Chapter

▶ Choosing baby's sex – and more

▶ Confronting the hardest decision – selective reduction

▶ Deciding what to do with leftover embryos

▶ Understanding cloning and deciding where you stand

▶ Imagining future issues in fertility treatment

· ·

*P*rimum non nocere' or 'above all do no harm' is part of the Hippocratic oath that all good doctors live by. In the field of fertility medicine, this notion is especially important because fertility patients may be childless but they're generally fit and well adults and need to stay that way. Everything done in the fertility clinic must be designed to help healthy couples have healthy babies (preferably one at a time!) with the minimum necessary level of intervention.

Technology is a double-edged sword. With every advance come questions about what technology *can* do versus what it *should be allowed to* do. And fertility treatment has been at the centre of some of the most intriguing debates about what should and shouldn't be done. From the early days of artificial insemination, to the first test-tube baby, to donor egg and sperm programmes and the use of frozen sperm to produce posthumous babies, doctors, patients, ethicists, politicians, actresses, and bishops have argued whether these advances are ethically or morally defensible. Fertility issues fill the tabloids, hit the headlines, and challenge the courts. Some of the newest advances – sex selection, preimplantation genetic diagnosis (PGD – designer babies), and stem cell research – have also come under heavy fire by ethicists and others concerned about the consequences of tinkering with potential human beings.

In this chapter, we look at some of the hottest fertility debates and how they affect you now; we also put on our visionary glasses to see what new advances may be available ten years from now.

Looking Down the Road: Long-Term Health Effects of Fertility Medication

Fertility medications, or *gonadotrophins*, are powerful stuff. Anyone who takes them through even one cycle can attest to the physical and emotional effects of having one's hormones surging at a much higher level than nature ever intended. Do people suffer long-term effects 2 or 20 years down the road? No one knows for sure, but here are the most recent conclusions on the safety of taking gonadotrophins.

Part of the difficulty in assessing the effects of fertility medication lies with the enormous emotional and personal significance of having fertility treatment in the first place. Couples reading this book have probably already had months or even years of 'trying': Of being prodded and poked; giving blood samples, semen samples, urine samples . . . So it's easy to understand how the side effects of the treatment, the physical effects of the drugs, the psychological effects of the stress, and the emotional side effects of *needing* treatment all get muddled up and produce symptoms. Tiredness, headaches, tearfulness, and loss of libido are all side effects of the drugs, but they're also side effects of being stressed, worried, anxious, and scared. In other words, that's what having fertility treatment is like!

Effects on the mother

At this time, experts have no solid proof that taking gonadotrophins has any long-term effect on women. Some studies have shown a possible link to clomiphene citrate, commonly known as Clomid (a medication which induces ovulation by making the pituitary gland make more follicle-stimulating hormone, or FSH), and ovarian cancer, but other studies have not supported these findings. In the UK, the recommendation is that no woman has more than 12 cycles of clomiphene treatment.

One thing most studies have agreed upon is that the risk of ovarian cancer is higher in all women who've never become pregnant, regardless of whether or not they've taken fertility medications. If you're found to have ovarian cysts then a blood test for CA 125 and a pelvic ultrasound scan can pick up problems while they can still be effectively treated. This testing is especially important if other women in your family have had ovarian cancer and/or breast cancer because doctors have established a genetic link for these types of cancer, among others.

Effects on the baby

No one is sure whether fertility medications will have a long-term effect on the children conceived through their use – many of the children born through high-tech methods such as in vitro fertilisation (IVF) aren't old enough yet. The oldest IVF baby, Louise Brown, and her younger sister (also an IVF baby) have both had healthy babies naturally and this news is enormously reassuring. Techniques such as ICSI and assisted hatching are even newer; they've only been used extensively since the 1990s.

Because research is ongoing even as children are being born, high-tech treatment has an element of risk, simply because the jury's still out on long-term effects. Some studies have indicated that high-tech babies have lower birth weight and developmental delays.

However, more twins and triplets are born to mothers using fertility medications, and multiples more commonly have low birth weight and developmental delays. Also, more babies are born to older mothers through high-tech treatment, and older women tend to have more complicated pregnancies than women under age 35.

Recent research has found that couples who are *sub*-fertile rather than *in*-fertile (they conceive naturally, but it takes them over a year) also tend to have babies with lower birth weight.

Because some men who need ICSI to conceive have part of their Y chromosome missing, which results in their infertility, some of their sons may have the same chromosomal abnormality and may also need to do ICSI (or whatever high-tech methods are available in 30 years) to have children. A higher incidence of sex chromosome abnormalities is found in the offspring of men with poor sperm who need IVF but only a tiny minority of births are affected. Men who need ICSI because they have had a vasectomy that can't be reversed are a useful 'control group' because they had normal natural fertility before the 'snip'. Their partner's pregnancies do not show this level of chromosome risk, and so we can be confident that the ICSI technique itself is not what causes the problem.

Selecting the Sex: When You Absolutely, Positively, Want a Boy Or a Girl

Whenever you ask a pregnant mum-to-be whether she's hoping for a boy or a girl, the usual answer is 'We don't mind as long as the baby is healthy!' This is how it should be as babies are gifts, not commodities. But if you already have five boys and would dearly love a girl, or if you carry a genetic link to a sex-determined disease, such as haemophilia, your answer may well be one in which you state a preference. Until recently, 50/50 odds were the best you could do, but newer advances have increased the odds of taking home the boy or girl you're hoping for.

You hear lots of old wives' tales about how to ensure that you conceive a boy rather than a girl. The ancient Greeks believed that 'boy' sperm was made in the right testicle and 'girl' sperm in the left and, therefore, if you wanted a boy you should tie a string around the left testicle . . . Ooch!

Sex selection is only legal in the UK if it's done for medical reasons such as avoiding sex-linked genetic diseases. In such cases 'sperm sorting' is done in conjunction with ICSI, IVF, and PGD (preimplantation genetic diagnosis). This method is a very effective, very expensive (about £5,000), and very high-tech type of fertility treatment, and may give you only a few embryos to test. Don't try this because you fancy a football team or an all-girls' choir!

Sperm sorting

Naturally, a sample of sperm contains a 50:50 mix of boy-making and girl-making sperm. Some methods claim to enrich or increase the 'concentration of the sperm sample for X (female) or Y (male) chromosome-bearing sperm that can then be used in IUI (intrauterine insemination) or IVF, but they're far from 100 per cent reliable.

Female sperm (carrying the Xs) are heavier (they contain 2.8 per cent more DNA) and slower swimming than male sperm (the Ys). Using techniques that increase the proportion of one type of sperm may slightly increase the chance of getting a baby of the gender you want: the X and Y chromosomes in sperm can be labelled or 'tagged' with a fluorescent marker that allows a very sophisticated machine called a flow cytometer to separate the sperm into 'boys' and girls'. The process is more efficient (90 per cent) at identifying 'girl' sperm. Remember, however, that no absolute guarantees come with this method, and IUI and IVF treatment is expensive and not very successful after all. The latest published data for this type of sperm sorting (in the US, where it's legal) gives a pregnancy rate of just over 10 per cent per cycle for IUI with 92 per cent of births being the 'desired' gender where a girl was wanted. Figures for boys are less successful.

The trouble with statistics like these is that they're a bit misleading. You have to remember that nature gives you odds of about 53 per cent to 47 per cent in favour of males, so a 65 per cent chance of a boy is only 12 per cent more than nature gives you already. Think how you (and the child of the 'wrong' sex) are going to feel if you go to all that trouble and it doesn't work out.

Saviour siblings

One important area for gene selection that causes ethical controversy is that of *saviour siblings*.

For many genetic disorders such as Blackfan-Diamond anaemia or diseases such as leukaemia, the only hope of a cure when conventional therapies have failed is a stem cell transplant from a perfectly genetically matched donor. If the parents or existing siblings of the sick child don't match, then if the mother undergoes IVF, the embryos can be 'screened' to see which ones can turn into babies that would be a perfect match, and the stem cells can be harvested from the baby's umbilical cord and used to save the life of its sick older sibling.

For some people creating one child to save the life of another sounds horrible, as if babies are being made 'to order' just to save someone else. Others argue that if the parents of the sick child are desperate to help were to have another baby anyway, and purely by chance the baby turned out to be a perfect genetic match for the sick sibling, then it would be wonderful piece of luck. So what's wrong with helping the parents to 'stack the odds' in their favour?

Preimplantation genetic diagnosis (PGD)

At the moment, the only absolute way to determine a baby's sex is to do *preimplantation genetic diagnosis* (PGD), in which a cell taken from an already created embryo can be analysed to see if the baby will be a boy or a girl. Right now, PGD is mainly used to screen for genetic diseases or to check for sex if the parents are carriers of a disease that affects only a child of one sex.

Currently, PGD can test for a wide variety of genetic diseases, including haemophilia, Huntington's disease, muscular dystrophy, sickle-cell disease, and Tay-Sachs, as well as chromosomal defects, such as Down syndrome and Turner's syndrome.

As genetic mapping advances, it's not hard to imagine parents screening embryos not only for sex or genetic diseases but also for hair and eye colour, intelligence, and personality traits. Although none of these traits will ever be able to be accurately determined by PGD because they're determined by multiple 'gene complexes', one day they may be. This possibility has ethicists concerned about where PGD is heading.

Ten years from today, will parents be routinely selecting the child of their choice, picking height, IQ, hair and eye colour, and left- or right-handedness? The potential for gene tinkering is limitless, after certain traits have been mapped out and identified. The positive aspect of such manipulation is the elimination of certain diseases or handicaps.

The negative side is that we could end up with populations skewed in one direction only, such as a nation full of tall, blonde, genius tennis players. Or we could find the male-to-female ratio off balance, as is happening in China with its one-child-only rule that has led to an excess of boys.

Although the potential for using gene selection for good purposes is high, the potential for abuse is just as high.

Selective Reduction: Making the Hardest Choice

Nature never intended women to have more than one baby at a time. Most women can carry two without serious complications, but triplet and higher pregnancies can be a disaster. Triplet and higher-order pregnancies (that can occur with ovulation induction) are dangerous for both the mother and the babies, and the incidence of prematurity, handicap, and neonatal death are high.

In the UK, a maximum of two embryos can be transferred to women unless they are 40 years or older. This policy has reduced the incidence of triplets. Sometimes, even with a two-embryo transfer, however, triplets can result because one of the embryos spontaneously 'twins'.

When faced with multiples, some parents consider *selective reduction*, in which one or more fetuses in a multiple pregnancy are eliminated. This decision is difficult to make, and few couples make it lightly, especially when they've tried so hard to get pregnant in the first place. Reduction is usually performed only to reduce triplets or higher, although some women with severe medical conditions may want reduction to a single baby.

Selective reduction isn't done too early in the pregnancy because of the risk that some of the fetuses won't continue to grow past five or six weeks. Usually, doctors wait until ten weeks or so to see what happens. The process in done under ultrasound guidance; the doctor tries to pick the fetus that appears least likely to grow well, such as the smallest. The doctor also tries to pick a fetus that's furthest away from another, to avoid losing both babies.

Potassium chloride is injected into the sac, and the fetus dies and is absorbed in the body. The miscarriage rate after reduction is low, less than 5 per cent. Some studies have shown that the remaining babies are born slightly earlier than the norm.

Dividing Up the Leftover Embryos

In an ideal world, couples would use up all their embryos, having one baby initially and then one or more a few years later. However, for various reasons, that often doesn't happen. Leftover embryos then become a huge emotional and legal headache for most IVF centres. Space is needed to store them and money is required to maintain the storage tanks. Few centres want to make decisions for potential human beings without some input from their parents, even if the parents haven't been seen or heard from in years.

When parents separate or divorce with embryos still in storage, frozen embryos can be fought over bitterly. In more than one case, divorcing couples have fought publicly over what should be done with their unused embryos. The situation can be even more traumatic when those frozen embryos represent the only chance for becoming a genetic parent.

Even in 1983, when IVF was a brand-new technology, frozen embryos made the news when their wealthy 'parents' were killed in a plane crash, leaving no heirs. Technically, their only offspring were two frozen embryos. Of course, many women offered to carry the embryos and raise them – as long as their inherited fortune came with them! In the end, the embryos were treated as property and were destroyed.

Some of the most important consent forms you're asked to sign are concerned with what happens to your frozen embryos (refer to Chapter 9 for an account of the HFEA regulations). You may have difficulty contemplating the three 'Ds' (death, divorce, and disability) but those forms do need to be completed, and this moment can be a good opportunity to talk about what are usually taboo subjects. Frozen embryos have been at the centre of other types of lawsuits.

Even if couples don't divorce or die, the decision of what to do with frozen embryos is a tough one, because the choices are limited. Couples can donate the embryos to research, donate them to another couple, or have them taken out of the cryostore and allowed to perish. Not liking any of the choices, many parents just keep the embryos in storage, postponing any decision on what to do with them. Some would rather the clinic just allowed them to perish when they got to the end of their legal storage period, but clinics have a responsibility to inform couples of their options.

Putting Old Genes into New Skins: Cytoplasmic Transfer

The DNA in the egg nucleus is what helps determine 'who' the baby will be, but the quality of the egg and its ability to turn into an embryo, and ultimately a baby, is determined by the cytoplasm of the egg. So scientists have tried taking the egg of an older woman and injecting a small amount of cytoplasm from a younger donor's egg into her egg.

Cytoplasm is found inside the shell of the egg but outside the nucleus, which contains the genetic material. So a woman who gets pregnant after cytoplasmic transfer has her own biological child.

Cytoplasm contains *mitochondria*, which are the energy cells of the body, and the spindles along which genes separate and divide. Some doctors believe that older eggs need extra 'energy' to divide and grow, and that their older spindles allow DNA to separate abnormally. So by injecting cytoplasm, they hope to energise and normalise call division in the egg.

Cytoplasmic transfer has a couple of potential pitfalls:

✔ The egg injected with cytoplasm has to be genetically normal, and the reason that many women over 40 don't get pregnant is that the majority of their eggs contain abnormal genetic material. The cytoplasm injected won't fix a genetically abnormal egg.

✔ The mitochondria transferred carries a little DNA from the donating egg with it, so the resulting baby has DNA from three people instead of two. Proponents of cytoplasmic transfer say that the extra DNA isn't harmful and occurs frequently in nature as spontaneous mutations. Opponents are concerned that the children created, even though they look normal at birth, may develop problems down the road from the extra DNA.

About 30 children have been born after cytoplasmic transfer. The main genetic problem found in the pregnancies was the rate of Turner's syndrome, a genetic abnormality where the female has only one X chromosome. The rate was about six times higher than normal.

Cytoplasmic transfer isn't permitted in the UK, and couples need to consider whether travelling abroad to get the treatment is a step too far while there is such uncertainty about long-term safety.

Posthumous Conception: Legal and Ethical Issues

You don't have to be married, you don't have to have a partner, you don't even have to be alive to become a parent in the Brave New World of cryobiology.

Posthumous collection of sperm – removing sperm from the testes after a man has died – has been done on just about every continent. The legal issues have been discussed almost as much as the ethical issues. And there's still little legal or moral consensus about using a deceased man's sperm to create a child.

The person using the sperm is usually the spouse or partner of the dead man. Sometimes, but not always, she has advance written permission to collect and use the sperm at the time of his death. Legal issues have revolved around inheritance of the dead man's property and the payment of welfare benefits to the children who are born after a man's death – more than 300 days after his death.

The waters become murkier when the man has given no written permission for the sperm extraction. Can a spouse or partner legally request this removal be done? How does she know that it's what the man would want done? Does it matter? Just a few of the posthumous conception scenarios that have occurred recently are listed here:

- ✔ One widow used a videotape in which her husband, who had been killed in a car accident, expressed a desire to have children someday as support for her request to have sperm removed at the time of his death.

- ✔ A case in which a man left frozen sperm to his fiancée came under scrutiny because she didn't want to use the sperm, but the man's parents did. They wanted to use donor eggs and a gestational carrier to create a child of their child, which they presumably would then raise.

- ✔ In England, a widower is trying to find a surrogate to carry embryos created right before his wife's death; she had an egg retrieval done while she was waiting for a heart-lung transplant.

- ✔ In another case of motherhood after death, the parents of a dead woman were searching for a gestational carrier to give birth to their dead daughter's children, created from their daughter's eggs and donor sperm.

The story of Diane Blood

In England, the case of Diane Blood brought all these issues to public attention. When Diane's husband lapsed into a coma following an attack of meningitis, she persuaded the medical team to extract some sperm so that she could have a chance of children. Technically the extraction was illegal, because he had not given written consent and so the fertility treatment that Diane needed wasn't allowed in the UK. Enormous public sympathy was felt for Diane and by a curious legal manoeuvre she was allowed to 'export' the sperm to Belgium where she was helped to conceive twice, producing a healthy son on each occasion. Happy ending. A further legal development now allows the deceased father to be named on the birth certificate of posthumous children born following fertility treatment.

So many cases crop up where children are unwanted, abused, and neglected that it may seem difficult to deny the wishes of those would-be parents or grandparents who are desperate to make a baby in order to have some aspect of a departed loved one to hang onto. But society needs to remember that babies grow up to be children and people in their own right; babies should not be 'made' to stop a widow being lonely.

Cloning and Human Concerns

People talk about cloning as if all cloning is the same thing. In reality, different types of cloning have been developed; some have been successful, some have been partially successful, and some haven't been done at all yet, as far as we know.

✔ **Using a healthy embryo:** The cloning causing the most controversy is the type that produced Dolly the sheep. It involves taking a healthy embryo, removing its DNA, and putting the DNA from another creature of the same species into the embryo. Most cells contain DNA, so obtaining DNA isn't difficult. If the embryo continues growing normally, it can be placed into a host uterus to develop.

Many concerns are raised over this type of reproductive cloning. Many of the offspring cloned so far have had serious abnormalities. 'Large calf' syndrome, in which the cloned offspring of cows have been so large that they cannot be delivered normally, has been used to justify a total ban on human reproductive cloning. The concern that cloned individuals may age much faster than normal because their DNA was obtained from a mature adult is also under scrutiny.

The creation of Dolly

The cloning technique that created Dolly, the well-known (and now dead) cloned sheep, involved taking a mammary cell nucleus from another sheep and putting it into a sheep embryo. (Dolly was named in honour of Dolly Parton in memory of which bit of sheep anatomy was used to harvest the cell!) The original genetic material was removed from the embryo, so that the only DNA was from the donor sheep, which was about 6 years old at the time. Dolly was the only successful clone born out of about 300 original attempts. Dolly started to develop arthritis when she was almost 6 years old, causing concern that she was aging faster than normal. In early 2003, Dolly had to be put down at the age of 6 after being diagnosed with a progressive lung disease. Sheep usually live to be 12 to 14 years old. Calf cloning has been mildly successful; 73 per cent of pregnancies end in miscarriage, and 20 per cent die soon after birth. Some are born oversized, with enlarged tongues, with immune deficiencies, or with diseases such as diabetes.

✔ **Using an embryonic cell:** Another type of cloning that could be used to create human beings has been done pretty successfully in animals. The process involves taking a cell from an embryo and allowing it to grow into a second, identical embryo. This way is how identical twins occur in nature.

The technique allows the possibility of giving birth to identical twins several years apart, which is done frequently in farming. The method also provides the option to do genetic testing on the 'cloned' embryo while freezing the original. If the clone passed the genetic tests, the 'original' can then be thawed and implanted.

People wanting an exact copy of themselves may be disappointed because cloned animals aren't totally identical. Environmental influences can change certain characteristics and alter appearance.

Saving Stem Cells for Research

Stem cells are cells that have the ability to develop into any type of tissue or organ. In other words, they're *pluripotent*. Human embryos are a good source of stem cells, and it could be possible to substitute DNA from a living person into a human egg after the egg's DNA has been removed. The egg could then be 'shocked' to get it to grow, and after two weeks or so, the stem cells would be removed, and the embryo would die. The stem cells would then be grown into whatever the adult needed – organs, skin, or other tissue. Because the genetic match would be exact, the person's body wouldn't reject the new organ or tissue.

People needing organ transplants or new skin after a burn may find this type of science valuable. Scientists have also suggested that stem cell technology may help people with degenerative diseases, such as Parkinson's or Alzheimer's, as neural tissues grown from stem cells could be injected into the brain to repopulate the areas that make the neurotransmitters that are deficient in these diseases.

Some doctors feel that the surplus of embryos destroyed every year should be used for stem cell development. Others feel that the potential life of the embryo shouldn't be sacrificed to save an already living person. Many people with frozen embryos would like to see something positive done with embryos that they donate for research, and would rather have them used for stem cell development than just be destroyed.

Fertility patients in the UK can donate their surplus frozen embryos for scientific research and can specify that they want to contribute to stem cell projects. Women may also donate eggs altruistically for scientific research but given the invasive nature of the process they are recommended for in-depth counselling, which is vital before committing themselves.

Stem cells can be obtained from other places besides human embryos. Many parents are now banking blood from their child's umbilical cord in case the child needs stem cells at a later date. In the UK, plans are being made to develop a national cord blood bank so that a stem cell match can be found for patients who needed it.

'Welfare of the Child': Asking Clinics to Decide Who's Fit to Parent

If you're fertile, you can become a parent anytime you want. No one is in your bedroom rating your ability to raise children. And after children are born, they're taken only from parents who've repeatedly demonstrated appalling parenting behaviour.

People who do IVF are no better or worse as parents than anyone else; the potential for child abuse or neglect exists just as it does in any other population. In fact, people who are prepared to put themselves through all the hoops and face the stress, the discomfort and the expense of IVF may be demonstrating rather better parenting intentions than usual. Doctors have no way of possibly identifying those who are psychologically unprepared to raise children.

At this time, most clinics set their own rules for evaluating patients. One prime example is the use of donor eggs or embryos for older women – older as in over 50. Many centres use 50 as an arbitrary cut off age. Why 50 and not

57? Some centres do strict testing on patients over 40 to make sure that they're healthy enough to carry a pregnancy. Yet some 45-year-olds are much healthier than some 25-year-olds.

The current Human Fertilisation and Embryology Act doesn't explicitly lay down rules about who can be accepted, or rejected, as a possible parent. Human rights and anti-discrimination legislation is encouraging a more 'open access' policy in many clinics and this ethic is to be encouraged. Individual clinics Web sites tell you if they offer the type of treatment that you need. Personal recommendation is valuable but you can always pick up the phone or drop the clinic an email. Being a parent is hard work and the work may start with finding the right clinic for you!

Making Mistakes in the Lab: When Saying You're Sorry Isn't Enough

A baby of one race being born to a couple of another race. Embryos misplaced while in storage. An embryologist found guilty of doing embryo transfers with 'empty' catheters because he had 'sold' the embryos to another clinic. These examples are just a few of the mistakes (whether accidental or intentional) that fertility clinics have made.

Strict regulations are in place to minimise the risk of mistakes in the lab. (In fact, IVF is very well regulated in the United Kingdom and the HFEA is held up as a model of a regulatory system.) Clinics are careful not to work on eggs or embryos belonging to two different people at the same time. They label everything that they're working with including the name, date of birth, and clinic number to prevent mix-ups, and every step where sperm, eggs, or embryos are moved or processed has to be 'double-witnessed'. Despite these precautions, mix-ups do sometimes occur.

When a clinic makes mistakes of this kind, saying sorry isn't nearly good enough. Most of the highly publicised cases of parents ending up with the wrong children have come to light only because the parents and children were of different races. It's hard to say whether similar errors have been made and not discovered because parents and children were all the same race.

In one instance involving black children and white parents, the error was made in the andrology lab; sperm from a black man was used instead of the sperm from the Caucasian spouse. In this case, the birth mother was also the biological mother, making the children genetically hers.

Safeguarding yourself against errors of this type is hard. The errors aren't made purposely; they're the result of fallible human beings making mistakes. You can help keep mistakes to a minimum by reading everything you're given to sign, and making sure that your name is properly spelled on everything. When you leave a semen specimen, make sure that it's labelled properly. When the embryologist hands your embryos over for transfer, make sure that she says your proper name.

If you have questions at any point about your eggs or embryos, ask them at that time. If there's any question of error, getting to the bottom of it right then is much easier than getting to the bottom of it nine months later. Monetary compensation is never going to be adequate to fix the heartbreak caused by an error in an embryology lab.

Where Is All This Leading? New Fertility Frontiers

Doctors are always breaking new ground in infertility treatment. In 1978 when Louise Brown, the first IVF baby in the world was born in the UK, egg retrievals and embryo transfers were major surgical procedures. Now, patients who have egg retrievals and transfers go home the same day and are back to work the next.

In 1992, the perfection of ICSI (check out Chapters 10 and 13) brought new hope of biological fatherhood to hundreds of thousands of men. A few years later, the development of blastocyst culture seemed like the chances for embryos to implant would be greatly increased. Now, ICSI and blastocyst transfer are routine, and the focus is on determining which embryos are most likely to implant, decreasing multiple pregnancies, and improving the chances for women over 40.

Preimplantation genetic diagnosis (PGD), discussed earlier in this chapter, may be routine in the next ten years. When only the best embryos are implanted, the pregnancy rates increase. This advance brings new concerns about destroying 'not-so-perfect' embryos.

If egg freezing becomes routine, women who wish to delay having children a decade or two will have no problem waiting. For those women who are already over 40, some new variation on cytoplasmic transfer may be developed in the next ten years.

Critics of fertility treatment may say that we live in an overpopulated world, but the thought provides no comfort to a childless couple in the UK to know that a mother in Africa is struggling to feed her seven children. Women are deferring starting a family not because they want to have it all, but often because matters of life and livelihood, jobs, and mortgages are just too pressing. Our society needs to make the process easier for women to try to have babies when they're more fertile, where Mother Nature is more likely to oblige. And where she won't then access to specialist help should be swift and preferably available on the NHS.

Fertility medicine is a fascinating, frustrating, and intensely moving branch of medicine. Usually in other branches of medicine or surgery, if everyone does everything right, treatment works 95 per cent of the time. In fertility medicine, it is reasonable to hope that we can offer the infertile the same chance of getting pregnant in a single treatment cycle as the normally fertile have in a month of 'trying' (about 35 per cent). Doctors, nurses and scientists working in the field share the frustration of patients who do everything right and yet never succeed in becoming genetic parents, but they also share the joy and wonder of couples who get to be parents against all the odds.

Part VII
The Part of Tens

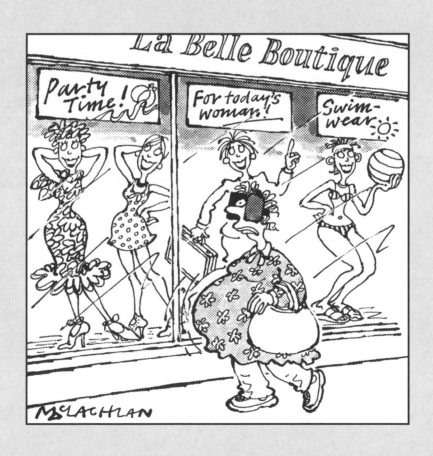

In this part . . .

In this part we offer you sound advice to get through the key stages of trying to conceive and going through assisted conception. We also describe the most frequently prescribed drugs used in fertility treatment. This is at-a-glance essential information at your fingertips!

Chapter 24

Ten Tips to Get You Through Treatment (and Keep You Sane!)

*T*his whole book is full of tips to get you through every stage of planning to have a baby and getting pregnant. But to help you, we've summarised the top tips for helping you through the assisted baby-making process.

Give Yourself Time

If you don't get pregnant within three months of trying, don't panic and assume that donor eggs and ICSI are the only ways you'll have a baby. Sometimes, even Mother Nature likes to take her time. Of every 100 couples trying to conceive naturally:

- ✔ 80 won't conceive within one month
- ✔ 30 won't conceive within six months
- ✔ 15 won't conceive within a year
- ✔ 10 won't conceive within 18 months
- ✔ 5 won't conceive within two years

Don't Panic

If you've been trying for a while and you're advised to consider assisted conception, again, don't panic! Remember that one in every six couples now needs help to conceive – you're not alone and nowadays there are many experts who can help.

Remember You're Not Alone

More than 2 million babies have been born worldwide after IVF treatment. That means that almost every year in every school in the UK probably has at least one 'test-tube baby' – and yours may join them in the future. In one local primary school, Mary, the archangel Gabriel and two shepherds were all IVF babies – who said there was no room at the lab?!

Don't Blame Yourself

A frustratingly high amount of both male and female infertility is still 'unexplained'. It's not your fault, you've done nothing 'wrong', it's not fair . . . but help is available to try to overcome it.

If you're part of a couple, don't blame your partner for his or her subfertility or infertility. Thinking this way won't help you emotionally and simply puts you under more stress, which can increase the risk of unsuccessful treatment. The clinic will treat you as a couple, so think of your infertility as a shared problem.

Listen to Friends – Occasionally

Don't be distracted by the 'helpful' advice of family and friends regarding apocryphal stories, and old wives' tales (check out Chapter 2). This is your fertility journey and it won't be influenced by folklore or the experience of a friend-of-a-friend.

Don't Delay Treatment

Don't keep delaying your appointments with your GP, specialist, or your clinic – especially if you're in your 30s. If you leave going through the process too long, those couple of extra years may have been when the treatment had a better chance of success.

Don't Freak about the Financing

A single cycle of IVF will not cost you a second mortgage and can make you pregnant. It's more affordable than you may think.

You may be lucky enough to live in an area where NHS funding is available for one or two cycles of treatment – check it out with your GP, before you start raiding your savings or flexing your plastic. Go to Chapter 9 for information on how to finance fertility treatment.

Don't Get Needled about Needles

Many people have a fear of needles and injections. But just remember that every time you stick a needle in your leg or tummy to down-regulate or stimulate those follicles, you're one step closer to realising your dream. You *can* do it! (A lump of ice or an ice-pop rubbed in the spot for a few minutes in advance of the injection can help – others swear by anaesthetic gel.)

Share Your Treatment Experience

Some couples choose to 'tell no one', but most, women especially, get through it by confiding in at least one good friend, a sister, or a colleague.

What if you feel like blowing a fuse because 'nothing's going right', 'no one understands' and feel as though your partner, friends, and family have had enough of fertility talk? Well, get on to a Web site forum, message board, or chat room to share your feelings with complete strangers who know exactly how you feel and understand where you are with your treatment. You'll get 24/7 support from these kindred spirits and never have to worry about over-burdening them with you fertility frustrations. Visit www.fertilityfriends. co.uk or www.infertilitynetworkuk.com or www.midlandfertility. com/forum. Real and lasting friendships are sometimes forged from these virtual support groups.

Coming to Terms with No Success

More to Life (MTL) is a national network, part of I N UK, dedicated solely to providing a support service to those who, involuntarily, remain childless. For more information visit the More to Life section of www.infertilitynetworkuk. com. Not being able to have a baby is not your fault. After unsuccessful attempts, review your treatment and your emotions with your fertility doctor, nurse, or counsellor and, if it's what you want, accept their 'permission' to stop trying. Taking this decision can be a positive step to a new life that may, or may not, include children.

Chapter 25

Ten (Okay, Seven) Groups of Fertility Medications and Where to Find Them

··

In This Chapter

▶ Sorting the drugs

▶ Locating what you need (and when you need it!)

··

*A*lthough fertility medications come with a bewildering array of names, they fit into only a few categories. The different names are brand-name-only differences, in most cases. In this chapter, we describe the different categories (known as generics) and list the most common brand names of each. We also tell you where to get your drugs (and make sure that you're not paying too much!)

Fertility medications are generally sold in boxes of five or ten vials or ampoules. The ones that come with rubber stoppers on the top are called *vials*, and the ones that have a glass 'nipple' that you need to break off are called *ampoules*.

Gonadotrophins

The most important (and most expensive) fertility drugs are the gonadotrophin injections that stimulate your ovaries to produce egg-containing follicles. Gonadotrophins (urinaries) are produced by purifying menopausal women's urine; they can also be *recombinant*, which means manufactured in the lab using genetic engineering technology.

Side effects of gonadotrophin include bloating, headache, and mood swings, as well as pregnancy (which also causes bloating, headache, mood swings, and great joy).

Your clinic teaches you how to mix up and administer your injections and supplies you with the syringes, mixing needles, injecting needles, and 'sharps bins' in which you need to dispose of your needles and syringes. These have to be taken back to your clinic or pharmacy for disposal because very strict rules prevent you just leaving them out for the dustman to take away. Some products are available in convenience devices, such as pens or prefilled syringes. However, these often require refrigerated transport and storage and can be expensive – you need to decide whether the extra expense and 'inconvenience' is worth avoiding the reconstitution process.

Unless you've led a somewhat rackety life in the drugs sub-culture (or have a relative with diabetes who takes insulin) the last time you probably ever saw a needle and syringe was when you had your tetanus booster age 12! Very few people are true needle phobics and you're soon going to feel quite cool about mixing up your injections and sticking a needle in yourself. If it stings a little, try holding an ice cube over the place you're planning to do your injection. Thigh, buttock, and tummy (below the waist) are the best sites for subcutaneous injections. Intramuscular injections are best done into the buttock or upper thigh.

Recombinant gonadotrophin

Recombinant drugs are 100 per cent lab created; they contain no proteins of human origin, they're highly purified, but the impurities they contain are from other sources. These drugs stimulate the early follicles and encourage the growth of many follicles rather than just one in an in vitro fertilisation (IVF) or stimulated cycle. Because they're pure and unlikely to cause a skin reaction (as with the highly purified urinary products), they can be given subcutaneously, with a very fine needle; women with a body mass index over 30 are better to give the drug intramuscularly for best absorption (or better still, diet before they start IVF). Two brands are currently available: GONAL-f (Serono) and Puregon (Organon).

- ✔ **Puregon:** Puregon is made by Organon, a large manufacturer of several fertility medications. Puregon is available in ready-mixed vials or in cartridges that can be loaded into a 'pen' for easy self-administration, but it does require refrigerated storage. The pen can be set to give any dose in increments of 50 IU (international unit) and this option is very convenient if your doctor needs to 'fine tune' your drug dosage.

- ✔ **GONAL-f:** GONAL-f is produced by Serono Labs, another large manufacturer of fertility medications. GONAL-f is also a ready-mixed solution supplied in cartridges for delivery via a pen system that must be stored in a refrigerator.

Urinary FSH

IBSA make a highly purified urinary FSH called Fostimon, which is available in ampoules containing 75 IU or 150 IU. It comes as a white powder and must be dissolved in 1 millilitre of diluent, which is supplied in other glass ampoules.

Mixing up the injections can be a little tricky to start with (but letting your partner help prepare your injections is great because it makes him feel like he's doing something useful!) Just like the recombinants, Fostimon can be given by subcutaneous injection. Storage is at room temperature.

hMG (human menopausal gonadotrophins) and urinary LH/FSH

hMG (human menopausal gonadotrophins) and urinary LH/FSH were the earliest gonadotrophins on the market. They're made from purified urine from menopausal women and contain nearly equal amounts of LH and FSH. Some doctors now believe that some LH is helpful in a stimulated cycle and may prescribe this hormone along with a pure FSH product.

Urinary gonadotrophins are supplied as powders and need to be mixed up prior to being given. They're generally much less expensive than recombinants, and are widely prescribed in the UK.

- ✔ **Merional:** Made by IBSA, Merional comes in 75 IU and 150 IU vials (which can be helpful if you're on a high dose). Up to 6 ampoules of powder can be mixed with 1 ampoule (1 millilitre) of diluent. Intramuscular injection is recommended, although in Europe it's used subcutaneously.

- ✔ **Menopur:** Manufactured by Ferring, Menopur is an hMG that's suitable for subcutaneous administration. It comes in 75 IU ampoules and it contains a 50/50 mix of FSH and LH and is widely prescribed.

GnRH Agonists

Gonadotrophin-releasing hormone agonists suppress the hormones LH and FSH and ensure that you become 'down-regulated', and ready to begin the stimulation phase of the cyclic or cycle. These medications can cause hot flushes, headaches, mood swings, and bone pain – in fact, all the symptoms your menopausal mother-in-law complains about. But don't worry, this 'mini-menopause' of yours *is* reversible.

GnRH agonists come in a bewildering array of formulations, but they all do the same basic job:

- ✔ **Short acting:** The 'short acting' agonists are intranasal sprays, which is great if you don't like needles. The two options are nafarelin (Synarel), which needs to be sniffed twice a day, and buserelin (Suprecur), which needs to be sniffed four times a day. You'll be doing this for a month in a 'long protocol' IVF cycle. Buserelin also comes as a subcutaneous injection called Suprefact and needs to be taken once a day. Buserelin is supplied in vials containing 5.5 millilitres, so each vial lasts 11 days.

> ✔ **Long acting:** The 'long acting' or 'depot' preparations last for a month so may be more convenient if you're the forgetful type. They produce a more profound 'down-regulation' (lower estradiol levels) so the side effects (such as hot flashes and night sweats) can be more severe. The brand names are Prostap SR, Decapeptyl SR (subcutaneous solutions), and Zoladex (subdermal pellet that must be administered by a nurse or doctor).

GnRH Antagonists

A newer category of medication called GnRH antagonists was designed to keep women from releasing eggs early during an IVF cycle without the suppressing effects of the agonists. Antagonists are manufactured by Organon as Orgalutran and by Serono as Cetrotide. Cetrotide is manufactured as a 3 milligramme depot (one-time) injection and also as a 0.25 milligramme daily injection; Orgalutran is sold as a daily 0.25 milligramme injection. The daily injection usually starts around day six of an IVF cycle. Orgalutran is sold in a prefilled syringe that requires no mixing. Cetrotide comes with a syringe prefilled with diluent, which needs to be injected into a powder; the mixture is then drawn back into the syringe and injected.

The development of the gonadotrophin-releasing hormone (GnRH) antagonists (cetrorelix and ganirelix) has dramatically shortened the 'delay period' before ovarian stimulation can start in a super-ovulation cycle, because these drugs allow ovulation induction to begin at almost any point in the cycle. Antagonists are very useful because they stop you ovulating before the embryologist is ready to collect your eggs. If you ovulate too early, the process of trying to find your eggs in a pool of fluid sloshing about in the bottom of your pelvis makes looking for a needle in a haystack seem like a pushover.

hCG (Human Chorionic Gonadotrophin) Intramuscular

Human chorionic gonadotrophin (hCG) is the 'magic bullet' that mimics the natural LH surge and ensures that ovulation occurs. Several different brands of hCG are sold; all contain 5000 IU of hCG. They're packaged as powder in ampoules and must be mixed with diluent. Depending on the brand they can be subcutaneous or intramuscular: Choragon (Ferring); Pregnyl (Organon); and Gonasi (IBSA).

hCG Subcutaneous Recombinant

Ovitrelle is a lab-manufactured subcutaneous dose of hCG packaged as 250 microgrammes equivalent to 10,000 IU, ready mixed. Serono makes Ovitrelle.

Progesterone

Progesterone can be given in intramuscular injections (painful but the best absorbed), vaginal pessaries, vaginal gel, or pills (the least absorbed):

- **Injections:** The intramuscular injection form of progesterone (gestone) requires deep intramuscular injections and it hurts! There's no evidence here for the Jane Fonda mantra 'If it's not hurting, it's not working!'

- **Vaginal pessaries:** These pessaries are made in several strengths (200 milligrammes and 400 milligrammes) and the brand name in the UK is Cyclogest (Allpharma). Think of them as tiny tampons. They contain progesterone in a waxy base and as they melt in the vagina, the progesterone is absorbed. Messy, but effective. They need to be inserted morning and evening and they're a vital part of the IVF process.

- **Gel:** Crinone is a gel manufactured by Serono; it comes in prefilled applicators of 90 milligrammes. Some patients have fewer problems with yeast (thrush) infections and irritation with Crinone than with vaginal pessaries but the pessaries are much less expensive.

- **Capsules:** These are manufactured as Uterogestan by Solvay and are available in 100 and 200 milligrammes. They can be taken orally (by mouth) or vaginally (or both!).

Clomiphene Citrate

Clomiphene citrate is an 'anti-oestrogen' and it works by fooling your pituitary gland into thinking that it has not made enough FSH and must make some more! This has the effect of stimulating regular ovulation in women with low FSH (women with PCOS) or producing multiple follicles in women having IUI or IVF. The 'brand name' is Clomid, and it's a 50 milligramme pill that usually is taken on day 2–6 of the menstrual cycle. Side effects include hot flushes, bloating, headache, and blurred vision. If blurred vision occurs, you must stop taking the tablets and contact your doctor.

Locating What You Need

If you're an NHS patient, your clinic or hospital should supply you with everything you need in the way of drugs, syringes, needles, and so on for your treatment cycles. If you're a private patient, life becomes a little more complicated!

Your clinic may issue a 'private prescription', which you can take or send to any chemist you choose. This part is where you must be a savvy shopper as getting that prescription filled at your high street chemist may cost twice what a specialist fertility pharmacy would charge for exactly the same drugs.

The average IVF drug bill is £600+, so talk to your GP first before you have your prescription filled at a private chemist! You may have a wonderful GP who wants to help you with your IVF treatment and only wishes that you could have it all on the NHS. He/she may be prepared to convert that private prescription into an NHS one and then you can get all your drugs for £10–£15.

Many private IVF units are located in private hospitals (BUPA, Nuffield, and so on), which have their own pharmacies, which can dispense the medicines you need. Some supply them at wholesale price and some put on a big mark up. No clinic should refuse to treat you just because you want to source your drugs elsewhere, so ask those difficult questions early on!

An exciting new development in the fertility world has been the arrival of the 'Homecare Companies'. These are postal/online pharmacies that can process your prescription directly from your clinic and then arrange to deliver your drugs (with syringes, needles, sharps bin, and so on) to your home or workplace at a time to suit you. They are usually able to source the products cheaper than high-street chemists, and specialise in these types of treatments, so their prices are always lower. Their staff are very knowledgeable about fertility treatment, and they know that you need your drugs on a certain day (not three days later after the Bank Holiday!). The major fertility homecare companies in the UK are:

- ✔ Pharmasure: 01923 233466 www.pharmasure.co.uk
- ✔ Healthcare at Home: 0870 600 1540 www.healthcare-at-home.co.uk
- ✔ Clinovia: 01279 456789 www.clinovia.co.uk

Index

• F •

• G •

• R •

Notes

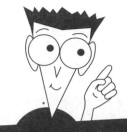

FOR DUMMIES

Do Anything. Just Add Dummies

PROPERTY

UK editions

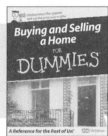

0-7645-7027-7

0-470-02921-8

0-7645-7047-1

PERSONAL FINANCE

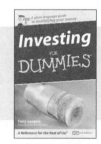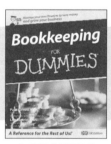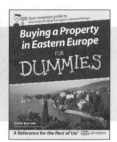

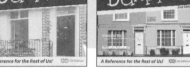

0-7645-7023-4

0-470-05815-3

0-7645-7039-0

BUSINESS

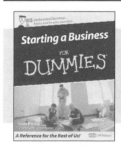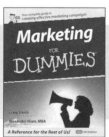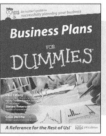

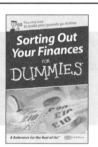

0-7645-7018-8

0-7645-7056-0

0-7645-7026-9

Answering Tough Interview
Questions For Dummies
(0-470-01903-4)

Arthritis For Dummies
(0-470-02582-4)

Being the Best Man
For Dummies
(0-470-02657-X)

British History
For Dummies
(0-470-03536-6)

Building Confidence
For Dummies
(0-470-01669-8)

Buying a Home on a Budget
For Dummies
(0-7645-7035-8)

Children's Health
For Dummies
(0-470-02735-5)

Cognitive Behavioural Therapy
For Dummies
(0-470-01838-0)

Cricket For Dummies
(0-470-03454-8)

CVs For Dummies
(0-7645-7017-X)

Detox For Dummies
(0-470-01908-5)

Diabetes For Dummies
(0-7645-7019-6)

Divorce For Dummies
(0-7645-7030-7)

DJing For Dummies
(0-470-03275-8)

eBay.co.uk For Dummies
(0-7645-7059-5)

European History
For Dummies
(0-7645-7060-9)

Gardening For Dummies
(0-470-01843-7)

Genealogy Online
For Dummies
(0-7645-7061-7)

Golf For Dummies
(0-470-01811-9)

Hypnotherapy For Dummies
(0-470-01930-1)

Irish History For Dummies
(0-7645-7040-4)

Neuro-linguistic Programming
For Dummies
(0-7645-7028-5)

Nutrition For Dummies
(0-7645-7058-7)

Parenting For Dummies
(0-470-02714-2)

Pregnancy For Dummies
(0-7645-7042-0)

Retiring Wealthy For Dummies
(0-470-02632-4)

Rugby Union For Dummies
(0-470-03537-4)

Small Business Employment
Law For Dummies
(0-7645-7052-8)

Starting a Business on
eBay.co.uk For Dummies
(0-470-02666-9)

Su Doku For Dummies
(0-470-01892-5)

The GL Diet For Dummies
(0-470-02753-3)

The Romans For Dummies
(0-470-03077-1)

Thyroid For Dummies
(0-470-03172-7)

UK Law and Your Rights
For Dummies
(0-470-02796-7)

Winning on Betfair
For Dummies
(0-470-02856-4)

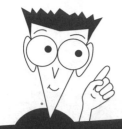

FOR DUMMIES®

Do Anything. Just Add Dummies

HOBBIES

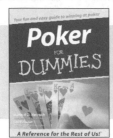

Poker
0-7645-5232-5

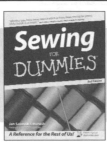

Sewing
0-7645-6847-7

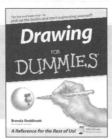

Drawing
0-7645-5476-X

Also available:

Art For Dummies
(0-7645-5104-3)

Aromatherapy For Dummies
(0-7645-5171-X)

Bridge For Dummies
(0-471-92426-1)

Card Games For Dummies
(0-7645-9910-0)

Chess For Dummies
(0-7645-8404-9)

Improving Your Memory
For Dummies
(0-7645-5435-2)

Massage For Dummies
(0-7645-5172-8)

Meditation For Dummies
(0-471-77774-9)

Photography For Dummies
(0-7645-4116-1)

Quilting For Dummies
(0-7645-9799-X)

EDUCATION

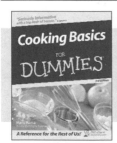

Cooking Basics
0-7645-7206-7

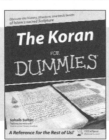

The Koran
0-7645-5581-2

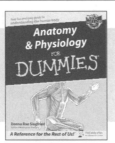

Anatomy & Physiology
0-7645-5422-0

Also available:

Algebra For Dummies
(0-7645-5325-9)

Algebra II For Dummies
(0-471-77581-9)

Astronomy For Dummies
(0-7645-8465-0)

Buddhism For Dummies
(0-7645-5359-3)

Calculus For Dummies
(0-7645-2498-4)

Forensics For Dummies
(0-7645-5580-4)

Islam For Dummies
(0-7645-5503-0)

Philosophy For Dummies
(0-7645-5153-1)

Religion For Dummies
(0-7645-5264-3)

Trigonometry For Dummies
(0-7645-6903-1)

PETS

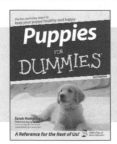

Puppies
0-470-03717-2

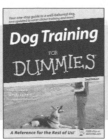

Dog Training
0-7645-8418-9

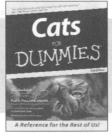

Cats
0-7645-5275-9

Also available:

Labrador Retrievers
For Dummies
(0-7645-5281-3)

Aquariums For Dummies
(0-7645-5156-6)

Birds For Dummies
(0-7645-5139-6)

Dogs For Dummies
(0-7645-5274-0)

Ferrets For Dummies
(0-7645-5259-7)

Golden Retrievers
For Dummies
(0-7645-5267-8)

Horses For Dummies
(0-7645-9797-3)

Jack Russell Terriers
For Dummies
(0-7645-5268-6)

Puppies Raising & Training
Diary For Dummies
(0-7645-0876-8)

Available wherever books are sold. For more information or to order direct go to www.wiley.com or call 0800 243407 (Non UK call +44 1243 843296)

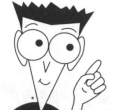

FOR DUMMIES®

The easy way to get more done and have more fun

LANGUAGES

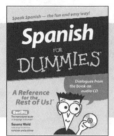
0-7645-5194-9

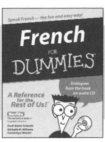
0-7645-5193-0

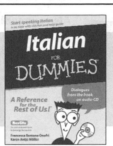
0-7645-5196-5

Also available:

Chinese For Dummies
(0-471-78897-X)

Chinese Phrases
For Dummies
(0-7645-8477-4)

French Phrases For Dummies
(0-7645-7202-4)

German For Dummies
(0-7645-5195-7)

Italian Phrases For Dummies
(0-7645-7203-2)

Japanese For Dummies
(0-7645-5429-8)

Latin For Dummies
(0-7645-5431-X)

Spanish Phrases
For Dummies
(0-7645-7204-0)

Spanish Verbs For Dummies
(0-471-76872-3)

Hebrew For Dummies
(0-7645-5489-1)

MUSIC AND FILM

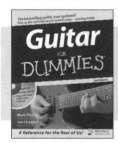
0-7645-9904-6

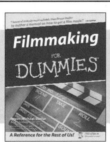
0-7645-2476-3

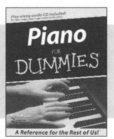
0-7645-5105-1

Also available:

Bass Guitar For Dummies
(0-7645-2487-9)

Blues For Dummies
(0-7645-5080-2)

Classical Music For Dummies
(0-7645-5009-8)

Drums For Dummies
(0-471-79411-2)

Jazz For Dummies
(0-471-76844-8)

Opera For Dummies
(0-7645-5010-1)

Rock Guitar For Dummies
(0-7645-5356-9)

Screenwriting For Dummies
(0-7645-5486-7)

Songwriting For Dummies
(0-7645-5404-2)

Singing For Dummies
(0-7645-2475-5)

HEALTH, SPORTS & FITNESS

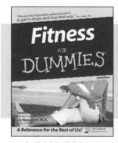
0-7645-7851-0

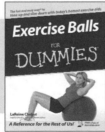
0-7645-5623-1

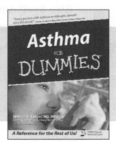
0-7645-4233-8

Also available:

Controlling Cholesterol
For Dummies
(0-7645-5440-9)

Dieting For Dummies
(0-7645-4149-8)

High Blood Pressure
For Dummies
(0-7645-5424-7)

Martial Arts For Dummies
(0-7645-5358-5)

Menopause For Dummies
(0-7645-5458-1)

Power Yoga For Dummies
(0-7645-5342-9)

Weight Training
For Dummies
(0-471-76845-6)

Yoga For Dummies
(0-7645-5117-5)

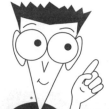

FOR DUMMIES®

Helping you expand your horizons and achieve your potential

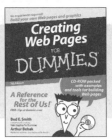
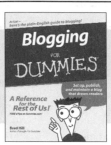
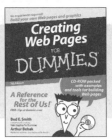
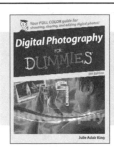
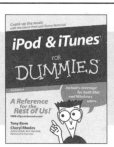
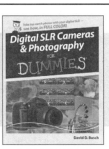
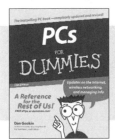
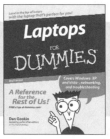
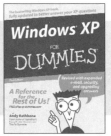